# Virtual and Augmented Reality in Mental Health Treatment

Giuliana Guazzaroni
*Università Politecnica delle Marche, Italy*

A volume in the Advances in Psychology, Mental Health, and Behavioral Studies (APMHBS) Book Series

IGI Global
DISSEMINATOR OF KNOWLEDGE

Published in the United States of America by
IGI Global
Medical Information Science Reference (an imprint of IGI Global)
701 E. Chocolate Avenue
Hershey PA, USA 17033
Tel: 717-533-8845
Fax: 717-533-8661
E-mail: cust@igi-global.com
Web site: http://www.igi-global.com



Library of Congress Cataloging-in-Publication Data

Names: Guazzaroni, Giuliana, 1968- editor.
Title: Virtual and augmented reality in mental health treatment / Giuliana Guazzaroni, editor.
Description: Hershey, PA : Medical Information Science Reference, [2019] | Includes bibliographical references.
Identifiers: LCCN 2018017840| ISBN 9781522571681 (hbk.) | ISBN 9781522571698 (eISBN)
Subjects: | MESH: Mental Disorders--therapy | Virtual Reality Exposure Therapy
Classification: LCC RC480 | NLM WM 450.5.V6 | DDC 616.89/1--dc23 LC record available at https://lccn.loc.gov/2018017840

This book is published in the IGI Global book series Advances in Psychology, Mental Health, and Behavioral Studies (APMHBS) (ISSN: 2475-6660; eISSN: 2475-6679)

British Cataloguing in Publication Data
A Cataloguing in Publication record for this book is available from the British Library.

# Advances in Psychology, Mental Health, and Behavioral Studies (APMHBS) Book Series

Bryan Christiansen
Global Research Society, LLC, USA
Harish C. Chandan
Argosy University, USA

ISSN:2475-6660
EISSN:2475-6679

## Mission

The complexity of the human mind has puzzled researchers and physicians for centuries. While widely studied, the brain still remains largely misunderstood.

The **Advances in Psychology, Mental Health, and Behavioral Studies (APMHBS)** book series presents comprehensive research publications focusing on topics relating to the human psyche, cognition, psychiatric care, mental and developmental disorders, as well as human behavior and interaction. Featuring diverse and innovative research, publications within APMHBS are ideally designed for use by mental health professionals, academicians, researchers, and upper-level students.

## Coverage

- Substance Abuse
- Mental Health & Disorders
- Treatment & Care
- Human Behavior
- Psychiatry
- Human Interaction
- Eating Disorders
- Developmental Disorders
- Socialization
- Personality Disorders

IGI Global is currently accepting manuscripts for publication within this series. To submit a proposal for a volume in this series, please contact our Acquisition Editors at Acquisitions@igi-global.com or visit: http://www.igi-global.com/publish/.

The Advances in Psychology, Mental Health, and Behavioral Studies (APMHBS) Book Series (ISSN 2475-6660) is published by IGI Global, 701 E. Chocolate Avenue, Hershey, PA 17033-1240, USA, www.igi-global.com. This series is composed of titles available for purchase individually; each title is edited to be contextually exclusive from any other title within the series. For pricing and ordering information please visit http://www.igi-global.com/book-series/advances-psychology-mental-health-behavioral/110200. Postmaster: Send all address changes to above address. 

## Titles in this Series

*For a list of additional titles in this series, please visit: www.igi-global.com/book-series*

*Scientific Concepts Behind Happiness, Kindness, and Empathy in Contemporary Society*
Nava R. Silton (Marymount Manhattan College, USA)
Information Science Reference • ©2019 • 321pp • H/C (ISBN: 9781522559184) • US $185.00 (our price)

*Handbook of Research on Psychosocial Perspectives of Human Communication Disorders*
Sanjeev Kumar Gupta (All India Institute of Speech and Hearing, India) and Srinivasan Venkatesan (All India Institute of Speech and Hearing, India)
Medical Information Science Reference • ©2018 • 465pp • H/C (ISBN: 9781522549550) • US $275.00 (our price)

*Deconstructing Stigma in Mental Health*
Brittany A. Canfield (Southern New Hampshire University, USA) and Holly A. Cunningham (CPES Inc., USA)
Medical Information Science Reference • ©2018 • 307pp • H/C (ISBN: 9781522538080) • US $225.00 (our price)

*Social, Psychological, and Forensic Perspectives on Sexual Abuse*
Rejani Thudalikunnil Gopalan (Gujarat Forensic Sciences University, India)
Information Science Reference • ©2018 • 374pp • H/C (ISBN: 9781522539582) • US $195.00 (our price)

*Raising Mental Health Awareness in Higher Education Emerging Research and Opportunities*
Melissa Martin (State University of New York at Plattsburgh, USA) Jean Mockry (State University of New York at Plattsburgh, USA) Alison Puliatte (State University of New York at Plattsburgh, USA) Denise A. Simard (State University of New York at Plattsburgh, USA) and Maureen E. Squires (State University of New York at Plattsburgh, USA)
Medical Information Science Reference • ©2018 • 136pp • H/C (ISBN: 9781522537939) • US $175.00 (our price)

*Web-Based Behavioral Therapies for Mental Disorders*
Sitwat Usman Langrial (Sur University College, Oman)
Medical Information Science Reference • ©2018 • 310pp • H/C (ISBN: 9781522532415) • US $255.00 (our price)

*Measuring the Psychological and Electrophysiological Attributes of Human Personality Emerging Research ...*
Sanja Tatalović Vorkapić (University of Rijeka, Croatia)
Information Science Reference • ©2017 • 242pp • H/C (ISBN: 9781522522836) • US $130.00 (our price)

IGI Global
DISSEMINATOR OF KNOWLEDGE

701 East Chocolate Avenue, Hershey, PA 17033, USA
Tel: 717-533-8845 x100 • Fax: 717-533-8661
E-Mail: cust@igi-global.com • www.igi-global.com

## Editorial Advisory Board



## List of Reviewers

# Table of Contents

**Preface** .......... xv

**Acknowledgment** .......... xxiii

**Section 1**
**Infrastructural, Therapeutic, and Cultural Contexts**

**Chapter 1**
Ubiquitous Bodies: A "Metrobodily" Transition From Real to Virtual .......... 1
*Giorgio Cipolletta, Università di Macerata, Italy*

**Chapter 2**
Impact of Virtual Reality in Healthcare: A Review .......... 17
*Anitha S. Pillai, Hindustan Institute of Technology and Science, India*
*Prabha Susy Mathew, Bishop Cottons Women's Christian College, India*

**Chapter 3**
Serious Games, Meditation, Brain-Computer Interfacing, and Virtual Reality (VR): Empowering Players to Discover Their Minds .......... 32
*Ryan Murdoch, The Glasgow School of Art, UK*

**Chapter 4**
Virtual Reality Therapeutic Environments in Autism Spectrum Disorder (ASD) and Alzheimer's: Treatment, Diagnosis, and Refinement .......... 51
*David W. Sime, Online Corporate Video Production Ltd., UK*

**Chapter 5**
Virtual Reality (VR) as Medical Prevention of Adverse Childhood Experiences (ACEs) .......... 60
*Anastasia Miron, Child Proof Yourself, USA*

**Chapter 6**
A SWOT Analysis of Virtual Reality for Seniors .......... 78
*Pooya Soltani, Aix Marseille University, France*

## Section 2
## Virtual and Augmented Reality in Mental Health Treatment: Pedagogy, Psychology, and Technology

**Chapter 7**
Virtual and Augmented Reality Mirrors for Mental Health Treatment: Analysis and Future Directions ........ 95
*Sergio Casas, University of Valencia, Spain*
*Cristina Portalés, University of Valencia, Spain*
*Lucía Vera, University of Valencia, Spain*
*José Vicente Riera, University of Valencia, Spain*

**Chapter 8**
The State of Virtual and Augmented Reality Therapy for Autism Spectrum Disorder (ASD) .......... 118
*Sinan Turnacioglu, Floreo, Inc., USA*
*Joseph P McCleery, Saint Joseph's University, USA & Children's Hospital of Philadelphia, USA*
*Julia Parish-Morris, University of Pennsylvania, USA & Children's Hospital of Philadelphia, USA*
*Vibha Sazawal, University of Maryland, USA*
*Rita Solorzano, Floreo, Inc., USA*

**Chapter 9**
Virtual Reality (VR) for School Children With Autism Spectrum Disorder (ASD): A Way of Rethinking Teaching and Learning ........ 141
*Giuliana Guazzaroni, Università Politecnica delle Marche, Italy*
*Anitha S. Pillai, Hindustan Institute of Technology and Science, India*

**Chapter 10**
Virtual Reality (VR) for Children Diagnosed With Autism Spectrum Disorder (ASD): Interventions to Train Social and Everyday Living Skills ........ 159
*Ali Adjorlu, Aalborg University – Copenhagen, Denmark*
*Stefania Serafin, Aalborg University – Copenhagen, Denmark*

**Chapter 11**
Autism Spectrum Disorder (ASD) and Attention-Deficit/Hyperactivity Disorder (ADHD) Children: From Users to Creators of Virtual Reality Learning Content ........ 176
*Giuliana Guazzaroni, Università Politecnica delle Marche, Italy*

**Chapter 12**
From Chat Therapy to Virtual Reality (VR): The Case of Idego – Digital Psychology ........ 199
*Simone Barbato, Idego – Psicologia Digitale s.r.l., Italy*
*Lorenzo Di Natale, Idego – Psicologia Digitale s.r.l., Italy*

**Chapter 13**
Uses of Virtual Reality (VR) for Chronic Pain ........ 221
*Bradley Chi, Zucker School of Medicine at Hofstra/Northwell, USA*
*Brian Chau, Loma Linda University Health, USA*
*Phillip Ta, Loma Linda University Health, USA*

**Chapter 14**
E-Learning and Augmented Reality (AR) for Chronic Wound Assessment: Promoting Learning and Quality of Care ........ 241
*Nelson Ribeiro Jorge, Universidade Aberta, Portugal*
*Lina Morgado, Universidade Aberta, Portugal*
*Pedro J. S. Gaspar, Instituto Politécnico de Leiria, Portugal*

**Chapter 15**
Look of Life: The Wonder Therapy ........ 262
*Vittoria Sichi, ANT Foundation, Italy*
*Giacomo Ercolani, ANT Foundation, Italy*
*Luca Franchini, ANT Foundation, Italy*
*Luca Golfari, ANT Foundation, Italy*
*Silvia Varani, ANT Foundation, Italy*
*Daniela Rizzoli, ANT Foundation, Italy*
*Raffaella Pannuti, ANT Foundation, Italy*
*Daniele Roganti, ANT Foundation, Italy*

**Compilation of References** ........ 271

**About the Contributors** ........ 321

**Index** ........ 327

# Detailed Table of Contents

**Preface** .......... xv

**Acknowledgment** .......... xxiii

**Section 1**
**Infrastructural, Therapeutic, and Cultural Contexts**

**Chapter 1**
Ubiquitous Bodies: A "Metrobodily" Transition From Real to Virtual .......... 1
*Giorgio Cipolletta, Università di Macerata, Italy*

While the digital era has provided us with an incredible amount of accessibility, availability, and speedy tools, it has also made us lose that sense of critical awareness that was once considered a rare and precious gift. The marking feature of the present is ubiquity, as in the loss of spatial and temporal coordinates and the gain of a presence-absence that new technologies allow us to live – both positively and negatively. The body is the core of this electronic, virtual, and increased involvement. In this phase we're living in, the author suggests we introduce the neologism "metrobody" to identify this new hybrid condition undertaken by the body. This expression allows the author to reconfigure and hypothesize a different level and a different meaning of corporeality.

**Chapter 2**
Impact of Virtual Reality in Healthcare: A Review .......... 17
*Anitha S. Pillai, Hindustan Institute of Technology and Science, India*
*Prabha Susy Mathew, Bishop Cottons Women's Christian College, India*

Virtual reality (VR) is the simulation of reality where the users would be immersed in an artificial/virtual environment that isn't there but creates an illusion as if it really exists. People using this technology get a feeling that they are performing everything in real time. This gives users a sense of satisfaction. Initially, VR technology was used for gaming purposes, but now it is used in many sectors, including healthcare. There are many situations wherein, when it is expensive or impossible to do something, in reality, a probable solution is virtual reality. An important area where it is explored is healthcare for training doctors, diagnosis, and treatment of various ailments. The main objective of this chapter is to shed light on the applications of VR in healthcare and to discuss some applications showing how the medical field has already started reaping the benefits of VR.

**Chapter 3**
Serious Games, Meditation, Brain-Computer Interfacing, and Virtual Reality (VR): Empowering Players to Discover Their Minds ........ 32
*Ryan Murdoch, The Glasgow School of Art, UK*

Brain-computer interfacing (BCI), the ability to interact with software and technology with our thoughts and feelings, presents an exciting new frontier for serious games and learning. This chapter outlines an approach to incorporating real-time brain-monitoring in educational games. Both outlining and suggesting how technically this can be achieved using affordable and accessible "off the shelf" consumer technology and the popular game engine Unity. By designing such experiences considering pedagogy and serious game theory, we can attempt to classify this new form of user interaction and its value for educational purposes. Specifically, this chapter looks to engage players with ideas of meditation by monitoring their "meditation" using BCI technology and visualizing it in engaging game worlds and experiences. As a valuable tool for addressing mental illness and personal wellbeing, meditation is worth exploring as a learning outcome within serious games.

**Chapter 4**
Virtual Reality Therapeutic Environments in Autism Spectrum Disorder (ASD) and Alzheimer's: Treatment, Diagnosis, and Refinement ........ 51
*David W. Sime, Online Corporate Video Production Ltd., UK*

This chapter is devoted to observing and analyzing the role of virtual reality environments in the therapeutic treatment, analysis, and ongoing treatment planning of autistic spectrum disorders (ASD), Alzheimer's, and dementia. Using live real-world examples of the above activities in action and a literature review, the chapter will examine the level of empirical data and pre-existing qualitative and quantitative research to support these ongoing approaches. Critical analysis will also be made of the current level of empirical research available highlighting areas that should be focused on for future research.

**Chapter 5**
Virtual Reality (VR) as Medical Prevention of Adverse Childhood Experiences (ACEs) ........ 60
*Anastasia Miron, Child Proof Yourself, USA*

This chapter identifies numerous cases on adverse childhood experiences (ACEs) and their link with post-traumatic stress disorders (PTSD). It explores the use of virtual reality (VR) as a clinical tool in diagnosis, prevention and treatment of ACEs. The emotional, physical, psychological and cognitive demands of a child going through ACEs are discussed using scientific researchers. The purpose of this chapter is to introduce the beneficial uses of virtual reality (VR) in the prevention, diagnosis, and treatment of ACEs.

**Chapter 6**
A SWOT Analysis of Virtual Reality for Seniors ........ 78
*Pooya Soltani, Aix Marseille University, France*

The population of older people is increasing. In this book chapter, the author reviewed some of the applications of virtual reality (VR) for seniors in form of a strengths, weaknesses, opportunities, and threats (SWOT) analysis. This approach is commonly used to assess and guide internal and external parameters to accomplish a mission. Some of the challenges that the elderly are facing were reviewed and the way VR can help in overcoming those challenges were discussed. A comparison of VR technologies was also presented. The results show that VR's feasibility and concept are linked to existing technologies and the characteristics of each system control immersion, interaction, and stimulation. VR interventions might have the potential to be used as ecologically valid e-health screening systems. Systems should be specifically designed and adapted for seniors and usability issues should be addressed. Ideally, VR interventions work best in addition to traditional methods. Future studies should use more subjects to ensure the efficacy of such interventions for seniors.

**Section 2**
**Virtual and Augmented Reality in Mental Health Treatment: Pedagogy, Psychology, and Technology**

**Chapter 7**
Virtual and Augmented Reality Mirrors for Mental Health Treatment: Analysis and Future Directions ........ 95
*Sergio Casas, University of Valencia, Spain*
*Cristina Portalés, University of Valencia, Spain*
*Lucía Vera, University of Valencia, Spain*
*José Vicente Riera, University of Valencia, Spain*

Virtual and Augmented Reality are technologies widely used in a variety of areas, including the medical sector. On the other hand, regular mirrors have been traditionally used as tools to aid in mental health treatment for a variety of diseases and disorders. Although it is possible to build Virtual and Augmented Reality experiences based on mirror metaphors, there are very few contributions of this kind in the medical sector. In this chapter, the great benefits that regular mirrors have brought for mental health treatment are addressed. In addition, a review on the state of the art in mirror-based Virtual and Augmented Reality applications is given, highlighting the potential benefits that these enhanced mirrors could bring for the mental health treatment.

**Chapter 8**
The State of Virtual and Augmented Reality Therapy for Autism Spectrum Disorder (ASD) .......... 118
*Sinan Turnacioglu, Floreo, Inc., USA*
*Joseph P McCleery, Saint Joseph's University, USA & Children's Hospital of Philadelphia, USA*
*Julia Parish-Morris, University of Pennsylvania, USA & Children's Hospital of Philadelphia, USA*
*Vibha Sazawal, University of Maryland, USA*
*Rita Solorzano, Floreo, Inc., USA*

Autism spectrum disorder (ASD) is a heterogeneous neurodevelopmental condition affecting a growing number of individuals across the lifespan. It is characterized by observable impairments in social communication, as well as repetitive behaviors and restricted patterns of interests. Early, intensive behavioral interventions improve long-term outcomes in ASD, but are often expensive and hard to administer consistently. This chapter describes a new approach to autism intervention, using highly motivating virtual reality (VR) and augmented reality (AR) technologies that could soon support traditional autism therapies across ages and ability levels. The chapter begins by reviewing the ASD phenotype, followed by a review of the current landscape of research on VR and AR in ASD. A discussion of ASD-specific benefits and risks is followed by a presentation of new, harnessed immersive VR technology from Floreo, Inc. Finally, we propose a series of future research directions.

**Chapter 9**
Virtual Reality (VR) for School Children With Autism Spectrum Disorder (ASD): A Way of Rethinking Teaching and Learning ........ 141
*Giuliana Guazzaroni, Università Politecnica delle Marche, Italy*
*Anitha S. Pillai, Hindustan Institute of Technology and Science, India*

Various medical and technological organizations are working on the development of unconventional solutions such as therapy and assistance for people with autism spectrum disorder (ASD). Different organizations, researchers and educators have been involved in the study and realization of virtual reality (VR) solutions to be used as therapy, training, and support for these individuals. Previous researches and experiments showed that it is possible to ameliorate the level of concentration, coordination, socialization, communication, self-awareness, and memory in school children treated with these tools. VR environments may offer a total physical involvement of the ASDs that may see the world through virtual immersion and active practice. This chapter presents a way of rethinking teaching and learning.

**Chapter 10**
Virtual Reality (VR) for Children Diagnosed With Autism Spectrum Disorder (ASD): Interventions to Train Social and Everyday Living Skills ........ 159
*Ali Adjorlu, Aalborg University – Copenhagen, Denmark*
*Stefania Serafin, Aalborg University – Copenhagen, Denmark*

Children and adolescents diagnosed with autism spectrum disorder (ASD) have significant difficulties with communication and social skills. Consequently, children diagnosed with ASD are often victims of social rejection and targets of bullying, which have an adverse impact on their emotional and mental wellbeing. Social anxiety, depression, and poor academic achievement are some of the consequences that can harm their whole lives. This chapter will begin with an elaboration of the challenges facing children and adolescents diagnosed with ASD. This will be followed by an introduction to virtual reality (VR) and its advantages for extending the capabilities of some of the traditional interventions developed to teach social and everyday living skills to children and adolescents diagnosed with ASD.

**Chapter 11**
Autism Spectrum Disorder (ASD) and Attention-Deficit/Hyperactivity Disorder (ADHD) Children: From Users to Creators of Virtual Reality Learning Content ........ 176
*Giuliana Guazzaroni, Università Politecnica delle Marche, Italy*

Autism spectrum disorder (ASD) is a serious neurological disorder. Using virtual reality (VR), researchers are exploring alternative solutions to treat ASD. Recent experiences show that VR can be a motivating platform to safely practice social and communication skills for children with ASD. It is also seen as an effective method to build empathy and help improve the general understanding of the condition. This study will focus on using and experimenting different 360-degree immersive learning environments for ASD and attention-deficit/hyperactivity disorder (ADHD) pupils and their schoolmates. The chapter will report on a few ASD students who use VR facilities to communicate, learn, improve self-awareness, autobiographical memory, and reduce school pressure, and a few ADHD students who enjoy a VR environment to improve concentration and self-esteem. Both the ASD students and the ADHD ones decided, during the trial, to become VR creators building their own content, with the help of a facilitator.

**Chapter 12**
From Chat Therapy to Virtual Reality (VR): The Case of Idego – Digital Psychology..................... 199
*Simone Barbato, Idego – Psicologia Digitale s.r.l., Italy*
*Lorenzo Di Natale, Idego – Psicologia Digitale s.r.l., Italy*

This chapter aims to highlight some aspects linked with the psychological interventions adaptability to the virtual setting, focusing on advantages, limits, and the effectiveness criteria of an online intervention, and of the virtual reality (VR) applications in the clinical psychology field. First of all, the authors will examine the characteristics of the web-based setting and of the online psychological counseling service, underling opportunities and risks of text talk-based chat therapy and the issues dealing with the role of the therapist. This will be followed by the analysis of Twende! Project, an online psychological counseling service created by the Italian company Idego – Digital Psychology s.r.l. The chapter will conclude with the presentation of VR systems as an e-therapy tool, considering their application scopes in order to treat mental disorders and showing their adaptability and operational effectiveness in several clinical psychology areas.

**Chapter 13**
Uses of Virtual Reality (VR) for Chronic Pain........................................................................... 221
*Bradley Chi, Zucker School of Medicine at Hofstra/Northwell, USA*
*Brian Chau, Loma Linda University Health, USA*
*Phillip Ta, Loma Linda University Health, USA*

Chronic pain affects many people worldwide with significant individual impact and societal cost. One such area involves the psychiatric co-morbidities associated with chronic pain. Despite its prevalence, the underlying mechanism of chronic pain is not fully understood although evidence suggests the importance of biologic, psychologic, and social factors in the perception of pain. Virtual reality has the potential to be a powerful therapeutic option for chronic pain. This may be due to its impact on attention, emotion, and potentially central nervous system plasticity. Virtual reality therapy has been used successfully for a variety of chronic pain conditions showing its potential. It has also been safely used in pediatric populations. However, the major current limitation is quality of evidence; therefore, future studies should aim to address this issue.

**Chapter 14**
E-Learning and Augmented Reality (AR) for Chronic Wound Assessment: Promoting Learning and Quality of Care.............................................................................................................. 241
*Nelson Ribeiro Jorge, Universidade Aberta, Portugal*
*Lina Morgado, Universidade Aberta, Portugal*
*Pedro J. S. Gaspar, Instituto Politécnico de Leiria, Portugal*

This investigation aimed to verify if augmented reality (AR) increases students' motivation and enhances the development of clinical decision-making skills in wound diagnosis and treatment. A quasi-experimental study was carried out with a sample of 54 nursing students. A comparative analysis of the progress of the control and experimental group was made using the data extracted from the simulator and a questionnaire. First, both groups used e-FER, a virtual simulator that simulates the diagnosis and treatment of virtual clinical cases. In the second moment, the control group continued using only e-FER, while the experimental group used e-FER combined with an AR application to observe the chronic wounds. The results showed that AR enhanced student performance, particularly in wound diagnostic parameters, with highly statistically significant differences (p<0,001), and registering high levels of motivation and simulator usability, even with the introduction of an additional device in the activity.

**Chapter 15**
Look of Life: The Wonder Therapy ........................................................................................ 262
*Vittoria Sichi, ANT Foundation, Italy*
*Giacomo Ercolani, ANT Foundation, Italy*
*Luca Franchini, ANT Foundation, Italy*
*Luca Golfari, ANT Foundation, Italy*
*Silvia Varani, ANT Foundation, Italy*
*Daniela Rizzoli, ANT Foundation, Italy*
*Raffaella Pannuti, ANT Foundation, Italy*
*Daniele Roganti, ANT Foundation, Italy*

The use of virtual reality (VR) shows promising results in improving the emotional wellbeing of cancer patients, reducing anxiety, depression, and pain symptoms. No data exist concerning the use of VR in cancer patients assisted at home. The ANT Foundation decided to conduct a pilot study to test the use of VR in cancer patients assisted at home. Fifty-eight ANT patients were randomized and assigned to a control group that didn't use VR devices and to an experimental group that used them. The primary objective of the pilot study was to determine whether VR device could be a viable instrument in homecare patients. Furthermore, the aim of the study was to discover if VR could have beneficial effects on patients' quality of life as well as discover which kind of videos were more effective. The innovative aspect of this study was to test the use of VR directly at home of patients, proposing a use of VR that is compatible with the needs and the daily rhythms of families, and investigating its effectiveness through appropriate validated psychometric questionnaires and semi-structured interviews.

**Compilation of References** .................................................................................................. 271

**About the Contributors** ....................................................................................................... 321

**Index** ..................................................................................................................................... 327

# Preface

## INTRODUCTION

Nowadays, various medical and technological organizations, mostly ICT, are working on the development of 'unconventional' solutions such as therapy and assistance for people with behavioral problems. In particular, autism, down syndrome, Alzheimer's disease, anxiety, phobias, learning difficulties etc. Different organizations have been involved in the study and realization of virtual reality (VR) and augmented reality (AR) solutions to be used as therapy and support for this kind of disabilities.

Previous researches and experiments (Rizzo, 2011; Radu, 2014) showed that it is possible to double or even quadruple the level of concentration in children treated with these tools. The history of these methodologies is recent, consequently it is not possible to state the durability of these therapies, for this reason it is necessary to proceed with a large-scale experimentation; there exists a need for an edited collection of original research in this area. VR is used in teaching and training ASD pupils. Different studies (Parsons & Cobb, 2011; Bellani et al., 2011; Rizzo & Kim, 2005) pointed out that this technology is advantageous for people with cognitive and perceptual impairments, including autism, because VR can support in planning, problem-solving and management of behaviour. Moreover, VR offers an effective communication help for children with limited language (Parsons & Cobb). The literature is progressively accepting the benefits of VR and AR facilities in teaching ASD individuals, especially related to social skills (Parsons & Mitchell, 2002; Bellani et al., 2011; Kandalaft et al., 2013; Didehbani et al., 2016; Newbutt et al., 2016; Saadatzi et al., 2018).

This book aims to provide relevant and innovative theoretical frameworks and the latest empirical research findings in the area of VR and AR for mental health treatment. It is written for professionals and educators who want to improve their understanding of the strategic role of VR and AR treatments in mental health.

The target audience of this book is composed of professionals, medical staff, educators and researchers working in the field of information technology, education and medicine, e.g. mental health, rehabilitation, library, information and communication sciences, education, adult education, sociology, computer science, and information technology. Moreover, the book provides insights and support professionals concerned with mental health treatments and/or teaching of students with special needs.

## ORGANIZATION OF THE BOOK

This book consists of 15 chapters, written by 35 authors, loosely grouped into two sections. The book chapters cover different themes, infrastructural, therapeutic, and cultural contexts; pedagogy, psychology and technology. The last group provides a collection of analyzed experiences and literature. While, the first group of contributions provides a cultural and a general reflection on the use of virtuality, immersive virtual experiences, therapeutic environments and augmented reality in mental health.

### Section 1: Infrastructural, Therapeutic, and Cultural Contexts

This section considers infrastructural, therapeutic, and cultural contexts regarding VR and AR for mental health. It includes virtuality and the human body, healthcare, empowerment and discover of one's own mind, therapeutic environments in Autism Spectrum Disorder (ASD) and Alzheimer's, Adverse Childhood Experiences (ACEs) and, lastly, a SWOT analysis of VR for seniors.

#### Chapter 1: "Ubiquitous Bodies: A 'Metrobodily' Transition From Real to Virtual" by Giorgio Cipolletta

The digital era has provided us with an incredible amount of accessibility, availability and speedy tools, but it has also made us lose that sense of critical awareness that was once considered a rare and precious gift. The marking feature of the present is ubiquity, as in the loss of spatial and temporal coordinates and the gain of a presence-absence that new technologies allow us to live - both positively and negatively. The body is the core of this electronic, virtual, and increased involvement. In this phase we're living in, a sort of "metrobody," a neologism to identify this new hybrid condition undertaken by the body. This expression allows people to reconfigure and hypothesize a different level and a different meaning of corporeality.

#### Chapter 2: "Impact of Virtual Reality (VR) in Healthcare: A Review" by Anitha S. Pillai and Prabha Susy Mathew

VR is the simulation of reality where people would be immersed in an artificial environment that isn't there but creates an illusion as if it really exists. People using VR gets a feeling that they are performing everything in real time. This gives users a sense of satisfaction. Initially, VR technology is now used in healthcare. There are many situations wherein when it is expensive or impossible to do something, in reality, then a probable solution is virtuality. An important area where it is explored is healthcare for training doctors, diagnosis, and treatment of various ailments. The main objective of this chapter is to throw light on the applications of VR in Healthcare and to discuss some applications showing how medical field has already started reaping the benefits of VR.

## Chapter 3: "Serious Games, Meditation, Brain-Computer Interfacing, and Virtual Reality (VR): Empowering Players to Discover Their Minds" by Ryan Murdoch

Brain-computer interfacing (BCI) is the ability to interact with software and technology with our thoughts and feelings. It presents an exciting new frontier for serious games and learning. This chapter outlines an approach to incorporating real-time brain-monitoring in educational games. Both outlining and suggesting how technically this can be achieved using affordable and accessible 'off the shelf' consumer technology and the popular game engine Unity. By designing such experiences considering pedagogy and serious game theory we can attempt to classify this new form of user interaction and its value for educational purposes. Specifically this chapter looks to engage players with ideas of meditation; by monitoring their 'meditation' using BCI technology and visualizing it in engaging game worlds and experiences. As a valuable tool for addressing mental illness and personal well-being, meditation is worth exploring as a learning outcome within serious games.

## Chapter 4: "Virtual Reality Therapeutic Environments in Autism Spectrum Disorder (ASD) and Alzheimer's: Treatment, Diagnosis, and Refinement" by David W. Sime

David W. Sime analyzes the role of VR environments in the therapeutic treatment, analysis and ongoing treatment planning of ASD, Alzheimer's and dementia. Using live real-world examples of the above activities in action, surrounding literature review, the chapter examines the level of empirical data and pre-existing qualitative and quantitative research to support these ongoing approaches.

## Chapter 5: "Virtual Reality (VR) as Medical Prevention of Adverse Childhood Experiences (ACEs)" by Anastasia Miron

Anastasia Miron identifies numerous cases on ACEs and their link with post-traumatic stress disorders (PTSD). the chapter explores the use of VR as a clinical tool in diagnosis, prevention and treatment of ACEs. The emotional, physical, psychological and cognitive demands of a child going through ACEs are discussed using scientific researchers. The purpose of this chapter is to introduce the beneficial uses of VR in the prevention, diagnosis, and treatment of ACEs.

## Chapter 6: "A SWOT Analysis of Virtual Reality (VR) for Seniors" by Pooya Soltani

The population of older people is increasing. Pooya Soltani reviewed some of the applications of VR for seniors in form of a SWOT (Strengths, Weaknesses, Opportunities, and Threats) analysis. The results show that VR interventions might have the potential to be used as ecologically valid e-health screening systems. Systems should be specifically designed and adapted for seniors and usability issues should be addressed.

## Section 2: Virtual and Augmented Reality in Mental Health Treatment – Pedagogy, Psychology, and Technology

This section considers pedagogical, psychological and technological issues. It offers a collection of analyzed experiences and relating literature regarding: VR and AR mirrors for mental health treatment, state-of-the-art of VR and AR therapy for ASD, VR as a way of rethinking teaching and learning, train social and everyday living skills for ASD children, VR learning materials for ASD and Attention-deficit/hyperactivity disorder (ADHD) students, VR for clinical psychology, VR for chronic pain, E-Learning and AR for chronic wound assessment and VR to reduce cancer patients' anxiety, depression and pain symptoms.

### Chapter 7: "Virtual and Augmented Reality Mirrors for Mental Health Treatment: Analysis and Future Directions" by Sergio Casas, Cristina Portalés, Lucía Vera, and José Vicente Riera

Regular mirrors have been traditionally used as tools to aid in mental health treatment for a variety of diseases and disorders. Although it is possible to build VR and AR experiences based on mirror metaphors, there are very few contributions of this kind in the medical sector. In this chapter, the great benefits that regular mirrors have brought for mental health treatment are addressed. In addition, a review on the state-of-the-art in mirror-based VR and AR applications is given, highlighting the potential benefits that these enhanced mirrors could bring for the mental health treatment.

### Chapter 8: "The State of Virtual and Augmented Reality Therapy for Autism Spectrum Disorder (ASD)" by Sinan Turnacioglu, Joseph P. McCleery, Julia Parish-Morris, Vibha Sazawal, and Rita Solorzano

This chapter describes a new approach to autism intervention, using highly motivating VR and AR technologies that could soon support traditional autism therapies across ages and ability levels. The chapter begins by reviewing the ASD phenotype, followed by a review of the current landscape of research on VR and AR in ASD. A discussion of ASD-specific benefits and risks is followed by a presentation of new, harnessed immersive VR technology from Floreo, Inc. Finally, the authors propose a series of future research directions.

### Chapter 9: "Virtual Reality (VR) for School Children With Autism Spectrum Disorder (ASD): A Way of Rethinking Teaching and Learning" by Giuliana Guazzaroni and Anitha S. Pillai

Different organizations, researchers and educators have been involved in the study and realization of VR solutions to be used as therapy, training and support for ASD individuals. Previous researches and experiments showed that it is possible to ameliorate the level of concentration, coordination, socialisation, communication, self-awareness and memory in school children treated with these tools. VR environments may offer a total physical involvement of the ASDs, that may see the world through virtual immersion and active practice. This chapter presents a way of rethinking teaching and learning.

## Chapter 10: "Virtual Reality (VR) for Children Diagnosed With Autism Spectrum Disorder (ASD): Interventions to Train Social and Everyday Living Skills" by Ali Adjorlu and Stefania Serafin

Children diagnosed with ASD are often victims of social rejection and targets of bullying, which have an adverse impact on their emotional and mental well-being. Social anxiety, depression, and poor academic achievement are some of the consequences that can harm their whole lives. This chapter begins with an elaboration of the challenges facing children and adolescents diagnosed with ASD. This is followed by an introduction to VR and its advantages for extending the capabilities of some of the traditional interventions developed to teach social and everyday living skills to children and adolescents diagnosed with ASD.

## Chapter 11: "Autism Spectrum Disorder (ASD) and Attention-Deficit/ Hyperactivity Disorder (ADHD) Children: From Users to Creators of Virtual Reality Learning Content" by Giuliana Guazzaroni

This study focuses on using and experimenting different 360-degree immersive learning environments for ASD and ADHD pupils and their schoolmates. Especially, the chapter will report of a few ASD students that use VR facilities to communicate, learn, improve self-awareness, autobiographical memory and reduce school pressure; of a few ADHD students that enjoy a VR environment to improve concentration and self-esteem. Both the ASD students and the ADHD ones decided, during the trial, to become VR creators building their own content, with the help of a facilitator.

## Chapter 12: "From Chat Therapy to Virtual Reality (VR): The Case of Idego – Digital Psychology" by Simone Barbato and Lorenzo Di Natale

This chapter aims to highlight some aspects linked with the psychological interventions adaptability to the virtual setting, focusing on advantages, limits and the effectiveness criteria of an online intervention, and of the VR applications in the clinical psychology field. First of all, the authors will examine the characteristics of the web-based setting and of the online psychological counseling service, underling opportunities and risks of text talk-based chat therapy and the issues dealing with the role of the therapist. This is followed by the analysis of Twende! Project, an online psychological counseling service, created by the Italian company Idego – Digital Psychology s.r.l.. The chapter will conclude with the presentation of VR systems as an E-therapy tool, considering their application scopes in order to treat mental disorders and showing their adaptability and operational effectiveness in several clinical psychology areas.

## Chapter 13: "Uses of Virtual Reality (VR) for Chronic Pain" by Bradley Chi, Brian Chau, and Phillip Ta

Chronic pain affects many people worldwide with significant individual impact and societal cost. One such area involves the psychiatric co-morbidities associated with chronic pain. Despite its prevalence, the underlying mechanism of chronic pain is not fully understood although evidence suggests the importance of biologic, psychologic and social factors in the perception of pain. Virtual reality has potential to be a powerful therapeutic option for chronic pain. This may be due to its impact on attention, emotion, and potentially central nervous system plasticity. Virtual reality therapy has been used successfully for a variety of chronic pain conditions showing its potential. It has also been safely used in pediatric populations. However, the major current limitation is quality of evidence, therefore future studies should aim to address this issue.

### Chapter 14: "E-Learning and Augmented Reality (AR) for Chronic Wound Assessment: Promoting Learning and Quality of Care" by Nelson Ribeiro Jorge, Lina Morgado, and Pedro J. S. Gaspar

This investigation aimed to verify if AR increases students' motivation and enhances the development of clinical decision-making skills in wound diagnosis and treatment. A quasi-experimental study was carried out with a sample of 54 nursing students. A comparative analysis of the progress of the control and experimental group was made using the data extracted from the simulator and a questionnaire. First, both groups used e-FER, a virtual simulator that simulates the diagnosis and treatment of virtual clinical cases. In the second moment, the control group continued using only e-FER, while the experimental group used e-FER combined with an AR application to observe the chronic wounds. The results showed that AR enhanced student performance, particularly in wound diagnostic parameters, with highly statistically significant differences, and registering high levels of motivation and simulator usability, even with the introduction of an additional device in the activity.

### Chapter 15: "Look of Life: The Wonder Therapy" by Vittoria Sichi, Giacomo Ercolani, Luca Franchini, Luca Golfari, Silvia Varani, Daniela Rizzoli, Raffaella Pannuti, and Daniele Roganti

The use of VR shows promising results in improving emotional well being of cancer patients, reducing anxiety, depression and pain symptoms. No data still exist concerning the use of VR in cancer patients assisted at home. The ANT Foundation decided to conduct a pilot study to test the use of VR in cancer patients assisted at home. 58 ANT patients were randomized and assigned to a control group which didn't use VR device and to an experimental group that used it. The primary objective of the pilot study was to determine whether VR device could be a viable instrument in home care patients. Furthermore, the aim of the study was to discover if VR could have beneficial effects on patient's quality of life as well as discover which kind of videos were more effective. The innovative aspect of this study was to test the use of VR directly at home of patients, proposing a use of VR that is compatible with the needs and the daily rhythms of families, and investigating its effectiveness through appropriate validated psychometric questionnaires and semi-structured interviews.

## CONCLUSION

The 15 chapters included in this book were selected from twenty-four original proposals submitted by different authors and researches worldwide. They embrace different subjects, group sizes and institutions. They are written by physicians, psychologists, engineers, ICT experts, educators, teachers, researchers etc. Professionals involved in the different topics (psychology, psychiatry, medicine, mental health, special education, engineering, technology, virtuality, etc.) proposed by this publication are actively involved in utilizing VR and AR therapeutic and learning environments and in proposing innovative practices in their specific field.

This book provides a state-of-the-art of best practices in the area of reference. It presents pros and cons of the value of using VR and AR technologies in mental health treatment. The target of this book includes professionals, physician, mental health staff, engineers, ICT experts, educators, special education teachers, researchers working in the field of information technology, education and medicine (mental health, rehabilitation, library, information and communication sciences, education, adult education, sociology, computer science, information technology etc.).

The book includes general themes regarding the human body, healthcare, empowerment and the discover of one's own mind using serious games, therapeutic environments in ASD and Alzheimer's, VR in special education, ACEs, analysis regarding the use of VR and AR. Moreover, it offers a collection of analyzed experiences about VR and AR mirrors, VR and AR therapy for ASD, VR to teach social and everyday living skills to students with ASD, VR learning content involvement for ASD and ADHD pupils, VR for clinical psychology, VR for chronic pain, AR and E-Learning for chronic wound assessment and VR for cancer patients, to relieve their anxiety, depression and pain.

## REFERENCES

Bellani, M., Fornasari, L., Chittaro, L., & Brambilla, P. (2011). Virtual reality in autism: State of the art. *Epidemiology and Psychiatric Sciences*, *20*(3), 235–238. doi:10.1017/S2045796011000448 PMID:21922965

Didehbani, N., Allen, T., Kandalaft, M., Krawczyk, D., & Chapman, S. (2016). Virtual reality social cognition training for children with high functioning autism. *Computers in Human Behavior*, *62*, 703–711. doi:10.1016/j.chb.2016.04.033

Kandalaft, M. R., Didehbani, N., Krawczyk, D. C., Allen, T. T., & Chapman, S. B. (2013). Virtual reality social cognition training for young adults with high-functioning autism. *Journal of Autism and Developmental Disorders*, *43*(1), 34–44. doi:10.100710803-012-1544-6 PMID:22570145

Newbutt, N., Sung, C., Kuo, H. J., Leahy, M. J., Lin, C. C., & Tong, B. (2016). Brief report: A pilot study of the use of a virtual reality headset in autism populations. *Journal of Autism and Developmental Disorders*, 1–11. PMID:27272115

Parsons, S., & Cobb, S. (2011). State-of-the art of virtual reality technologies for children on the autism spectrum. *European Journal of Special Needs Education*, *26*(3), 355–366. doi:10.1080/08856257.2011.593831

Parsons, S., & Mitchell, P. (2002). The potential of virtual reality in social skills training for people with autistic spectrum disorders. *Journal of Intellectual Disability Research*, *46*(5), 430–443. doi:10.1046/j.1365-2788.2002.00425.x PMID:12031025

Radu, I. (2014). Augmented reality in education: A meta-review and cross-media analysis. *Personal and Ubiquitous Computing*, *18*(6), 1533–1543. doi:10.100700779-013-0747-y

Rizzo, A., & Kim, G. J. (2005). A SWOT analysis of the field of virtual reality rehabilitation and therapy. *Presence (Cambridge, Mass.)*, *14*(2), 119–146. doi:10.1162/1054746053967094

Rizzo, P. (2011). *Accuracy of self-perceptions in children and adults with ADHD* (Unpublished doctoral dissertation). University of Zurich, Switzerland. Retrieved April, 7 2018, from http://www.zora.uzh.ch/id/eprint/52775/1/RizzoFinales_Manuskript_dez_2011.pdf

Saadatzi, M. N., Pennington, R. C., Welch, K. C., & Graham, J. H. (2018). Small-Group Technology-Assisted Instruction: Virtual Teacher and Robot Peer for Individuals with Autism Spectrum Disorder. *Journal of Autism and Developmental Disorders*. doi:10.100710803-018-3654-2 PMID:29926295

# Acknowledgment

I wish to thank all the authors for having shared their precious research, work and experiences.

I wish to express sincere thanks to Nigel Newbutt for having shared his passion and commitment for the themes proposed in this publication. I also thank all the Editorial Advisory Board members, in particular Anitha S. Pillai, Sergio Casas and David Alberto Murolo for their support.

I also thank all the reviewers who prepared accurate evaluations of the chapters and helped me with their constructive reviews.

A special thanks goes to my previous professor, Tommaso Leo, for his brilliant advice during my PhD years at Università Politecnica delle Marche and for having inspired me with his vision of innovation and research.

My heartfelt thanks go to Daisaku Ikeda, philosopher and educator committed to individual empowerment, social engagement and dialogue for peace, for having enlightened me with his words.

Finally, a very special thank you goes to all my family and friends for their loving encouragement to complete this work.

*Giuliana Guazzaroni*
*Università Politecnica delle Marche, Italy*

# Section 1

# Infrastructural, Therapeutic, and Cultural Contexts

# Chapter 1
# Ubiquitous Bodies:
## A "Metrobodily" Transition From Real to Virtual

**Giorgio Cipolletta**
*Università di Macerata, Italy*

## ABSTRACT

*While the digital era has provided us with an incredible amount of accessibility, availability, and speedy tools, it has also made us lose that sense of critical awareness that was once considered a rare and precious gift. The marking feature of the present is ubiquity, as in the loss of spatial and temporal coordinates and the gain of a presence-absence that new technologies allow us to live – both positively and negatively. The body is the core of this electronic, virtual, and increased involvement. In this phase we're living in, the author suggests we introduce the neologism "metrobody" to identify this new hybrid condition undertaken by the body. This expression allows the author to reconfigure and hypothesize a different level and a different meaning of corporeality.*

## INTRODUCTION

*Visible and mobile, my body is a thing among things;*

*I caught in the fabric of the world,*

*and its cohesion is that of a thing.*

*But, because it moves itself and sees,*

*it holds things in a circle around itself.*

*Merleau-Ponty (2003)*

The anthropological change that the digital era has brought about opens a gap between existing images and the reality they should be a reflex of, a gap between what we believe they are and what they really are. This paradoxical experience in the digital age can be extended at a global level. While our nervous

DOI: 10.4018/978-1-5225-7168-1.ch001

system is allowed to ingest a vast quantity of information and intangible data, our own Self increases the condition of solitude. We are predominantly alone in front of the screen when we are connected; but at the same time, we also take part into the greatest social sharing. The relationship with the machine carries with it the risk of altering our nervous system by causing sensory amputations. Anyways, it is no longer possible to grow apart from our technological system because we need it since our bodies now blend naturally with the artificial and electronic environment. Instead, our interiority is in danger of easily swapping with the exterior of the screen: rather than 'the medium is the message', perhaps today it is the body itself that tends to become message, as in it becomes medium for accessing the world. In the virtual space lays the opportunity for *every-body* to become a *no-body* once and for all. But instead of aspiring to becoming no one, we shall consider Luigi Pirandello's formula "one, none, and a hundred thousand" as an opportunity to multiply ourselves in the "cross-narrative" circuit of the Net. Moving over Luigi Pirandello's disillusionment, we are actually heading towards Marinetti's multiplied man or McLuhan's global man. Therefore the theme of the body is again the central "core" because there's a need to rethink it again, now considering its expanded potential. The body expands at the borders of the virtual dimension and loads itself with new meanings. The contemporary body represents a changing and transitory reality defined by the context and connected to virtual and simulated reality practices. In this panorama, the creative process requires to deal with multiple and contemporary levels of complexity and various timescales.

## Ascott's Cyberception

Many artists working with electronics are interested in the new possibilities created by telecommunication technology and seem to be researching around inventing and extending it. We shall be optimistic about the potential meanings of these developments. Roy Ascott, a longtime pioneer in this works, writes that the art of our time is one system, process, behavior, interaction: indeed, this is the very potential of telematic system. English artist and theorist Roy Ascott was the first to have applied to art the cybernetic theories – defined by Norman Wiener in 1948 as the scientific study of communication between animals and machines – and telematics, the term used since 1978 to indicate the convergence of communication and computers. His theories found their practical environments in an experiment destined to be a historical point of reference exactly thirty years ago. In 1983 Ascott was invited by Frank Popper to take part in the Electra. Electricity and Electronics in the Art of the XX Century exhibit that was being held at the Musée d'Art Moderne de la Ville in Paris. Here the English artist displayed his trailblazing project *La Plissure du Texte / The Pleating of the Text: A Planetary Fairytale*, also known by its acronym *LPDT.* The title is an explicit reference to an essay by French critic Roland Barthes that was published ten years earlier with the title *Le Plaisir du Texte* (1973), a popular essay discussing, among many other things, on authorship and on the role of reader as a writer of the text. Ascott foresees multiple authors and readers. Artists and authors from eleven different countries and continents scattered around the globe(including the United States, Canada, Europe and Australia) were called together to contribute to the creation of the "planetary fairytale" for the *La Plissure duTexte*. The narrative text of one was a continuation of another from a remote position with the same spirit as the one found in the surrealist game of *Cadavere exquis* (Exquisite corpse), as media theorist Edmond Couchot remarked. Ascott drew upon all the potential offered by the network and telematics of the time to put his concept of "distributed authorship" into practice. This project has become an historical reference but its origin precedes this date. In regard to this point, we would like to mention his essay *The Construction of Change* published in 1964 in "Cambridge Opinin.41. Modern Art in Britain". This was the first published article by Ascott that redefined art in light of Wiener's cybernetics. His immediate understanding of the impact cybernetics was to have on society and art's eventual role in the interception of these changes meant that he was capable of projecting and anticipating a new definition of artistic interest through information, behaviour and interaction. Conceiving and structuring a work as a combination of relations in which comprehending the interactivity – change and considering art in its educational role – meant bringing its programming and behavioural aspects to the forefront, placing them before the final result (Rossi, 2018). In 2010, *The Plissure du Texte was* revised and redeveloped in Second Life by the author in collaboration with Max Moswitzer, Selavy Oh and Elif Ayiter. It is from here that the two new versions LPDT2 LPDT3 and take off: structured with the architecture and textual geography placed between worlds and dimensions – where autonomous robots intervene as communicative junctions among narrators and where visitors in physical space can interact by (among other things) sending text messages and tweeting. The undisputed figure of Ascott today has brought researchers and curators to reconsider his group of groundbreaking analogical works in which he prefigures his theories on the network and telematic interaction. A series of projects like those carried out between 1963 and 1970 was presented by Plug In ICA, with Video Pool Media during the summer of 2013 (Rossi, 2018).

The breadth of Ascott's vision, fed also by his continuous educative commitment which is still extremely active with his International research platform I-Nodes, is what has guided the intuition and foresight of this artist and theorist towards the ongoing anticipation and vision of the variety of ways in which technology is interwoven with humankind – in its physical and social organization. Among these, the singling out of our need to re-create new nature – *Natura II* – which belongs to a world that is neither digitally dry nor biologically wet. In short, a "moist media". This is what is derived from his interest in quantum physics and techno-ethics and the direction in which his scientific commitment to the most current research is heading, coherently moving from his pioneering work (Ascott, 2004).

*Figure 1. LPDT2*
*(Flickr, 2010)*

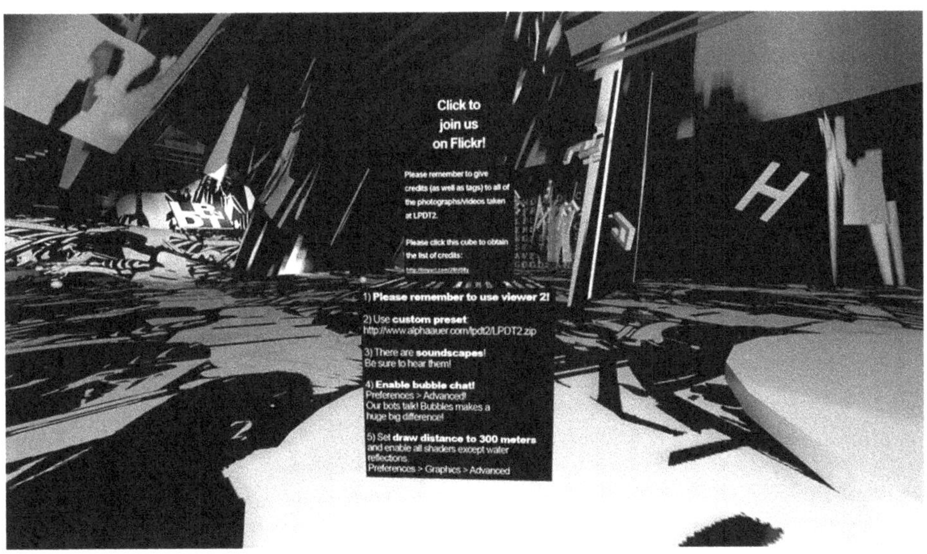
Click to
join us
on Flickr!
Please remember to give
credits (as well as tags) to all of
the photographs/videos taken
at LPDT2.
Please click this cube to obtain
the list of credits:
1) Please remember to use viewer 2!
2) Use custom preset
http://www.alphaauer.com/lpdt2/LPDT2.zip
3) There are soundscapes!
Be sure to hear them!
4) Enable bubble chat!
Preferences > Advanced!
Our bots talk! Bubbles makes a
huge big difference!
5) Set draw distance to 300 meters
and enable all shaders except water
reflections.
Preferences > Graphics > Advanced

With electronic media, its flows of images and texts, and the ubiquitous connectivity of telematic system, this isolation and separateness of humans shall eventually disappear, and new architectural structures and forms of cultural association shall emerge. In this panorama we are assisting to new art practices, with new strategies and theories, new form of public accessibility, new method of presentation and display, new learning network, - quoting Ascott - "whole new cultural configurations". According to the British artist, we are looking at a culture in which intelligence is spilling out of our brains to fill every nook and cranny of the world, every environment, every tool, every product. The dry world of computational virtuality and the wet world of biological systems are converging to produce a new substrate for creative work, "moistmedia", consisting of bits, atoms, neurons, and genes. There is also a convergence of three VRs. According to Ascott (2004) - who considers the space and state of our consciousness- our mind pivots on the triangulation between three poles that he refers to as the Three VRs: *Virtual Reality*, *Validated Reality* and *Vegetal Reality*.

Ascott (2004) describes *Virtual Reality* as the one that allows the viewer to simultaneously see the internal dynamics and the external features of an object of study. Therefore Virtual Reality changes the way we see ourselves, our behaviour, and the environments we wish to inhabit. Instead, *Validated Reality* is the authorised reality with narrow confines that restrict the sense of what we are or what we could be. It controls the coordinates of our daily life, dictates protocols of behaviour, and provides an illusion of coherence in a contingent universe. It is precisely the *Validated Reality* that has 'created' Nature as in an array of objects set in the Euclidean space, rather than a dynamic network of processes and relationships. The third VR, *Vegetal Reality*, can be understood as the transformation of consciousness by plant technology. The canon of practice and insight in this technology is archaic in its human application and known to us mainly through the largely visionary work of shamans, often operating in a context of healing which is extremely distant from the *Validated Reality* of Western medicine. However, frequently during the past century we have seen the appropriation and synthesis of shaman's knowledge of plants by the pharmaceutical industry. This ancient knowledge allowed us to have some of the most spectacular products of modern medicine (Ascott, 2001). There is a fourth VR, that Ascott calls *Variable Reality*, which is the syncretic reality. One of the conditions we can assume in *Variable Reality* is "cyberception".

So, according to Ascott, "cyberception" is the convergence of perceptive and conceptual processes in which the connectivity of telematic networks plays a constructive role (Ascott, 1999). We are computer-mediated and computer-enhanced. These new ways of conceptualising and perceiving reality involve more than simply some sort of quantitative change in how we see, think and act in the world. They constitute a qualitative change in our being, a whole new faculty, the post-biological faculty of "cyberception". In other words - Roy Ascott explains us - the post-biological technologies enable us to become directly involved in our own transformation and are bringing about a qualitative change in our being. The emergent faculty of "cyberception" - i.e. our artificially enhanced interactions of perception and cognition - affects the transpersonal technology of global networks and cybermedia. Cyberception" not only implies a new body and a new consciousness but a redefinition of how we might live together in the interspace between the virtual and the real (Ascott, 1994). Finally Ascott (2013) sums up:

*the way we are now!*

*our planet is telematic*

*our media is moist*

*our mind is technoetic*

*our modeling is cybernetic*

*our sensorium is extended*

*our identity is multiple*

*our body is transformable*

*our art is syncretic*

*our substrate is nano*

*our reality is variable.*

In summary, each of us when connected to the Net is transformed into a plurality of individuals who interface with each other. This new way of relating to, looking at and perceiving reality is what I call the metrobodily condition, an ubiquitous condition of the body in virtual reality.

## Virtual Condition

Many authors have addressed the concept of the virtual highlighting different conditions of "presence". Virtual Reality (VR) applies the progress in speed computing, graphics display, sensor sciences, and programming techniques in order to provoke in a participant an immersive experience inside a computer generated space that we call a virtual world. Virtual worlds may or may not be analogous to our physical

*Figure 2. 4th VR by Roy Ascott*
*(© Copyright 2012, Roy Ascott. Used with permission)*

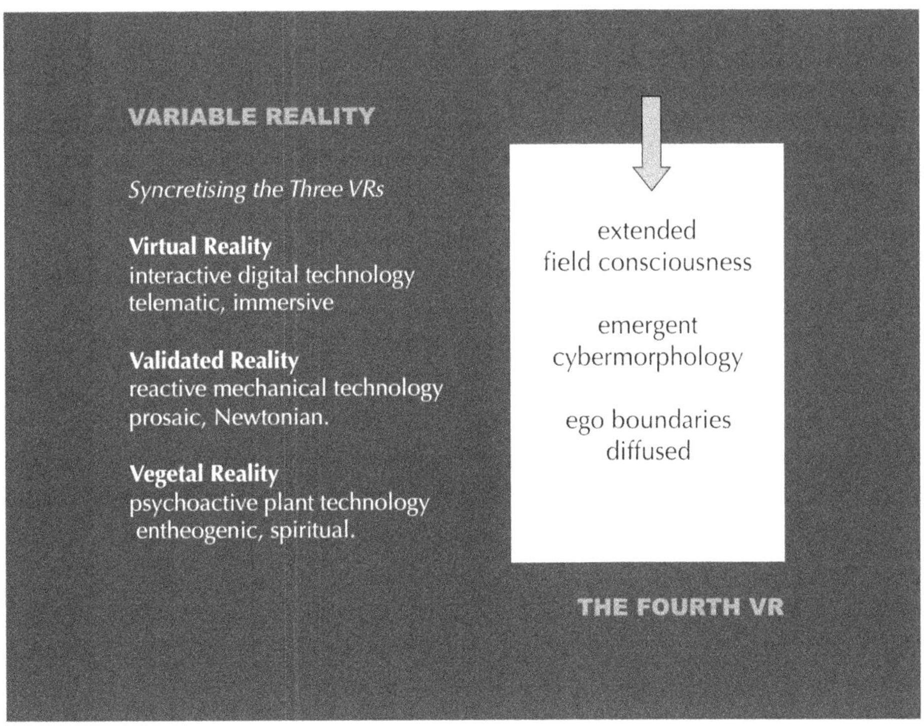

space; virtual environments may be realistic, extrasensory, telepresent or hybrid. The sensation of immersion is accomplished by peripheral devices wearable on the head such as visual and auditory displays with motion trackers. Therefore, by the term 'virtual body' we refer to any of the many realizable and realized possibilities of the real body's extensions, including the one in a uni-directional relation to the real world. The body becomes an image, that is an algorithm in binary format turned into a *phenomenon* in the interaction between a user and another user. Hence, since the body in Virtual Reality is first and foremost an interactive digital image, it can interact through the peripheral devices of a computer: it can even interact with a real biorobotic prosthesis, thus provoking an extremely high degrees of "immersion". The virtual body acts as an intermediary between us and what is beyond the screen. It is not unique, it multiplies and escapes the dichotomy between "internal" and "external". These multiple bodies are neither a simple cognitive product of consciousness, nor consciential images. The user is aware of experiencing 'another' reality. It is not the bodies that are produced, but rather body-images (bodies&images) that become "events" in the happening of the interaction, as Italian theorist Roberto Diodato (2012) explains According to Diodato (2012), the perception of the body-image is established by the interaction. Hence, the virtual body cannot be conceived as mere resistance and inertia to interaction since it only exists in the virtual environment of a network which is never individual, it's always an interaction. Therefore, the individual is defined as an algorithm of one of the possible phenomenal actualizations. This new communicational dynamic creates a symbiosis between man and machine: the body keeps its central position while it acquires a new body dimension.

The body disseminated on the Net can be a very powerful instrument of communication, because it allows both an enhancement and an increase of the individual's capacities, and a real collective dimension, in real time, not only of abstract intelligences, but of the whole of man's bodily functions and activities. Therefore, as the body turns virtual and becomes a body-image, it acquires a double meaning: on one hand it represents the digital images in our computer monitors; on the other hand the body-image interacts with our augmented body. Virtual body is not a simply copy of the body but it is an autonomous object able to introduce us to new perceptive and cognitive possibilities. The virtual body is indeed an interaction, an object-event: an action (relation of interaction) (Diodato, 2018). The body does not disappear (Kroker, 1996), it certainly modifies and carries out a dissemination (Caronia, 2011) in the networks and in the immaterial virtual spaces of the digital machines. Through new media, the displacement of the reality operated by the image has created a process of virtualization of both space and body, both involved in the development of media re-mediation through which multiplying the body itself. The body can be seen through TV or film screens. Moreover, the same categories of space and time are radically re-established, while realities continuously take on different forms. French philosopher Pierre Lévy (1997) talks about the virtual, too. He writes about the process of virtualization that it 'produces a deterritorialization, through which the multiplication of spaces makes us a new kind of nomad: instead of following the wandering and migrating lines within a certain extension, we jump from one network to another, from one proximity system to the next'. According to Levy, the real resembles the possible; the present, instead, is not at all similar to the virtual: it responds to it. The virtualization process corresponds to a production of new identities. Again, Deleuze (1968) uses the term virtual in the meaning of what is powerful and not in action. The virtualization process represents the transition, the elevation to power of an entity. The idea of a virtual body refers to what tends to actualize itself and is distinguished from the idea of the possible as what is realized. The qualitative difference between current and real consists in the fact that if the updating is a creative response to virtuality, which in turn is the elevation of an entity to the general state of a problem, the real is already inscribed in the possible as happening of a possible predefined. Deleuze (2002) writes:

*It is by virtue of their mutual inextricability that virtual images are able to react upon actual objects. From this perspective, the virtual images delimit a continuum, whether one takes all of the circles together or each individually, a spatium determined in each case by the maximum of time imaginable. The varyingly dense layers of the actual object correspond to these, more or less extensive, circles of virtual images. These layers, whilst themselves virtual, and upon which the actual object becomes itself virtual, constitute the total impetus of the object. The plane of immanence, upon which the dissolution of the actual object itself occurs, is itself constituted when both object and image are virtual. But the process of actualization undergone by the actual is one which has as great an effect on the image as it does on the object. The continuum of virtual images is fragmented and the spatium cut up according to whether the temporal decompositions are regular or irregular. The total impetus of the virtual object splits into forces corresponding to the partial continuum, and the speeds traversing the cut-up spatium. The virtual is never independent of the singularities which cut it up and divide it out on the plane of immanence. [...] The actual is the complement or the product, the object of actualization, which has nothing but virtual as its subject. Actualization belongs to the virtual. The actualization of the virtual is singularity whereas the actual itself is individuality constituted. The actual falls from the plane like a fruit, whist the actualization relates it back to the plane as if to that which turns the object back into a subject (pp. 149-150).*

From Deleuze's and Levy's philosophical point of view, virtualization represents a vector of reality. In technological development, instead, the concept of the virtual is reversed through the description of a process of disembodiment and dematerialization. This process modifies the relationship with materiality and the substantial loss of reality. Following a perspective of the virtual, according to French philosopher Baudrillard (1981) we enter the realm of simulacra and simulation. According to him, "simulation is no longer that of a territory, a referential being or a substance, but the generation of models of a real without origin or reality: a hyperreal" (pp. 166-167). Baudrillard sees in the electronic copy a substitution of reality, while Levy believes that the virtual does not subtract something to the world, rather it enriches it by adding a new dimension. For Baudrillard, the shift from the real to the hyperreal occurs when representation gives way to simulation. One could argue that we are standing at the brink of such a moment, marked primarily by the emerging presence of a virtual world (Nunes, 1995). From the neurobiological point of view, Chilean biologist Humberto Maturana keeps the distinction between perception and illusion. In other words, according to him, we reduce the reality generated by VR systems in terms of virtual reality by considering the daily experience in the 'real reality' as a validation term. In everyday life we live the experiences offered by VR systems as real and as these indistinguishable from ordinary ones. Neuroscientist Francisco Varela together with Maturana (1980) reminds us that there is no world, except what we experience through the processes that are given to us and that make us what we are. When we are inserted into virtual worlds we are conscious of our condition as beings determined by a biological structure, because only the human structure makes possible the enactment of a virtual reality and it validates its experience. The so-called 'reality effects' are nothing more than the product of the involvement of our sensory-motor structure, of our body, in actions and perceptions according to this structure. If the virtual world and the real world have something in common, that is the common enactive brand: the human structure. As Italian theorist Capucci (1993) explains, the point of view - as it is a foundation of the subject - shall be replaced by the *point d'être*: the artificial reality would then become 'presence upon the body', in contact with the existing reality and with the psychosensory indivisibility of the subject. Consequently, virtual bodies are neither just images, nor just bodies, but rather image-bodies. It can perhaps be said that, in its capacity as an emerging hybrid structure, the virtual body elides the two sides of the interactive relation: both the merely physical-material meaning of 'external' and the merely cognitive-personal meaning of 'internal'. Diodato (2018) explains: 'the virtual body is therefore configured as a subjective-objective chiasm. In a virtual body-environment, in which space itself is the result of an interaction, the world does not occur in terms of a process of distancing, but in the sense-feeling of immersion, and the body, inasmuch as it is perceived as other, takes on the sense of its reality, of its effectuality, as a pathic and imaginary incision. Thus the virtual body-environment is primarily an intermediary between inner and outer experience, a place in which the border becomes territory' (pp. 64-65). Media theoritian Flusser (1996, 1997) explains the topic in other words. According to him, the real/virtual category has now lost all meaning, since the worlds virtually produced can no longer be distinguished from the 'real' world. In fact we compute, we compose, and the escape from linearity produces a virtual objectivity. We no longer imagine that we perceive reality, rather that we build or process the perceived as reality. Therefore, we do not change anything that has already been given, we are not subjects wearing themselves out on objects. Instead, we tend to just realize given possibilities: we no longer get the change of reality, we have the realization of possibilities. Flusser (2004) writes: 'the digital world picture as it is being suggested to us by the sciences and presented to our eyes by computers [...] whether we like it or not [... and] this imposes on us not only a new ontology, but also a new anthropology. We have to understand ourselves – our 'self' – as such a 'digital distribution', as a realization of possibilities thanks to dense distribution' (p. 244).

The procedures of digital simulation, the virtual disguise of the body in the Net have led to a new understanding of the relationship with the world and with our body that does not disappear; above all what does not disappear is its symbolic function, that is a body immersed in another territory. The VR produces both a replica and an invasion of its own body until it determines a dissemination in the Net.

## Beyond the Virtual

At this point the question is: how many bodies do we have?

Canadian philosopher Brian Massumi answers this question stating that the obsolescence of the body is the condition of change, obsolescence is its vitality. He calls this condition 'body without an image', whereas Portuguese philosopher Jose Gil (1998) talks about the 'infra-linguistic body' and Deleuze and Guattarì (1983, 1987) develop the idea of the body without organs. In the VR you don't keep your body, but you leave it at the entrance of the 'world that opens beyond the interface', while your mind wanders without obstacles inhabiting an uncontaminated virtual body in cyberspace. The virtual reality represents the third space that lies between the object seen and the sensation felt. An important step of VR technology is the one going beyond the limits of the body itself, which in relation to the medium makes the subject 'disembodied'. In other words the body is virtual and the virtual is actual. This short circuit combines a sort of a potential process where the virtuality of the body is an emergence, and this emergence is a critical point where the transition happens.

The advent of microprocessors and VR systems has offered numerous advantages in terms of storage and modification of digital information. In this context of dispersion and immersion of the body, the body presence is less in favour of another presence which is located there, beyond, elsewhere. So *where am I?*

The mind turns out to be a system to generate continuous models, and through integration and sensorial manipulation the presence thus becomes its instrument. If the 'Self' finds itself having the sensation of being immersed in a situation (being there), this means that the mind has activated that particular cognitive-sensory mechanism called presence.

The development of these technologies has brought the recipient to be aware of being located in an environment other than the physical, outside of the same digital action. We can think of virtual presence as a mental state in which the user believes he is physically present in a visual, auditory and tactile space generated by a computer. The definition of presence is precisely the way in which the relationship between 'reality' and 'virtuality', between objective space and simulated space is conceived. The sensation of presence depends very much on the level of interaction that users experience in both real and simulated environment. In the latest years, with the further development of these virtual systems, cognitive sciences have tried to give a further answer to the concept of presence, defining it as a selective and adaptive mechanism that allows the 'Self' to define the boundary of action between internal and external in a sensory flux. According to this new perspective, the presence can be understood as the sensation of "being" inside a real or virtual environment, resulting from the ability to implement one's intentions through the affordances it offers. Virtual reality, telepresence and augmented systems have the ability to enable people to act within themselves through multimodal interaction, where the senses are embedded in a single experience that enables a complete immersion. The new body is immersed in pixels, social networks, databases, geographic coordinates, QR-Code (two-dimensional bar codes), augmented realities and ubiquitous technologies. This mutation created by the virtual condition goes beyond the concept of species. Technologies can be integrated into the body creating whole new perspectives through which roles, relationships and interrelationships of the world's inhabitants in all their forms can be reconsidered. The relationship between body and environment, and between body, environment and urban space, implies technology combining with the body itself in a continuous dialogue between virtualization and possibility. For example, virtual reality allows us to enter into three-dimensional spaces, while the connection to a network transforms the screen into a window through which we can access distant places. Following Massumi's thought, surely the body becomes a resonating vessel for the force of information to which it is now singularly sensitized. The Canadian philosopher Massumi (1998) explains: 'when I think of my body and ask what it does to earn that name, two things stand out. It/eels. In fact, it docs both at the same time, It moves as it feels, and it feels itself moving. Can we think a body without this: an intrinsic connection between movement and sensation whereby each immediately summons the other?' (pp. 1-2). We can talk about a sort of a 'new nature' that profoundly transforms social spaces, relationships, identity, memory, utopias, even human biology. A new imaginary opens up to a different gaze that is confused with reality made by photography, cinema, video, up to images obtained with the computer and Virtual Reality.

## Ubiquitous Bodies

In this transition from real to virtual, the body - the protagonist of this immersion - becomes an essential parameter of the contemporary and it can represent the world in a new multi-centric vision. The platforms will thus be the new virtual terrain where bodycodes will live and share, while flesh will be the place where technology will become a host (bodyhost) and the body will be the place 'of hospitality'. The one artist we shall mention then is Stelarc. His work also combines manifold artistic disciplines. In his work, performance art subsumes choreography, music, audiovisual arts and sculpture. Communicativeness, hybridity and virtuality become the essential properties of this artist's output, which is tantamount to stating that they become the principal attributes of his body, regarded as an artistic medium. Therefore, in this context I suggest we can introduce the neologism "metrobody" to identify this new hybrid condition undertaken by body. This expression allows me to reconfigure and hypothesize a different level and a different meaning of corporeality. When we establish the connection with the digital space, the shape and image of our body perception are 'embedded' and re-configurate itself while reacting to the presence of our body with a corporeal-feedback. This consists of a complex, distinct, decomposed and hybrid image. It is exactly at this stage of re-configuration that the condition of the "metrobody" comes to existence. It works as a filter between our lived body (Merleau-Pounty, 2003, 1968, 1962) as it is interacting (in connection) with digital space. Our bodies are virtually embodied in multiple functional identities marked with distinctive passwords and nicknames (avatars). "metrobody" is therefore thought as a metrics for the body under post-digital condition. Here the body becomes a device, an interface, a tool, a piece of art, while emphasizing its transitional state. In other words, I suggest that nowadays natural sciences shall open to the playfulness inherent in artistic practices, especially the playful nature that the arts apply in toying with scientific observations. Moreover, this transdisciplinary approach could promote interesting ways of thinking. One of these is for instance metaphor. In this new digital panorama, art is rethought as a process where science and technology are integrated, and intersect various fields of knowledge in a communication system, eventually understanding and recognizing the complex natural process of evolution of art (Cipolletta, 2014). This reflection could be an interesting and powerful model against dehumanization; also, it is a call for a re-aestheticization of technology and science (and of the human being).

An important example in the artistic field to mention is that of French artist, Organ (born Mireille Suzanne Francette Porte). In the surgical-operation-performances of early nineties, her identity research is 'reincarnated to present the climax of a long cognitive process. ORLAN transformed the operating room into an artist's studio where an artwork was produced, thus inaugurating the mutating paradigm of contemporary art – a progressive return to 'bodily' themes – in a direct relationship with new technologies and biotechnologies, a new trend where the French artist once again appears at the front. The appropriation of plastic surgery as a creative art form, both as subject and object of the performance in which the 'oeuvre-action' integrates the artist's body, marks the passage of *Body Art* into *Carnal Art* in ORLAN's work. In 1998 Orlan starts on a virtual tour of the world in search of aethestic standards of other civilizations. The portraits of the series "Self-Hybridisation" represent a fusion of criteria that belong to our epoch as well as to pre-columbian times (which saw a culture with various bodily deformations). Each generated image, digitally processed, corresponds a statue or a certain old mask. In the Self-Hybridization series (Pre-Colombian, African and the more recent ones on Native Americans), ORLAN continues and extends her journey through infinity of possible physical identities. By using various canons of beauty and aesthetics from different times and places, the artist creates 'living' totemic figures, almost tangible in their virtuality, fascinating in their disturbing appearance and seductive in their artificial otherness.

Another ubiquitous body (in a different way from the above example) that we can mention is that of Salvatore Iaconesi in the project *One Avatar.* The artwork is an installation/performance. The installation space features from two to four computers placed on black exhibition blocks, and connected to form a network. In the center of the space stands the performer wearing a *OneAvatar's* wearable device (suite). The visitors can use the computers to play a 3D game in which they hunt the performer's avatar in a virtual world. When they eventually catch and shoot him, the performer gets an electric shock,

*Figure 3. Orlan par Fabrice Lévêque 1997.*
*(Wikimedia Commons, 2016)*

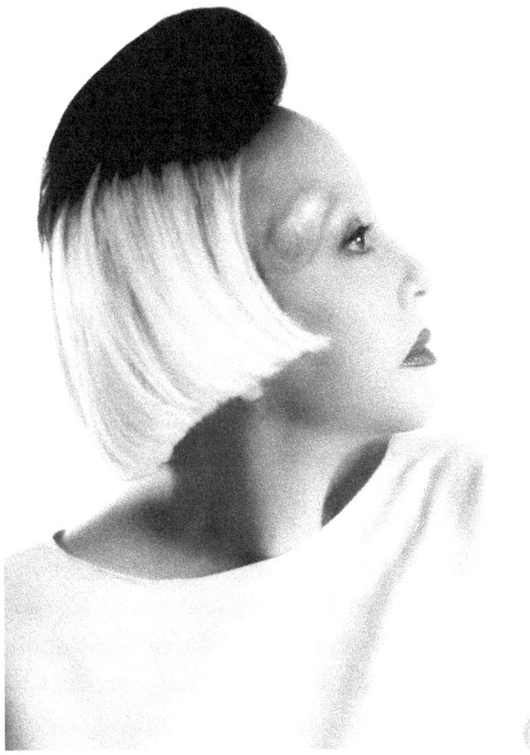

*Figure 4. OneAvatar @ Milano in Digitale*
*(Flickr, 2008)*

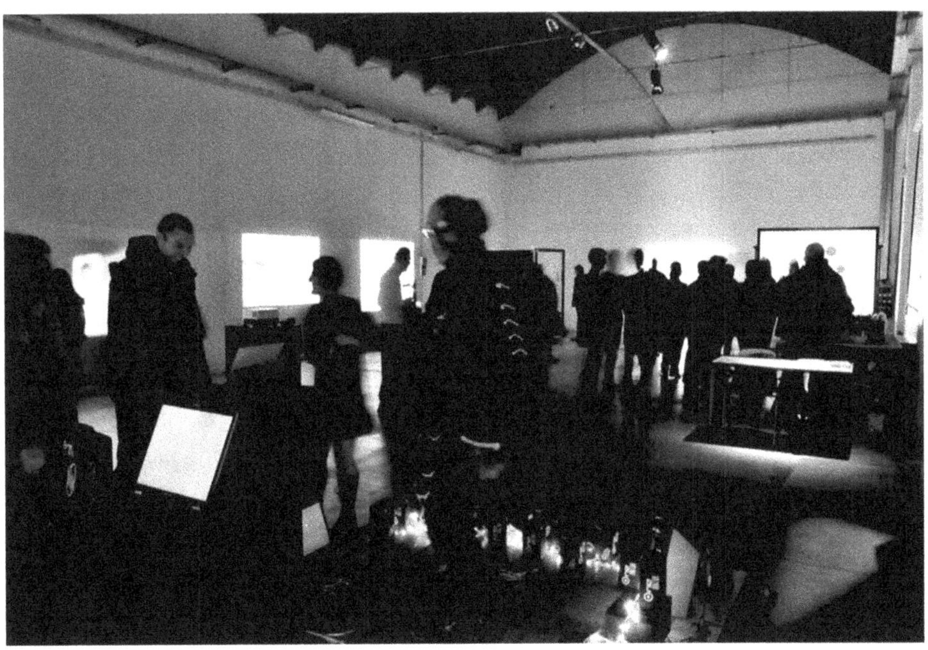

transmitted to the affected parts of the body of the avatar trough the electric circuit fit in the *OneAvatar suit*, placed in contact with the performer's body. When this happens, the sound of an electric shock is played and the led lights disseminated throughout the device/suit are illuminated through an electronic circuit, producing visual effects running through the body of the performer. During the performance the sound is three dimensional, providing an immersive experience, and a set of one or more video projections are played on the sides of the installation, displaying the in-game point of view of the performer's avatar and - if more than one projection is available - two info-aesthetic visualizations of the game's parameters and of the avatar/performer's body conditions (generative graphics controlled by body sweat, muscle fatigue and tension, body movement). Thus, the visitors are placed in front of a game which implements a bridge between virtual and real worlds: what happens in the virtual world has repercussions in the real one, under the form of the physical effects on the performer's body and of the multisensorial environment created in the installation's space. Iaconesi explains as the virtual Worlds such as Second Life and World of Warcraft address people's perceptions and sensorial domains in specific ways. By using (living) these worlds users experience emotions, sensations and perceptions to which they are used to or of completely new kind. Both types are 'new' in the fact that they are created in the users by means of technological devices and digital communications related practices. This is a major trend of contemporary technology. Bridges across information, architectures, processes and the body are constantly being created at sensorial or even physical levels. Interactive systems, wearable technologies, prosthetics, technologies that are embedded into objects and locations, domotics, robots, artificial intelligences. All of these things go towards eliminating the possible dualities intermediating between what is organic and inorganic, of what is body and what is architecture, what is thought or memory and what is external information flow, what is a physical product and what is an immaterial service. As the Italian anthropologist Massimo Canevacci (2012) explains: 'ubiquity is beyond any dualism of space and time male and female, material and immaterial, nature and culture, labor and work, body and soul. Ubiquity is the ontology of the sacred spreading out in the air of pixel' (pp. 256-257). In other words, the condition of ubiquity is the central concept of everyday experiences, based on digital revolution, transforming the traditional compact identity in an ubiquitous subject.

## For a Metrobodily Transition

The concept of "metrobody" represents the idea of a new metrics of the body, conceived both as a mutant parameter and a transitive variable. It does not measure, it is not measure, but is measured in relation to the physical and digital environment at the same time, losing even the limits of reality. From this point of view, the body becomes similar to a landscape and it vibrates into metrobodily transition. Smartphones, sensors, services of all kinds, interactive screens, urban screens, media façades, augmented realities, social networks, natural interaction systems are activated by gesture, voice and movement of the body. These and other devices, interfaces and services add up to even more common and widespread others that allow us to transform each action in data and information, whether we are aware of it or not. The life of these data and information is complex. Some of them are archived - according to various modalities and degrees of persistence- until they are needed. Others are directly used - to execute services and processes. This complex scenario generates a multitude of different ways in which these types of information can be transformed into opportunities for interaction with citizens and other human beings.

Furthermore, the information can be recombined in infinite different ways, to produce infinite different geographies, opportunities for interaction, services, games, artworks and more. We find ourselves in a digital Third Space, a more inclusive space in which information is not only attached to places, spaces, bodies and objects, but it is constantly recombined, remixed, recontextualized. In this interlude new emotional, linguistic, semantic, relational geographies arise. The body is willing to accept the challenge. It is 'placed on' the device. This 'body disposition' in the digital world opens up a new model of existence, a new way of living, and a new human ecosystem. Bodies narrate themselves by "dipping" into the technological narration surrounded by a multi-sensorial context. This sophisticated approach to the role of embodiment in our digital age reveals the "metrobody" as a very promising concept in addressing the constant creation of meaning we face today both on the virtual and analog side of media technology. The body opens up the process of subjectivation in the post-digital age for an existential understanding of our mediated sense of presence. This methodology allows the merge of classical and contemporary perspectives on the body between the natural and artificial in a very innovative way, where the body is placed between the analog and the virtual space. The data body is a virtual body which is composed of all the files connected to an individual. The virtual character of the data body means that social regulation that applies to the real body is absent. In other words, "metrobody" is a mental expression for describing this spherical mutation, where the ubiquitous bodies are interconnected for a living, hybrid and hyperconnected planet. Information systems, distributed computing, peer to peer networks, cryptography, steganography, software, are all tools that can be used to create new immaterial spaces and bodies. Augmented reality, wearable computing, location based technologies, ubiquitous communications, pervasive media and interactive architectures are all tools that can be used to colonize physical spaces and bodies, turning them into something new and emergent. Bodies are everywhere, absent and present at once. We have many bodies: physical, virtual, extended, multisensorial (Cipolletta, 2014). Art and science mix together for creating a new vision and re-thinking humanity in its evolution. Everyday we extend our senses through digital devices and our body turns into a device itself. The "metrobody" exceeds reality going further beyond Krueger's 'Artificial Reality' (1983) and Langton's 'Artificial Life' (1997) towards a psychopathic space that leads reality towards a hallucinatory satisfaction of desire at the war cry of 'virtual reality everywhere' (Weibel, 1993, p. 216). In other words, virtuality connects imaginary and reality in a sort of a faded bridge. Technology, simulates a new interactive bodily space and it is even the spirit that becomes a virtual system in the machine of the physical body. (pp. 219-221). The body acts on the spirit and the spirit acts on the body. In the dynamics of virtuality, all this merges in a simulated dream. Here we are at the end of a path where the body moves with its physical and conscious content through a technological variation. It has been investigated, searched, surpassed and modified, scanned: in other words, hybridized. The ""metrobody"" becomes a bodily vehicle of a new metrics of the body, with the body as a mutant parameter. The "metrobody" is invisible, absent; it resides in a "non-border" and mobilizes its functions filtering reality to connect to the virtual reality. The "metrobody" could be a geography of the virtual (in terms of potentiality, what can a body do?). The re-virtualization of bodies is the condition of amplification and modification of the very human nature. We are all experience of an hybrid conditions of being, our blood and flesh intertwining with economic growth and technological development. In other words, the condition of hybridism of human beings with the technology, tackles the relationship between human biology and culture in the imaginary, virtual and real life. The Hybrid Age is therefore the transitional period between the Information Age - as in the "third wave" for Toffler (1980) - and the moment of technological singularity, when machines surpass human intelligence (Kurzweil, 2005). The Hybrid Age is a phase in which we cross the threshold on to a new mode of arranging global society. It is a new socio-technical era currently unfolding as technologies merge with each other while humans merge with technology itself. Sciences and technology have enormous effects on the ways in which we perceive our body, our interconnection with the rest of the world – whether human or non-human – our health and well-being. We are all ubiquitous bodies.

## REFERENCES


Ascott, R. (1988). Art and Education in the Telematic Culture. *Leonardo*, (1), 7-11.

Ascott, R. (Ed.). (1999). *Reframing Consciousness: Art, Mind and Technology*. Bristol, UK: Intellect.

Ascott, R. (2001). *When the Jaguar lies down with the Lamb: speculations on the post-biological culture.* Paper presented at CAiiA-STAR Symposium: 'Extreme parameters. New dimensions of interactivity', Barcelona, Spain. 10.7238/a.v0i1.677

Ascott, R. (2013). *Interstitial Creativity Art/Mind/Technology.* Paper presented at COST Arts & Technologies Workshop - CAT, Zagreb, Croatia.

Baudrillard, J. (1980). *Simulacres et simulation*. Paris: Galilée.

Canevacci, M. (2012). Digital Auratic Reproducibility: Ubiquitous Ethnographies and Communicational Metropolis. In *An Ethnography of Global Landscapes and Corridors*. Retrieved July 8, 2018, from http://www.intechopen.com/books/an-ethnography-of-global-landscapes-and- corridors/digital-auratic-reproducibility

Capucci, P. L. (1993). *Realtà del Virtuale. Rappresentazioni tecnologiche, comunicazione, arte*. Bologna: CLUEB.

Caronia, A. (1996). *Il corpo virtuale. Dal corpo robotizzato al corpo disseminato nelle reti*. Padova: FrancoMuzzio Editore.

Cipolletta, G. (2014). *Passages metrocorporei. Per un'estetica della transizione.* Macerata: eum.

Deleuze, G. (1968). *Spinoza et le problème de l'expression*. Paris: Les Editions de Minuit.

Deleuze, G., & Guattarì, F. (1983). *Anti-Oedipus*. Minneapolis, MN: University of Minnesota.

Deleuze, G., & Parnet, C. (2002). *Dialogues II*. New York: Columbia University Press.

Deluze, G., & Guattarì, F. (1987). *A Thousand Plateaus*. Minneapolis, MN: University of Minnesota.

Diodato, R. (2012). *Aesthetics of the Virtual*. New York: Suny Press.

Diodato, R. (2018). Virtual. In *International Lexicon of Aesthetics. Spring 2018 Edition*. Retrieved July 8, 2018, from https://lexicon.mimesisjournals.com/archive/2018/spring/Virtual.pdf

Flickr. (2008). *OneAvatar @ Milano in Digitale*. Retrieved from https://www.flickr.com/photos/xdxd_vs_xdxd/3033590996/in/photostream/

Flickr. (2010). *Torley*. Retrieved from https://www.flickr.com/photos/torley/5054603928

Flusser, V. (1996). *Kommunikologie*. Frankfurt am Main, Germany: Fisher Taschenbuch Verlag.

Flusser, V. (1997). *Medienkultur*. Frankfurt am Main, Germany: Fischer Taschenbuch Verlag.

Flusser, V. (2000). *Towards a Philosophy of Photography*. London: Reaktion Books.

Gil, J. (1998). *Metemorphoses of the Body*. Minneapolis, MN: Minnesota University Press.

Hansen, M. B. N. (2006). *Bodies in code. Interface with digital media*. New York: Routledge Taylor & Francis Group.

Khanna, P. A. (2012). *Hybrid Reality. Thriving in the Emerging Human-Technology Civilization*. TED Books.

Kroker, A., & Weinstein, M. (1995). *Data Trash*. Montreal: New World Perspectives.

Krueger, M. W. (1983). *Artificial Reality*. Boston: Addison-Wesley.

Kurzweil, R. (2005). *The Singularity Is Near: When Humans Transcend Biology*. New York: Viking Books.

Langton, G. L. (1997). *Artificial Life*. Boston: MIT Press.

Massumi, B. (1998). From Hypersurface Architecture. *Architectural Design*, *68*(5/6), 16–24.

Massumi, B. (2002). *Parables for the virtual: movement, affect, sensation*. Durham, NC: Duke University. doi:10.1215/9780822383574

Maturana, R. H., & Varela, F. (1980). *Autopoiesis and Cognition. The Realization of the Living*. Dordrecht: Reidel Publishing Company. doi:10.1007/978-94-009-8947-4

McLuhan, M. (1964). *Understanding Media*. New York: Graw-Hill Book Company.

Merleau-Ponty, M. (2003). *Nature: Course Notes from the Collège de France*. Evanston, IL: Northwestern University Press.

Merleau-Pounty, M. (1962). *Phenomenology of Perception*. London: Routledge and Kegan Paul.

Merleau-Pounty, M. (1968). *The Visible and the Invisible*. Evanston, IL: Northwestern University Press.

Nunes, M. (1995). Jean Baudrillard in cyberspace: Internet, virtuality, and postmodernity. *Style (Fayetteville)*, (29), 314–327.

Rossi, E. G. (2018). *Roy Ascott. Esperienze telematiche*. Retrieved July 8, 2018, from http://www.arshake.com/roy-ascott-esperienze-telematiche/

Spinoza, B. (2007). *Opere*. Milano: Mondadori.

Toffler, A. (1980). *The Third Wave*. New York: William Morrow & C.

Weibel, P. (1993). Mondi virtuali: i nuovi corpi dell'imperatore. In P. L. Capucci (Ed.), *Realtà del virtuale* (pp. 196–224). Bologna: CLUEB.

Wikimedia Commons. (2016). *File:Orlan par Fabrice Lévêque*. Retrieved from https://commons.wikimedia.org/wiki/File:Orlan_par_Fabrice_L%C3%A9v%C3%AAque_1997-2.jpg

Wilson, S. (2010). *Art +Science Now*. London: Thames & Hundson.

## KEY TERMS AND DEFINITIONS

**Cyberception:** This term was coined by Roy Ascott. It describes the convergence of perceptive and conceptual processes in which the connectivity of telematic networks plays a constructive role.

**Fourth VR (4VR):** Ascott calls it a variable reality, which is the syncretic reality.

**LPDT (*La Plissure du Texte*/The Pleating of the Text: A Planetary Fairytale):** The title is an explicit reference to an essay by French critic Roland Barthes that was published ten years earlier with the title *Le Plaisir du Texte* (1973), a popular essay discussing, among many other things, on authorship and on the role of reader as a writer of the text. Ascott foresees multiple authors and readers.

**Metrobody:** It is a neologism for representing the idea of a new metrics of the body, conceived both as a mutant parameter and a transitive variable. It does not measure, it is not measure, but is measured in relation to the physical and digital environment at the same time, losing even the limits of reality.

**Moistmedia:** Another term coined by Roy Ascott. It represents where art is now: representing a multiplicity of media, configured and manipulated in an infinite number of ways by distributed authorship, publication, and distribution. Moist represents a convergence of silicon, dry computational systems and wet biological processes, tremendously extending the sensorium of the self.

**Three Virtual Realities (3VRs):** According to Roy Ascott, who considers the space and state of our consciousness, our mind pivots on the triangulation between three poles that he refers to as the Three VRs: Virtual Reality, Validated Reality, and Vegetal Reality.

**Ubiquitous Bodies:** The condition of ubiquity is the central concept of everyday experiences, based on digital revolution, transforming the traditional compact identity in a ubiquitous subject.

**Virtual Reality (VR):** It applies the progress in speed computing, graphics display, sensor sciences, and programming techniques in order to provoke in a participant an immersive experience inside a computer-generated space that we call a virtual world. Virtual worlds may or may not be analogous to our physical space; virtual environments may be realistic, extrasensory, telepresent or hybrid. The sensation of immersion is accomplished by peripheral devices wearable on the head such as visual and auditory displays with motion trackers.

# Chapter 2
# Impact of Virtual Reality in Healthcare:
## A Review

**Anitha S. Pillai**
*Hindustan Institute of Technology and Science, India*

**Prabha Susy Mathew**
*Bishop Cottons Women's Christian College, India*

## ABSTRACT

*Virtual reality (VR) is the simulation of reality where the users would be immersed in an artificial/virtual environment that isn't there but creates an illusion as if it really exists. People using this technology get a feeling that they are performing everything in real time. This gives users a sense of satisfaction. Initially, VR technology was used for gaming purposes, but now it is used in many sectors, including healthcare. There are many situations wherein, when it is expensive or impossible to do something, in reality, a probable solution is virtual reality. An important area where it is explored is healthcare for training doctors, diagnosis, and treatment of various ailments. The main objective of this chapter is to shed light on the applications of VR in healthcare and to discuss some applications showing how the medical field has already started reaping the benefits of VR.*

## INTRODUCTION

### Overview of the Chapter

This chapter provides state of art review of the use of VR in Healthcare. Right from training medical doctors, it is used in treatment of various ailments and to aid in surgery. The use of VR in each of these areas is treated separately. The case studies presented in the chapter cover various VR applications in healthcare such as physical rehabilitation and physiotherapy, cognitive rehabilitation, reducing preoperative anxiety and pain management. The main idea is to put forth the advancements VR has brought in Healthcare and to prove its usefulness by presenting some case studies.

DOI: 10.4018/978-1-5225-7168-1.ch002

1. **Background:** This section provides the readers with the Introduction to VR, definition, various Components and the essential Software used in developing VR applications.
2. **Benefits of VR in Healthcare:** This section highlights the various areas of healthcare where VR is in use namely
    a. VR in Medicine
    b. Training Medical Practitioners
    c. Reducing Stress and Pain
    d. Counseling
    e. Cognitive Rehabilitation
    f. Physical Therapy
3. **VR Diagnostics and Treatment:** The objective of this section is to give an understanding to the users as to how VR has been used in the diagnostics and treatment of some health conditions. Benefits of VR in Surgery is also presented, the topics discussed under this section are:
    a. VR in Dentistry
    b. VR in Autism
    c. VR in Mental Health
    d. VR in Surgery
4. **Case Study:** There are many real time Healthcare applications where VR was used. In order to familiarize the readers with these works various case studies performed by doctors/ Healthcare professionals and researchers are presented.
5. **References:** The journal papers, books, proceedings and Websites referred in writing the chapter are mentioned in the Reference section.

## Background

Virtual Reality (VR) is a technology that makes it possible to experience anything, anywhere, anytime by actually convincing the human brain that something which is not actually there exists. Head mounted displays are used with headphones and hand controllers to provide a fully immersive experience. VR is emerging leaps and bounds as many large companies like Facebook, Google and Microsoft are investing billions of dollars into this area. There are a number of adventurous activities which we might dream of doing – going to Mars, swimming in an ocean, playing with elephants etc. But with the advancement of VR all these dreams are possible by sitting at home. VR actually simulates an imaginary world using high performance computers and sensory equipment like headsets, position tracker and a set of wired gloves. VR is not used only for entertainment but also to train pilots, physicians and for a scientist/ researcher to figure out complex problems.

The first actual VR head-mounted display (HMD) was created in 1968 by computer scientist Ivan Sutherland (Daniel Freeman & Jason Freeman,2017).From its development the essential elements of VR haven't changed greatly over the years — a computer generates an image, a display system presents the sensory information, and a tracker feeds back the user's position and orientation in order to update the image — but what's new is the sophistication and affordability of the technology (Freeman & Freeman,2017).

Some of the definitions of VR: Virtual Reality is electronic simulations of environments experienced via head mounted eye goggles and wired clothing enabling the end user to interact in realistic three-dimensional situations(Coates,1992). Virtual Reality is an alternate world filled with computer-generated images that respond to human movements. These simulated environments are usually visited with the aid of an expensive data suit which features stereophonic video goggles and fiber-optic data gloves (Greenbaum, 1992).

Special VR headset is used to experience virtual reality. Most VR headsets are connected to a computer (Oculus Rift) or a gaming station (Playstation VR) or stand alone device (Google Cardboard). Most standalone VR, work by inserting a smart phone on the headset to immerse in the virtual reality (Forbes contributors, 2018).

While VR is used across many industries, technologies such as Augmented Reality and Mixed Reality are also being used to support and enhance user experience. Unlike VR where the user completely immerses in the virtual world, in AR user interacts with the enhanced real world where digital information is added to it. MR on the other hand is merging of real and virtual worlds providing new environment. Some of the popular applications of AR are Pokemon Go, Instagram face filters, Apple's ARkit (Hsieh & Lee, 2017).

Major components of VR are as follows: (Chandra & Tang, 2017)

- **Hardware:** Human motions like button press, click, controller movements, eye and other body part movements are captured using sensors. The receptor of the sensors collects the energy and converts it into a signal from an electrical circuit. The hardware products are required for the VR technology to happen.

VR devices:

- **Personal Computer/Smartphone:** Computers are used to process inputs and outputs sequentially. In order to create and produce content, computing resources are required. Since users view and perceive the VR content its production on a good computer is very essential.
- **Output Devices:** These mainly include visual, auditory or haptic devices used to stimulate a sense organ by presenting the VR content or environment to the users and generate an immersive feeling.
- **Software:** It manages the input, output devices, analyzes incoming data and provides correct feedback. It is equally important as the input and output devices. Since these applications run on real time Software must be able to process the input data and send response to the output devices promptly so that the correct feelings of the users are captured in real time.

Some of the VR tools for application development in Windows (Bitner, 2017).

- **Unity 3D:** Unity 3D developed by Unity Technologies is one of the most ubiquitous of tools being used today for VR development. It has a direct VR mode and can preview the work in a Head Mounted Display which can aid in productivity. Unity is quickly becoming the default tool for VR development due to its ease of use and ability to quickly prototype VR applications with it (Bitner, 2017).Unity supports 2D, 3D graphics, functionality for drag-and-drop and scripting using C#.
- **Unreal Engine (UE4):** This is one of the main competitors of Unity 3D which has a gaming engine with VR integrations, an asset store, and great documentation. It has excellent graphics which is advanced and realistic and the learning curve is similar to Unity. Many of the VR demos built with UE4 are much more life-like and smoother to navigate within (Bitner, 2017).

- **Maya:** Different softwares of Maya 3D like animation, modeling, rendering etc provides very good, powerful toolset for animation, motion graphics, virtual reality and character creation. It has been found that many of VR applications are developed using this.
- **Blender:** It is a free and open source software written in Python and is available for Windows, Mac, and Linux. It is used for 3D modeling, has an add on for virtual reality "BlenderVR" and "Fire".
- **SketchUp:** Google's SketchUp is a basic modeling application with a very low learning curve and anyone can understand and learn it soon. Users will be able to develop applications in a short amount of time as it is easier to learn.

## BENEFITS OF VR IN HEALTHCARE

### VR in Medicine

Nowadays VR is not just associated with the entertainment or gaming genre. It is used in various sectors like manufacturing industries, Product design, real estate and of course in Healthcare too. VR has made a huge impact in Healthcare sector and is being used for surgery simulation, treatment of various conditions like phobia, autism, mental health, pain etc, robotic surgery and Medical skills training. Advancement in medical sector is demanding access to the latest technology. This in turn demands continuous learning of new skills. The main advantage of VR technology is that it allows healthcare professionals to learn new skills as well as refresh existing ones in a safe and conducive environment. And of course it allows all this without causing any danger to the patients. Medical specialists found the use of VR in handling stress disorder, phobia, relieving pain, assisting during surgery. Headsets, 3D glasses and special video screens are being used for this. Growth in computational power has made it easy to simulate, analyze various organs and also perform virtual surgery. Several systems have been developed and tested for physical or mental rehabilitation and for supporting mental health therapy by exposing the patient to appropriate experience or illusion (Székely & Satava,1999).

### Training Medical Practitioners

Several companies are exploring the use of 3D technologies i.e virtual reality and augmented reality in health care. The main stakeholders in healthcare are: doctors, nurses, caregivers and the patients. For doctors and other caregivers, these technologies are driving big leaps forward in training and education and for patients, it's all about greater engagement and enhanced healing, rehabilitation, and comfort (Mogk, 2017). Medical students are learning using these 3D models as it is easy to use and learn as against the pictures in a textbook or Website. Students can easily move, explore and understand the models easily. This would give them excellent hands on training without any risk. This helps in better understanding of concepts and improves retention of the students. VR provides such a convincing interface that users believe they are actually present in a three-dimensional world and navigate and interact with it in real time where their actions and reactions are experienced in the present moment (Villani, Riva, & Riva, 2007).

Proper training of doctors and nurses to perform well in their work is very essential. This of course is expensive, time consuming and getting qualified trainers for conducting training is also very difficult.

VR has really been a boon to do this type of training and it is used to study the anatomy of human body, Colonoscopy, endoscopy and also in performing virtual surgery.

AccuVein a start-up company uses Augmented Reality (AR) technology for its vein viewing system. With AccuVein vein finder, finding of a vein on the first stick is said to be 3.5 times more likely. It is a handheld scanner that can project the vasculature on the surface of the skin, making lives of both nurses and patients much easier. It solves a real world problem of finding the patient vein using augmented reality and reduces the number of misses. Such techniques improve quality of patient care and enhance patient experience (Carson, 2015).

## Reducing Stress and Pain

Stress is the feeling which most of us experience when we are put under pressure or when something unpleasant happens in our life. Some people are able to come out of this situation where as some people might require proper medical treatment. A certain amount of stress can be good, helping to motivate, however too much stress can cause mental and physical problems. Research has proved that stress can lead to many health issues like depression as a result of that productivity of individuals decline. According to the authors (Villani, Cipresso & Repetto, 2014) among the different interactive media to handle stress and strain the traditional method is Virtual Reality Exposure Therapy (VRET).In this approach, the users are immersed within a computer-generated simulation within a contextually relevant setting. The rationale for this view typically derives from early evidence that VRET produces better outcomes than imaginable exposure, provides equivalent outcomes and is a pragmatically attractive alternative to in vivo exposure, such as the real-world confrontation of feared stimuli (Villani, Cipresso & Repetto, 2014).

Villani et al. (2014) developed a VR system to aid sufferers by providing a means of relaxation in combination with other stress management techniques. The VR system was used to exploit the presence capabilities of virtual environments. The realism of the relaxing environment was used to relieve the participant of stress. The system presented a 3D immersive video with an audio narrative. The participants' heart-rate was monitored in addition to their respiration and their subjective opinion through questionnaires. From their measurements, they found that the VR and audio narrative did affect their emotions in a positive manner.

Rizzo, Difede, Rothbaum, Reger, Spitalnick, Cukor, and McLay (2010) developed a VR system called 'Virtual Iraq'. Within the system, the patient is exposed to visual, auditory, olfactory and tactile stimuli corresponding to the event that originally triggered their symptoms. Twenty military personnel were used in a trial of the VR system, with positive results.

A number of training cum rehabilitation centres are using VR to train and also engage patients to deal with things like pain, aging, and anxiety. One of the maximum medical complaints among patients is pain. The brain is so busy processing signals from VR that it has a hard time processing other signals, like pain (Heeti, 2018).

VR has proven to be effective in reducing procedural pain, as almost invariably observed even in patients subjected to extremely painful procedures, such as patients with burn injuries undergoing wound care and physical therapy (Indovina, Barone, Gallo, Chirico, Pietro, & Antonio, 2018).Moreover, Even in cancer related symptoms and also in patients undergoing chemotherapy VR showed promising results in cutting down the pain or uneasiness.

Having patients conscious and feeling pain during medical procedures or surgery is very difficult to handle. This is even worse in case of pediatric treatments. Because of pain even anxiety increases in children and becomes very difficult to control. Fortunately, psychological treatments can be used to help reduce pain and anxiety (Atzori, et al., 2018).Virtual Reality is one such painkiller or analgesic. There is a growing literature showing the potential of immersive virtual reality as a psychological pain control technique that can be used in addition to traditional pain medications the patient is already receiving (Atzori et al., 2018). Pain distraction VR has also been used as a distraction technique to reduce the levels of pain experienced by patients. The level of presence within a VR system can distract an individual from the pain that they are experiencing, for example, during a medical procedure.

Gold, Kim, Kant, Joseph, and Rizzo (2006) conducted a study to evaluate the effectiveness of pain distraction using VR to divert children's attention for intravenous (IV) placement. The study was conducted on twenty children requiring IV for undertaking magnetic resonance imaging/computed tomography, and was conducted in two conditions, one condition with no distraction and one with the VR used as distraction (playing a game). The children experienced more pain without distraction than those using VR for pain distraction. The children reported that they were less anxious about the IV procedure than those that received no distraction. The children also did not experience any motion sickness.

Hoffman et al. (2007) examined the analgesic effects in the use of VR with the introduction of thermal pain simulation on 9 subjects. VR and opioid (morphine like substance) were evaluated for pain relief, the pain was measured through a subjective rating and blood oxygen level-dependent assessments of brain activity in five specific, pain-related regions of interest (using magnetic resonance imaging). The results indicated that VR significantly provided pain relief for the participants in terms of a subjective rating and their brain activity (Hoffman et al., 2007). Literature survey also reported the successful use of VR to distract burn patients from pain while receiving daily wound care and during physical therapy following skin grafts.

Magora, Cohen, Shochina, and Dayan (2006) produced a study to assess the use of VR to control ischemic pain (insufficient blood flow for the needs of the organ). The study consisted of twenty healthy participants who would experience pain through the use of a blood pressure cuff. The duration of their tolerance of the pain was a measured as well as a subjective questionnaire concerning their experience of the pain. Results of this study showed that there was a significant difference between those with VR exposure and those without.

Ortiz-Catalan, Sander, Kristoffersen, Håkansson, Bo., and Brånemark (2014) introduced a non-invasive technique for treating Phantom limb pain (PLP). By decoding myoelectric signals, the technique predicts motion intents which are given as inputs to virtual reality (VR), augmented reality (AR) and gaming. VR allows interactive gaming challenging patients with different difficulty levels, wider range of motion and rehabilitation exercises. AR enhances the illusion of the restored limb. Compared to the conventional Mirror Therapy, this technique allowed full range of motion and direct volitional control of the virtual limb and provides motivational benefits of gaming and progress tracking by computerized systems. Patient treated using this technique had considerable PLP relief as opposed to conventional treatment.

## Counseling

One main area where VR has been effectively used is in treating fear of public speaking. Here virtual environment with a large audience is created and the sufferer is made to speak to overcome the fear and also to improve communication as well as interpersonal skills.

People who suffer from post traumatic stress disorder (PTSD) were also treated by teaching them a number of techniques for dealing with their condition. A six-session virtual reality treatment was associated with reduction in PTSD diagnoses and symptoms in Iraq and Afghanistan veterans, although there was no control condition for the virtual reality exposure (Rothbaum et al., 2014).

AR apps can provide post discharge support to patients as well as their care givers by demonstrating them the physiological processes and explaining things happening within the body. These apps can remind patients to take medications, encourage them to follow discharge guidelines thereby contributing in their quick recovery (Levski, n.d.).

## Cognitive Rehabilitation

Many times it is observed that Patients with brain injury from trauma or stroke find it very difficult to carry out their day to day activities. By creating a virtual environment different tasks could be assigned to these patients to monitor how they handle the situations and the progress in handling complex situations can also be assessed. Such activities help to speed up recovery and also help patients to regain a better level of cognitive function. They also help doctors or care takers in identifying if the patient has memory loss, reduced attention or difficulty in taking correct and proper decisions. Studies proved the positive impact of VR in neuropsychological rehabilitation. Usually paper and pencil exercises and tests are used as traditional methods for neuropsychological rehabilitation of particular cognitive functions that have become impaired as a result of stroke. Literature survey presented by Schultheis, Rizzo, and Himelstein, (2002) points out that VR-based rehabilitation methods have several important benefits when compared to traditional methods: Setting up of VR can be done at the patient's place of stay and real time monitoring with dynamic feedback is also possible. Training is also easy as repetition is possible based on the needs of the user and depending on the learning customization can be done to suite the user requirements.

## Physical Therapy

The use of virtual-reality technology in the areas of rehabilitation and therapy continues to grow, with encouraging results being reported for applications that address human, physical, cognitive, and psychological functioning (Rizzo & Kim, 2005)

Hoffman et al. (2000) performed a study where twelve patients aged 19 to 47 years performed range of motion exercises of their injured extremity under an occupational therapist's direction. Here each patient spent 3 minutes of physical therapy with no distraction and 3 minutes of physical therapy in VR All patients reported less pain when distracted with VR, and the magnitude of pain reduction by VR was statistically significant (e.g., time spent thinking about pain during physical therapy dropped from 60 to 14 mm on a 100-mm scale) (Hoffman, Hunter, Patterson, David, Carrougher, & Gretchen, 2000)

# VR DIAGNOSTICS AND TREATMENT

## VR in Dentistry

Virtual reality (VR) surgery using Oculus Rift and Leap Motion devices is a multi-sensory, holistic surgical training experience (Shah & Chong, 2018). A realistic VR surgery environment was developed using 360 degree videos, three-dimensional interaction, and stereoscopic videos. The innovation allows trainees to interact with the individual components of the maxillofacial anatomy and apply surgical instruments while watching close-up stereoscopic three-dimensional videos of the surgery (Shah & Chong, 2018). In this study, a novel training tool based on immersive virtual reality (iVR) was developed and validated by seven consultant oral and maxillofacial surgeons. The results confirmed the clinical applicability of VR for delivering training in orthognathic surgery (Shah & Chong, 2018).The adoption and adaptation of recent advances in digital technology, such as three-dimensional (3D) printed objects and haptic simulators, in dentistry have influenced teaching and/or management of cases involving implant, craniofacial, maxillofacial, orthognathic and periodontal treatments (Shah & Chong, 2018)

## VR in Autism

Autism spectrum disorders (ASD) are characterized by core deficits in three domains, i.e. social interaction, communication, and repetitive or stereotypic behavior (Bellani, Fornasari, Chittaro, & Brambilla, 2011)

It is very important to develop intervention strategies to help individuals with autism, their caregivers and educators in daily life. To this purpose, Virtual Reality (VR), i.e. a simulation of the real world based on computer graphics, can be useful as it allows instructors and therapists to offer a safe, repeatable and diversifiable environment during learning. This mini review examines studies that have investigated the use of VR in autism (Bellani et al., 2011). Virtual reality offers the potential to regulate an artificial computer environment to better match the expectations and needs of individuals with these problems (Strickland, 1998).

Use of VR in autism has been summarized by Strickland (1998):

1. **Controllable Input Stimuli:** The input stimuli can be simplified depending on the needs of the user's. Whenever a child faces attention problem, the level of stimulation and interaction can be raised to improve the attention level.
2. **Modification for Generalization:** With minimum modifications to similar scenes, the child learns to generalize easily. For example if the child has been taught to cross the road in one virtual road and if another similar road is shown, then the child generalizes the previous learning to the current situation. Initially the child should be given scenes with minimum differences and later it could be increased to teach cross recognition.
3. **Safer Learning Situation:** It is quite safe as mistakes are less catastrophic and virtual environment can be modified from simple to complex depending on the progress.
4. **A Primarily Visual/Auditory World:** Studies have proved that sight and sound are very effective in teaching concepts

5. **Individualized Treatment:** The training needs vary between individuals with these disorders. Personalized training depending on the needs of these individuals is possible with the help of VR.
6. **Preferred Computer Interactions:** The complexity of social interaction can interfere when teaching individuals with social disorders (Strickland, 1998). Literature studies reveal the use of computers from 1968 to assist language development therapy for children with autism. Advantages of computer learning aids have been reported in multiple studies for both autism and attention disorders (Strickland, 1998).
7. **Trackers:** In VR by means of head and body trackers the physical activities of an individual can be monitored allowing the machine to adjust according to the actions of the patients. It is seen that most of the individuals with autism never learn to communicate or there is a delay. Interactions in virtual reality using hand controls seem to be more effective than the verbal training given by a teacher.

## VR in Mental Health

Enthusiasm is growing among clinicians and researchers around the world about the potential that virtual reality offers to improve the assessment and treatment of mental and physical health problems (Valmaggia, 2017).

The main fields of research in virtual reality and psychosis are: safety and acceptability of the technology; neurocognitive evaluation; functional capacity and performance evaluation; assessment of paranoid ideation and auditory hallucinations; and interventions (Rus-Calafell, Garety, Sason, Craig, &, Valmaggia, 2018) The studies reviewed indicate that virtual reality offers a valuable method of assessing the presence of symptoms in ecologically valid environments, with the potential to facilitate learning new emotional and behavioural responses (Rus-Calafell, et al., 2018).In assessing neurocognitive deficiency and for the study of relevant clinical symptoms VR has shown promising results. Researchers also suggest that it can be applied for various treatment of psychosis like cognitive rehabilitation, social skills training interventions and virtual reality-assisted therapies.

Specific use of VR and AR becomes interesting for both social and functional rehabilitation whether it originates from traumatic situations and injuries or from pathologies known to show from neuromuscular disturbances to decay (Benyoucef, Lesport, & Chassagneux, 2017). As per Statistics, one out of four people has already or will develop a mental disorder during their lifetime according to the World Health Organization (WHO2001). Because virtual reality allows for a wide range of applications, this cutting-edge technology could find its place as a neuromodulator to target a panel of states from wellbeing to mental diseases and pain management (Benyoucef et al., 2017).

## VR in Surgery

VR and AR are used in Pre-operative planning as it helps surgeon to understand the finer details of complex structures. The challenge mainly for the surgeon is how he is able to integrate real and virtual environments. And if the challenges are overcome then it provides an opportunity for a safer and more efficient operation.

Virtual reality has an ability to transport users from one physical location to another location far away.

In the medical field, this has paved the way for treating / operating patients by virtually transporting the doctor to the location where the patient is. Many times it has been observed that people have been losing lives just because they did not have access to the right doctor at the correct point in time. With the help of virtual surgery senior and expert surgeons can help patients without stepping out of their operation room. With the help of head-mounted display and haptic gloves a surgeon can easily transport themselves to an operating room which is miles away where the patient resides. This is a great boon to healthcare sector as all patients would have the services / treatment of expert doctors.

Mostafa, Ryu, Chan, Takashima, Kopp, Sousa, and Sharlin (2017) describes the contribution of NeuroSimVR, a stereoscopic virtual reality spine surgery simulator which helps that allows novice surgeons to learn and practice a spinal pedicle screw insertion (PSI) procedure by using simplified interaction capabilities and 3D haptic user interfaces. By collaborating with medical experts and following an iterative approach, they provide characterization of the PSI task, and derive requirements for applying this procedure in a 3D immersive interactive simulation system (Mostafa et al., 2017). According to the authors surgical trainees can use this simulator to improve their surgical skill in PSI as it is very essential for neurosurgeons and orthopedic surgeons. They also suggest how medical experts can illustrate performing surgery without causing injuries to the spinal cord. In neurosurgery, the introduction of three-dimensional fusion imaging, in which multiple types of medical imaging datasets are fused, has boosted the development of virtual three dimensional surgery enabling interactive evaluation of surgical procedures (e.g., craniotomy), as well as easy acquisition of detailed anatomical information in the expected surgical field (Kin, Nakatomi, Shono, Nomura, Saito, Oyama, & Saito, 2017).

## CASE STUDY

Morrongiello, Corbett, Foster and Koutsoulianos (2018) used a fully immersive and interactive virtual reality (VR) pedestrian environment to evaluate how observing peers affects the behavior of child pedestrians. Street crossing behavior of about 55 children between the ages of 8-10 years old was measured both before and after exposure to a same-sex peer model that demonstrated either riskier or safer street crossing behavior compared to the participant's initial crossings. There was no difference in initial crossing behaviors across groups. However, children who observed peers of risky pedestrian behavior subsequently crossed in significantly riskier inter-vehicle gaps than those in the control group (Morrongiello et al., 2018).

Scapina, Guaniloa, Fuculo, Gonçalvesa, Rochaa, and Coimbraa, (2018) applied VR using three-dimensional features and video games. The findings showed the impact of VR with increased enjoyment and the reduction of pain, anxiety and stress during dressing changes, physical rehabilitation and physiotherapy.

Gamito, Oliveira, Coelho, Morais, Lopes, Pacheco, Brito, Soares, Santos, and Barata (2015) did a study to prove that use of virtual reality in cognitive rehabilitation offers cost benefits and other advantages. In order to carry out the study to test the effectiveness of VR for neuropsychological rehabilitation, a cognitive training program using VR was applied to stroke patients. Cognitive training using VR games was used, with attention and memory tasks consisting of their day to day activities. Out of the 20 stroke patients, few were exposed to the training program in which VR was added. It was observed from the study that patients exposed to the VR training module showed significant improvements in attention and memory functions compared to the other group who were not exposed to the VR training.

The findings of the authors provided very good support for the use of VR cognitive training applications in neuropsychological rehabilitation.

Esguerra and Johnson (2017) proved VR as an innovative technology in the assistance of physical therapy (PT). Authors present a case study wherein they explored the use of VR with a patient who suffered from unilateral vestibular hypofunction (UVH) .The 50-year old patient was referred to physical therapy following a vehicle accident. The patient had an acute left UVH, accompanied by dizziness, imbalance and gait disturbances which disturbed him in his construction work. The patient was examined two to three times a week for 40-minutes and was also advised an individualized home exercise. His treatment included vestibular rehabilitation exercises, balance training, gait training, and VR. VR was included to improve postural balance by including task specific simulations, exposure therapy to reduce anxiety, and static balance improvisation through smooth eye pursuits. Questionnaires such as the Activities-Specific Balance Confidence survey and the Dizziness Handicap Inventory (DHI) and functional tests like the Sensory Organization Test, Motor Control Test, and the Functional Gait Assessment (FGA) was used to measure the outcome. These measurements were performed at initial visit, at the 10th visit, and again at discharge. Notable improvements were seen on DHI and FGA scores (Esguerra & Johnson, 2017).Authors also observed that Dizziness, confidence, balance, and gait improved following vestibular rehabilitation combined with VR. With this they concluded VR in conjunction with vestibular rehabilitation therapy is effective in improving deficits of unilateral vestibular hypofunction. They also concluded after their study that the use of VR can be an effective tool for intervention to facilitate patient-specific goals.

Robertson et al. (2017) conducted a study to determine if preoperative anxiety in patients undergoing arthroscopic knee surgery could be reduced using VR immersion. The idea was to distract the patients and check if that reduced the pain. The study was carried out in Sixty patients by randomly dividing them into 3 groups: Standard care group, VR group and iPad group. Anxiety scores (Hospital Anxiety and Depression Scale), Galvanic Skin Response (GSR), heart rate and blood pressure were measured pre and post intervention (Robertson et al., 2017). The Standard care group did not receive any intervention, iPad group watched a video slideshow of beaches around the world and the VR group were made to immerse in a virtual beach . Guided relaxation audio content (via headphones) was replicated across VR and iPad groups (Robertson et al., 2017).GSR measures for the Standard care group increased by 54 per cent from time 1 to time 2 and the VR and iPad groups reduced slightly, demonstrating an ameliorating effect on anxiety levels (Robertson et al., 2017). There was only a marginal difference between the Standard care group and VR group in anxiety change scores. One of the observations was that although the VR condition reduced anxiety more than Standard care in both GSR and Anxiety change score measures, it did not provide major advantage over iPad condition. In conclusion, distraction using VR and iPad temporarily reduces self reported anxiety levels and GSR measures compared to standard care in patients prior to knee arthroscopy (Robertson et al., 2017).

Vázquez, Vaca, Wiederhold, Miller and Wiederhold (2017) conducted a study where Forty-four 44 women participated was split into two groups. One group received the virtual reality intervention, while the other group did not receive any pain distraction intervention. The VR group ranged from 18 to 73 years of age and the non-VR group ranged from 18 to 61 years old. The study revealed that throughout the gynecological procedures, the VR group reported significantly lower pain during the procedure than the non-VR group.

## CONCLUSION

From the applications of VR in healthcare it is very clear that VR can be used as a complimentary treatment to cure many of the disorders and diseases. From the Literature reviews we can conclude that few psychological disorders like psychosis, depression, self-harm, suicidal thoughts and obsessive compulsive disorders (OCD) can be treated to a great extent using VR. For better results it is always advisable to get the opinion of medical Practitioner while developing and using these systems for treatment.

## REFERENCES


Al-Heeti, A. (2018). *VR could be your next painkiller.* Retrieved from https://www.cnet.com/news/virtual-reality-at-hospitals-could-be-your-next-painkiller/

Bellani, M., Fornasari, L., Chittaro, L., & Brambilla, P. (2011).*Virtual reality in autism: state of the art.* Retrieved from https://www.ncbi.nlm.nih.gov/pubmed/21922965

Benyoucef, Y., Lesport, P., & Chassagneux, A. (2017). *The Emergent Role of Virtual Reality in the Treatment of Neuropsychiatric Disease.* Retrieved from https://www.ncbi.nlm.nih.gov/pmc/articles/PMC5591848/

Bitner, J. (2017). *11 Tools for VR Developers.* Retrieved from: https://www.lullabot.com/articles/11-tools-for-vr-developers

Carson, E. (2015). *6 cool uses for augmented reality in healthcare.* Retrieved from https://www.techrepublic.com/article/6-cool-uses-for-augmented-reality-in-healthcare/

Chandra, G., & Tang, S. (2017). *Virtual Reality:Components.* Retrieved from http://web.tecnico.ulisboa.pt/ist188480/cmul/devices.html

Coates, G. (1992). *Program from Invisible Site—a virtual sho.* San Francisco, CA: Performance Works.

Esguerra, S., Ben, J., & Johnson, K. (2017). Improving Balance through Virtual Reality and Physical Therapy Integration. *International Journal of Clinical Medicine*, *8*(5). doi:10.4236/ijcm.2017.85030

Forbes. (2018). *The Difference Between Virtual Reality, Augmented Reality And Mixed Reality.* Retrieved from https://www.forbes.com/sites/quora/2018/02/02/the-difference-between-virtual-reality-augmented-reality-and-mixed-reality/#7f235f002d07

Freeman, D., & Freeman, J. (2017). *Why virtual reality could be a mental health gamechanger.* Retrieved from: https://www.theguardian.com/science/blog/2017/mar/22/all.AnesthAnalg

Gamito, P., Oliveira, J., Coelho, C., Morais, D., Lopes, P., Pacheco, J., ... Barata, F. A. (2015). Cognitive training on stroke patients via virtual reality-based serious games. *Disability and Rehabilitation*, *39*(4), 385–388. doi:10.3109/09638288.2014.934925 PMID:25739412

Gold, J.I., Kim, S., Kant, J.A., Joseph, H.M., & Rizzo, A. (2006). Effectiveness of Virtual Reality for Pediatric Pain Distraction during IV Placement. *CyberPsychology & Behavior, 9*(2), 207-212.

Greenbaum, P. (1992). The lawnmower man. Film and Video, *9*(3), 58-62.

Hoffman, H.G., Patterson, D.R., & Carrougher, G.J. (2000). Use of Virtual Reality for Adjunctive Treatment of Adult Burn Pain During Physical Therapy: A Controlled Study. *The Clinical Journal of Pain, 16*(3), 244-250.

Hoffman, H. G., Richards, T. L., Van, T. O., Coda, B. A., Jensen, M. P., Blough, D. K., & Sharar, S. R. (2007). The analgesic effects of opioids and immersive virtual reality distraction: Evidence from subjective and functional brain imaging assessments. *Anesthesia and Analgesia*, *105*(6), 1776–1783. doi:10.1213/01.ane.0000270205.45146.db PMID:18042882

Hsieh, M. C., & Lee, J. J. (2018). Preliminary Study of VR and AR Applications in Medical and Healthcare Education. *Journal of Nursing and Health Studies, 3*(1).

Indovina, P., Barone, D., Gallo, L., Chirico, A., Pietro, D. G., & Antonio, G. (2018). Virtual Reality as a Distraction Intervention to Relieve Pain and Distress During Medical Procedures: A Comprehensive Literature Review. *The Clinical Journal of Pain.* Ahead of Print. Doi:10.1097/AJP.0000000000000599

Kin, T., Nakatomi, H., Shono, N., Nomura, S., Saito, T., Oyama, H., & Saito, N. (2017, October 15). Neurosurgical Virtual Reality Simulation for Brain Tumor Using High-definition Computer Graphics: A Review of the Literature. *Neurologia Medico-Chirurgica*, *57*(10), 513–520. doi:10.2176/nmc.ra.2016-0320 PMID:28637947

Leviski, Y. (n.d.). *AR and Healthcare: The Future Is Now.* Retrieved from https://appreal-vr.com/blog/augmented-reality-for-healthcare/

Magora, F., Cohen, S., Shochina, M., & Dayan, E. (2006). Virtual reality immersion method of distraction to control experimental ischemic pain. *The Israel Medical Association Journal*, *8*(4), 261–265. PMID:16671363

Mogk, C. (2017, June). *Virtual Reality in Health Care Makes Medical Reality Easier to Endure*. Retrieved from https://www.autodesk.com/redshift/virtual-reality-in-health-care/

Morrongiello, B. A., Corbett, M., Foster, A., & Koutsoulianos, S. (2018). *Using Virtual Reality to Examine the Effects of Peer Modeling on Child Pedestrian Behavior.* Retrieved from https://trid.trb.org/view/1494797

Mostafa, A. E., Ryu, W. H. A., Chan, S., Takashima, K., Kopp, G., Sousa, C. M., & Sharlin, E. (2017). *Designing NeuroSimVR: A Stereoscopic Virtual Reality Spine Surgery Simulator.* Retrieved from https://prism.ucalgary.ca/handle/1880/52230

Nepal, C. G., & Tang, S. (2017). *Virtual Reality Components*. Retrieved from http://web.tecnico.ulisboa.pt/ist188480/cmul/about.html

Ortiz-Catalan, M., Sander, N., Kristoffersen, B. M., Håkansson, Bo., & Brånemark, R. (2014). *Treatment of phantom limb pain (PLP) based on augmented reality and gaming controlled by myoelectric pattern recognition: a case study of a chronic PLP patient*. Retrieved from https://www.frontiersin.org/articles/10.3389/fnins.2014.00024/full

Rizzo, A., & Kim, J.G. (2005). A SWOT Analysis of the Field of Virtual Reality Rehabilitation and Therapy. *Presence, 14*(2), 119–146.

Rizzo, A. S., Difede, J., Rothbaum, B. O., Reger, G., Spitalnick, J., Cukor, J., & McLay, R. (2010). Development and early evaluation of the Virtual Iraq/Afghanistan exposure therapy system for combat-related PTSD. *Annals of the New York Academy of Sciences, 1208*(1), 114–125. doi:10.1111/j.1749-6632.2010.05755.x PMID:20955333

Robertson, A., Khan, R., Fick, D., Robertson, W. B., Gunaratne, D. G. R., & Yapa, S., … Rajan, R. (2017). *The effect of Virtual Reality in reducing preoperative anxiety in patients prior to arthroscopic knee surgery: A randomised controlled trial.* Paper presented at IEEE 5th International Conference on Serious Games and Applications for Health (SeGAH), Perth, Australia. 10.1109/SeGAH.2017.7939282

Rothbaum, O. B., Price, M., Jovanovic, T., Norrholm, S. D., Gerardi, M., Dunlop, B., … Ressler, J. K. (2014). *A Randomized, Double-Blind Evaluation of d-Cycloserine or Alprazolam Combined With Virtual Reality Exposure Therapy for Posttraumatic Stress Disorder in Iraq and Afghanistan War Veterans.* Retrieved from https://ajp.psychiatryonline.org/doi/abs/10.1176/appi.ajp.2014.13121625

Rus-Calafell, M., Garety, P., Sason, E., Craig, T. J. K., & Valmaggia, L. R. (2018, February). Virtual reality in the assessment and treatment of psychosis: A systematic review of its utility, acceptability and effectiveness. *Psychological Medicine, 48*(3), 362–391. doi:10.1017/S0033291717001945 PMID:28735593

Scapina, Q. S., Echevarría-Guaniloa, M. E., Fuculo, P. R. B., Jr., Gonçalvesa, N., Rochaa, P. K., & Coimbraa, R. (2018). *Virtual Reality in the treatment of burn patients: A systematic review*. Retrieved from https://www.sciencedirect.com/science/article/pii/S030541791

Schultheis, M. T., Rizzo, A. A., & Himelstein, J. (2002). Virtual reality and neuropsychology: Upgrading the current tools. *The Journal of Head Trauma Rehabilitation, 17*(5), 378–394. doi:10.1097/00001199-200210000-00002 PMID:12802250

Shah, P., & Chong, B. S. (2018, March). 3D imaging, 3D printing and 3D virtual planning in endodontics. *Clinical Oral Investigations, 22*(2), 641–654. doi:10.100700784-018-2338-9 PMID:29330656

Strickland, D. (1998). Virtual Reality for the Treatment of Autism. In G. Riva (Ed.), *Virtual reality in neuro-psycho-physiology* (pp. 81–86). Amsterdam: IOS Press.

Székely, G., & Satava, R. M. (1999). *Virtual reality in medicine.* Retrieved from: https://www.ncbi.nlm.nih.gov/pmc/articles/PMC1129082/

Valmaggia, L. (2017). *The use of virtual reality in psychosis research and treatment*. Retrieved from https://www.ncbi.nlm.nih.gov/pmc/articles/PMC5608845/

Vázquez, J., Vaca, V.L., Wiederhold, K.B., Miller, T.I., & Wiederhold, D.M. (2017). Virtual Reality Pain Distraction During Gynecological Surgery—A Report of 44 Cases. *Surgical Research Updates, 5,* 12-16 Doi:10.12970/2311-9888.2017.05.02

Villani, D., Cipresso, P., & Repetto, C. (2014). Coping with stress and anxiety: The role of presence in technology mediated environments. In Interacting with Presence: HCI and the Sense of Presence in Computer-Mediated Environments (pp. 139-151). De Gruyter Open Ltd. Doi:10.2478/9783110409697.9

Villani, D., Riva, F., & Riva, G. (2007). New technologies for relaxation: The role of presence. *International Journal of Stress Management*, *14*(3), 260–274. doi:10.1037/1072-5245.14.3.260

## KEY TERMS AND DEFINITIONS

**Augmented Reality (AR):** It is a technology that uses real world environment and enhances it by overlaying digital information on top of it. Example of AR are *Pokemon Go* and *Vein* finding system.

**Fusion Imaging:** It is a technique that uses data from two different imaging modalities such as magnetic resonance image (MRI), computed tomography (CT), positron emission tomography (PET), etc. to improve the quality of information for increased diagnostic accuracy.

**Immersive Interactive Simulation System:** It is a system that provides state-of-the-art interactive environment that blurs the line between the real and virtual world.

**Mixed Reality (MR):** It is also known as hybrid reality. It merges the real and digital environments that co-exist and interact with each other to produce new environment for the user to explore and manipulate. Examples of MR is Microsoft's HoloLens.

**Virtual Reality (VR):** It provides the user with computer-generated simulation of a real-life environment or situation. The headset gives the user a fully immersive experience, where what a user sees is a generated or an artificial environment and nothing of it is in the real world. Example of VR is gaming consoles.

**Virtual Reality Exposure Therapy (VRET):** It is a virtual reality-based exposure therapy for treating post-traumatic stress disorder (PTSD) as well as severe phobias. The goal of VRET is to expose the patient to stimuli by combining advanced computer graphics, 3D visual displays, and body-tracking technologies to create realistic virtual non-threatening environment so that their mind and body can learn not to become alerted when they are exposed to similar stimuli in real life.

**Virtual Surgery:** It is a virtual reality technique that simulates surgical procedures without the need of a patient or cadaver instead it allows the surgeons to practice surgery on 3D models. It helps the surgeons to have clear understanding of the outcome.

# Chapter 3
# Serious Games, Meditation, Brain-Computer Interfacing, and Virtual Reality (VR):
## Empowering Players to Discover Their Minds

**Ryan Murdoch**
*The Glasgow School of Art, UK*

## ABSTRACT

*Brain-computer interfacing (BCI), the ability to interact with software and technology with our thoughts and feelings, presents an exciting new frontier for serious games and learning. This chapter outlines an approach to incorporating real-time brain-monitoring in educational games. Both outlining and suggesting how technically this can be achieved using affordable and accessible "off the shelf" consumer technology and the popular game engine Unity. By designing such experiences considering pedagogy and serious game theory, we can attempt to classify this new form of user interaction and its value for educational purposes. Specifically, this chapter looks to engage players with ideas of meditation by monitoring their "meditation" using BCI technology and visualizing it in engaging game worlds and experiences. As a valuable tool for addressing mental illness and personal wellbeing, meditation is worth exploring as a learning outcome within serious games.*

## INTRODUCTION

Today technology marches forward at an ever accelerating pace. Computers that once took up whole floors of buildings now fit snuggly in our pockets, the internet connects people around the globe almost instantaneously to one another and to a nearly endless wealth of information. What impact does this acceleration have on us? Without a doubt it has massive and positive implications for mankind, but so too does it create new issues. This concept of human progress as a double edged sword is not new. Perhaps one of the most powerful speeches ever given on the subject was that of John F. Kennedy at Rice Uni-

DOI: 10.4018/978-1-5225-7168-1.ch003

versity (1962); his famous speech about putting a man on the moon. With regards to mankind's progress he noted that: 'This is a breathtaking pace, and such a pace cannot help but create new ills as it dispels old, new ignorance, new problems, new dangers'. These words still hold profound truth today. In an ever more connected world what happens to our idea of privacy? In an age of instantaneous gratification, endless media, data and content what happens to the length of our attention? What impact will the endlessness of the digital world have on us and our mental health? In a time with such advanced medicine to fortify our bodies and cure our physical ails, perhaps our mental well-being has been overlooked. The human mind as an unexplored vista is as enticing and mysterious as space to Kennedy, and the world, in the 1960s. This chapter aims to examine the technological tools and innovations that can let us explore and quantify this nebulous space, this space within each of us: the human mind. Since the beginning of time the human mind and understanding it has been one of man's greatest mysteries and challenges. It was often thought that what we now consider the mind; the element of a person that allows the gifts of thought, feelings and consciousness, was one and the same with the soul. In Aristotle's work De Anima he describes the mind as 'the part of the soul by which it knows and understands', in fact Aristotle believed it was human nature to long for knowledge and understanding (Shields, 2016), Thousands of years later our longing to understand the mind has led to many great discoveries; we can now peer into its workings, understanding the brain and mind through the lenses of neurology and psychology. However being able to read the mind is just the beginning, what if we could use that read data to inform computers and technology? That is the premise of Brain-Computer Interfacing (BCI); the science of communicating with machines using brain activity and thought. This chapter hopes to separate the science from the fiction that surrounds this exciting technology. Furthermore it aims to look past the novelty of BCI, to examine its potential in 'serious' or educational games and experiences. Providing an exploration of the unique feedback that can be provided by monitoring the brain, in an attempt to engage users with concepts of meditation and regulation of the mind. Because, even though science has worked hard to separate the mind from the soul, to understand our minds is still to understand ourselves. 'Serious Games do not simply teach their rules, narrative, fictions, metaphors or goals, but they teach the players something about the world, themselves and their own values, beliefs and behaviours' (Mitgutsch, 2011).

## Serious Games

'When we think of games, we think of fun. When we think of learning we think of work. Games show us this is wrong' (Gee, 2005). Serious games are games that have scope beyond recreation. They can be for training, teaching and propagating information, in fact games create uniquely customizable environments that excel in all of these areas. So the study of 'serious games', a seeming oxymoron in itself, spans multiple disciplines. From user psychology and pedagogy, the study of learning, to game art, design and narrative (Lim et al., 2014). The virtual world of games offer more than just flexibility with respects to learning, it offers a rich and fun way to present information to new audiences. Games naturally are designed to be fun, but they are also designed to be learned, a good game guides the player, teaching them seamlessly as the game progresses. It is these qualities that serious games draw on to create effective new ways to teach. Mitgutsch (2011) describes serious games using the famous song from 'Mary Poppins' (1964): 'A Spoonful of Sugar'. Which, according to the song, 'helps the medicine go down'. Mitgutsch goes on to describe serious games as: "'esigning a spoonful of sugar and filling it with serious content'.

## Meditation

Meditation is the practice of focusing or drawing attention to ones thoughts in order to relax, 'clear the mind' or find peaceful or mindful states. 'Meditation can be defined to include any of a family of practices in which the practitioner trains an individual to consciously calm his/her mind in order to realize some benefit or achieve inner peace or harmony' (Chen, 2011). Serious games require a problem area to be addressed, with intended learning outcomes. So is it possible to teach meditation and mental well-being with serious game approaches? Meditation is a particularly interesting area to attempt to engage learners with, it is very much an experiential phenomena and as tacit knowledge it is hard to verbalize or write about the experience of meditation. This creates a problem when trying to share and 'transfer' knowledge, the key goal of serious game approaches. Additionally as meditation has ancient roots in religious practice it often has a kind of 'mysticism' and associated stigmas. Despite this it has grown increasingly as an academic area of interest, with notable and measurable benefits to those who practice meditation. Despite increased enthusiasm that benefits from developing understandings of psychology and neurology (thanks to brain monitoring approaches), there is still much inconsistency within research across disciplines. Heinz (1981) notes: 'In reviewing the amassed psychological research on meditation, a consistent picture of meditation's purpose and defining features does not readily emerge'. Is it possible to use serious games and brain-computer interfacing technology to engage users with meditation in new, engaging and experiential ways?

## Brain-Computer Interfacing (BCI)

Brain-Computer Interfacing is the science of using measurable brain signals to communicate with technology and computers. The term was coined and discussed by Jacque Vidal in his 1973 paper 'Towards Direct Brain-Computer Communication', in his work he asked if 'observable electrical brain signals could be put to work as carriers of information in man-computer communication'. Considering the possibilities of BCI he went on to ponder if such approaches could be used to control 'prosthetic devices or spaceships'. Today prosthetic limbs are indeed being controlled by BCI (Coffey, 2014) and BCI is very much alive in science fiction and popular culture. Aired in 1991 'The Nth Degree', an episode of Star Trek: The Next Generation, featured a popular representation of Brain-Computer Interfacing. Lt. Barclay, a shy and fairly average engineer, is knocked unconscious by a probe. When he awakes he finds his knowledge expanded and influenced by an alien civilization, the Cytherians. Eager to fully utilize the Enterprise's computers he develops a 'neural-scan interface', to interact with the ships computers with greater speed, using his thoughts directly. However the new interface puts the life of not only Lt. Barclay, but the whole crew in danger. Today many approaches for monitoring the brain exist, but these technologies date back as far as the 1920's. The polygraph or lie detector exists as an early example of brain-machine communication and was invented in 1921. There are several possible brain-monitoring techniques that can be considered when creating brain-computer interfaces. Many of these techniques have benefits and draw backs, in particular approaches often trade off on spatial vs. temporal resolution. All brain monitoring approaches that will be discussed are unintrusive; requiring no surgery, as this chapters focus is on exploring accessible educational tools for mental health. In this chapter we will explore the potential of Brain-Computer Interfacing as an educational tool, informed by serious game theory and enhanced using the immersive potential of virtual and augmented reality. Focusing on the history of Brain-Computer Interfacing technology and examining case studies; from teaching meditation and wellbeing to creating useful interventions for attention disorders and even autism. Technology does not always have to serve as a distraction, but instead, as this chapter will show, can act as a means to learn about, reflect upon and combat mental illness in engaging and meaningful ways.

## BACKGROUND

Brain-Computer Interfacing (BCI) is the science of using measurable brain signals to communicate with technology and computers. It was coined and discussed by Jacque Vidal in his 1973 paper 'Towards Direct Brain-Computer Communication', in his work he asked if 'observable electrical brain signals could be put to work as carriers of information in man-computer communication'. Considering the possibilities of BCI he went on to ponder if such approaches could be used to control 'prosthetic devices or spaceships'. Today prosthetic limbs are indeed being controlled by BCI (Coffey, 2014) and BCI is very much alive in science fiction and popular culture. Today many approaches for monitoring the brain exist, but these technologies date back as far as the 1920's. The polygraph or lie detector exists as an early example of brain-machine communication and was invented in 1921. There are several possible brain monitoring techniques that can be considered when creating brain-computer interfaces. Many of these techniques have benefits and draw backs, in particular approaches often trade off on spatial vs. temporal resolution. All brain monitoring approaches discussed are unintrusive; requiring no surgery. Intrusive approaches are considered inappropriate within the context of this research.

### Functional Magnetic Resonance Imaging (fMRI)

Functional magnetic resonance imaging or fMRI is a neuroimaging approach that uses magnetic resonance imaging to monitor the change in blood as it flows around the brain. This unintrusive approach causes the subject no harm and does not require direct contact with the scalp. First used in the experiments of Roy and Sharrington (1980) it can produce immensely detailed pictures of brain activity with a high spatial resolution. However it can take between 2 and 10 seconds to capture this data, resulting in a sluggish temporal resolution (Kim & Uĝurbil, 1997).

### Electroencephalogram (EEG)

EEG or electroencephalogram is a method of using electrodes placed on the scalp to measure electrical brain activity, pioneered by Hans Berger in 1924. When neurons in the brain communicate information to one another the small electrical signals can be detected, together some 10^6 neurons create a measureable reading of a few microvolts that can be monitored this way. Despite being filtered by the meninges, skull and scalp there is a latency of less than a millisecond in this method of monitoring (Woodman, 2010). Giving it a much higher temporal resolution than that off fMRI. EEG is a particularly useful technique in that it is not intrusive, it 'has become one of the most useful tools in the diagnosis of epilepsy and other neurological disorders' (Miranda & Brouse, 2005). Various methods of EEG analysis exist including Hjorth, power spectrum and spectral centroid analysis, these methods take the frequency of the EEG and extrapolate readings from them often using FFT or similar approaches. EEG has some downfalls however; eye movement, eye blink and heartbeat can all cause artefacts in the EEG readings many modern methods of EEG monitoring use algorithms to account for this kind of bodily noise that is introduced. Additionally EEG is not capable of capturing the detailed images of brain function that can be captured with high spatial resolution of fMRI. EEG is the more affordable of the two approaches and EEG is used in almost all consumer BCI solutions.

## Event-Related Potential (ERP)

ERP or event-related potential uses EEG to monitor the brains response to specific stimulus. Using this technique specific internal or external events can be measured. It is usually measured using multiple electrodes across the scalp using a few milliseconds temporal resolution (Otten & Rugg, 2005).

This technique is popular for brain-computer interfacing, it allows users to 'think' a specific command that is then monitored and recorded. This command, such as 'up' can then be used to interact with other devices. This approach is used in the consumer Emotiv EPOC EEG headset which has been used experimentally with digital games (Badcock et al., 2013).

## Optical Imaging and Mixed Approaches

Several emerging approaches hope to address the failings of existing brain monitoring techniques. Combinations of fMRI and EEG approaches can allow for high spatial and temporal resolutions when gathering data. Additionally there is ongoing research into 'optical imaging', with this approach photons are fired into regions of the brain to gather information. This new approach is being researched in Facebook's 'Building 8' by leading researchers and a former DARPA director. Facebook intends to release a prototype in two years for an unintrusive consumer device that will allow users to type one hundred words a minute using BCI.

## BCI in Video Games

With BCI solutions, in particular those that make use of EEG and ERP, becoming increasingly accessible and affordable to developers there has been an increase in the research into BCI in video games over the last twenty years. Examples include 'Brainball' (Hjelm & Browall, 2000) which allowed to players to relax to move a metal ball on a game table, with a visualization of their relaxation as measured by EEG displayed to the players on a projected screen. Krepki et al. (2007) created a series of simple 2D BCI controlled games. Player's wore multi-electrode caps and their EEG feedback was used to allow them interact with various game scenarios. Exploring BCI's 'path towards multimedia applications'. Bos et al. (2010) explored using user focused human-computer interaction approaches in the domain of BCI games. Discussing the increasing availability of BCI solutions and its possible use in games and new mediums. 'Recently, the focal point has shifted to a new group of potential users: the general population. From a commercial perspective, such a large target group could be a very lucrative endeavour. Especially gamers are great potential users, as they are early adopters, willing to learn a new modality if it could prove advantageous' (Bos et al., 2010). Bonnet et al. (2013) experimented with multiuser BCI games, finding that a multiplayer element improved player's engagement in the game and reflecting on the trend of moving from more medical BCI uses towards games and media over the proceeding decade. It can be seen that BCI in video games is an increasing area of academic interest, providing for technical and artistic creativity through the medium of video games.

## Consumer BCI and the Age of Neurotechnology

Affordable brain-computer interfaces have seen a significant increase since the start of the millennium. In 2004, Neurosky's two electrode headset can monitor EEG data. InteraXon a company original working with Neurosky's technology released their own 'Muse' EEG headset in 2007. With Emotiv producing a similar product, but with the addition of ERP capabilities in 2011. 2017 has been heralded as the year of 'brain tech' (IEEE Spectrum, 2017). With investment in the technology from the likes of Facebook and Elon Musk causing increasing interest in the field. Significant progress has been made towards creating a platform for games and virtual reality, with Neurable releasing a modified HTC Vive headset with EEG and ERP monitoring capabilities. Promisingly this device supports Unity which is a highly accessible engine, popular amongst game developers.

## Neurofeedback: A Tool for Learning

Neurofeedback is the process of providing visual or sonified feedback to a user of their brain activity. This previous use of BCI was limited to experimental use in medical fields, displaying potential in treating ADHD in children (Duric, 2012) and epilepsy (Sterman & Egner, 2006). With a notable increase in interest for BCI, and so neurofeedback, in multimedia applications there has been criticism from the more established fields. "However, the ease in the development of new software programs for feedback functionality and displays, together with the entry into the field of a diverse group of professionals and semi-professionals, has led to an unfortunate lack of consensus on methodology and standards of practice. In turn this has contributed to reluctance by the academic and medical communities to endorse the field." (Sterman, 2006). Despite the criticism of the more creative side of neurofeedback, meaningful work has been carried out within the domain of serious games. Friedrich et al. (2015) created a serious game focused on neurofeedback for children with autism spectrum disorder, monitoring the MU signal via EEG and creating a neurofeedback game. Parents reported improved behaviour in the day to day life of the young participants, support neurofeedback as a powerful learning tool with potential in serious games.

Hinterberger (2010) combined EEG feedback with electrocardiogram (ECG) heart monitoring to create 'The Sensorium: A multimodal Neurofeedback Environment'. Projecting a biofeedback augmented light show onto the walls of the test room of the 'Sensorium' accompanied by a reactive soundscape. This visual and sonified neurofeedback was created to help users interact with their physiological functions, participants reported "An increase in contentment, relaxation, happiness and inner harmony" after using the neurofeedback experience. 'MeditAid' is a wearable neurofeedback devices that provides audio feedback on states of meditation developed by Sas and Chopra (2015). It used dynamic audio to aid users in the practice of deep meditation, using 'binaural beats' a method of brain entrainment that creates a psychoacoustic frequency to encourage similar frequencies neurologically. Brain entrainment methods have been shown to be beneficial for those suffering from cognitive functioning deficits, stress, pain, headache/migraines, PMS, and behavioural problems (Huang-Storms, 2008). MeditAid was shown to benefit the 'deepening of meditative states', helping users engage with meditation and mindfulness (Sas and Chopra, 2015).

## METHOD AND DESIGN

The aim of this research is to explore neurofeedback as a tool for serious games. To do this a simple neurofeedback experience was created using a Unity game engine, with design drawing on learning and pedagogical theory. Namely experiential and situated learning. This section will address how brain-computer interfacing can be contextualized within educational game frameworks, game design methodology and importantly how we can attempt evaluate this experience in these given frameworks.

### Research Questions

1. Can useable EEG BCI experiences be sufficiently designed using the described approach?
2. Can such an experience support learning, or more specifically the kind of valuable 'transformational' or 'deep' learning described in serious game literature?
3. What insight into this kind of approach can we gather from qualitative analysis of participant experience, does it support potential and future use of BCI and neurofeedback in serious games?

### Experience Design and Development

When designing a serious game there are many things to consider. Of course the learning outcomes, in this case engagement with ideas of meditation and its practice, take pride of place in considerations and so do the pedagogical theories that support those outcomes. It could be argued however that something often overlooked in the literature is the quality of the game or experience itself. Today gamers, which is almost everyone and not just young 'digital natives' (Selwyn, 2009), hold games and digital media to a very high standard. Game experiences need to at least attempt to adhere to the high levels of graphical, audio and user-experience quality players are familiar with. An underpinning concept of serious games is that they are fun; this idea of a 'spoonful of sugar'. An obstacle to user engagement and fun, and one that is increasingly becoming a tall order, is creating games of the quality players expect.

#### Defining Gameplay

When defining gameplay it is important to define player interaction, a player interacts with a game through 'mechanics'. For instance an attack mechanic could consist of a user pushing a button and his/her on screen avatar performing an attack move. When using BCI as a means of gameplay interaction there are no buttons, only the players mind. So how can we define player interaction within mechanics and therefor gameplay? The gameplay classification work carried out by Djaouti et al. (2007) proposes a simple set of 'game bricks' to represent types of game mechanic, by classifying mechanics we can identify them in other games and implement them knowingly in our own games. For example move, shoot and destroy are represented as individual 'mechanic' bricks, if we put these elements together we can imagine a game similar to 'Space Invaders' where the player moves, shoots and destroys alien spaceships to complete game outcomes. In the designed experience: 'Aurora - Mind over Matter' there is no moving shooting or destroying, so how can we classify the experiences elements? The input from brain-computer interface systems can be erratic, unpredictable and frustrating to manage if high demands are put on the player. For example having to meditate or relax enough to perform an attack in-game would not be a suitable form of gameplay, the spontaneous nature of pressing a button on a game controller is not shared by EEG neurofeedback. ERP methods, as mentioned previously, could more accurately realize this kind of 'cognitive button press'. Two 'game bricks' in particular stand out when trying to suggest mechanics for EEG BCI (Huster et al., 2014). Those are 'manage' and 'match'. The manage mechanic supports the idea of a player managing a resource to perform an action, usually this suggests managing ammo to fire a weapon or resources to build units. Can we consider user meditation a kind of in-game resource? One to be managed in order to achieve the desired outcome? Perhaps more accurate would be the 'match' brick, which requires the player to keep an element in a particular state to achieve outcomes, such as checkmate being achieved by the 'elements' being in the right place to check the enemy king. So perhaps it is better to consider player mediation as an element to be matched to a particular state, rather than resources meant to be managed to allow particular outcomes. To create a neurofeedback 'match' mechanic the experience was designed in such a way that when the players 'meditation' value reached a high enough threshold the game would react positively to the users input. This simple and minimalistic approach meant there were no additional mechanics or game interactions for the player to focus on, the sole purpose of the experience was to encourage the player keep their 'meditation' at the required state.

## Challenge, Reward, Growth

Having chosen to use a 'match' mechanic as the means of user interaction, we can then consider how that interaction will affect the gameplay. Games can generally be summarised to have a simple kind of 'gameplay loop' or cycle. Generally this is a challenge, a reward and subsequent growth. For instance the player overcomes a challenge, such as defeating an enemy, they are rewarded perhaps with treasure that enemy had. These rewards allow the player to advance and grow within the context of the game.

So what is the gameplay loop regarding the designed experience using a 'match' mechanic? In the designed experience the player must undergo the challenge of matching their 'meditation' as read in real time using BCI to a certain threshold. Upon completing this challenge or task the player is rewarded by a visual and sonic change in the game environment, acknowledge the players successful interaction and achievement of matching the required state. This success allows the player to achieve knowledge of what strategies, actions or approaches allowed them to achieve this meditative state, with the intention of letting them hone their meditation 'skills' within the context of the game and letting their understanding of the practice grow.

## Feedback and Heuristics

To support the player's interaction with the gameplay there must be understandable feedback given to the player, confirming their actions within the game. Here neurofeedback and game feedback cross paths. The feedback provided in neurofeedback allows players to understand and reflect on their cognitive functions, similarly feedback in games supports a player's understanding of their place in the game.

This is done through heuristics. There are two kinds of heuristics to be considered in relation to a game or experience. Positional heuristics that let the player know if they are winning or successfully completing the challenge and directional heuristics that allow the player to understand what strategy or approach to take to progress towards completing the given challenge. In the experience designed players are given directional heuristics through a score displayed on an in-game screen. This score represents their 'meditation' level as input through the BCI system and shows players the level of their meditation and how close they are to triggering the match mechanic. A change in game environment acts as a positional heuristic visually alerting players to their success at overcoming the match mechanic.

## Level Design

The game changes between two environments this is, as described above, to assist in showing the player via heuristics their progress and success in the game. This feedback is important to play the game and so learn its outcomes. Additionally with reference to situated learning the environments where created to inforce experiential learning. It also creates a subtle narrative to the game, where by the player clearing their mind, meditating and becoming peaceful causes the virtual environment of the game to mimic that action, and so reinforce it. The starting environment is a plain and mundane room, similar to the situation a player may choose to practice meditation in real life. Compared to the relaxing outdoor environment representing successful meditation.

## Importance of Soundscapes

Depending on whether the player chooses to practice deep meditation or mindfulness the players may choose to close their eyes. Therefor it is important that not only should the environment reflect their success when they open their eyes, the audio of the game should provide strong feedback to assist the player. The first bedroom environment has the sound of humming computers and screens and a beeping sound representing the player being 'plugged into the machine', attempting to draw on familiar schemas around BCI, like those in the Matrix. The second environment on the other hand has the sound of the vast outdoors; wind, trees creaking and distant animals. Additionally reaching very high levels of meditation triggers dynamic music, which fades in and out to provide feedback and a relaxing soundtrack for the player.

## Creating Flexibility and Encouraging Exploration

To allow players to find a 'meditation threshold' comfortable for them a difficulty setting was created, the difficulty between 1 and 5 is displayed on an in-game screen. Players could adjust this setting to make the 'match' mechanic more or less difficult to suit their own ability. This was intended to reducing the sometimes erratic nature of neurofeedback and make the game more engaging and playable, giving the players the potential to customize the experience. Additionally it was intended to allow the player to try and move between difficulties encouraging experimentation and reflection on their chosen approaches and strategies. Exploration helps facilitate learning within serious games, and engagement in general.

## Summary

In summary the experience created could be described as an interactive EEG BCI based neurofeedback experience that uses a customizable match mechanic to allow players to challenge themselves and learn experientially. With underpinning narrative and heuristics supported by visual and audio feedback in 3D situated learning environments.

## Testing

Testing was carried out to evaluate the usefulness of the developed approach and to analyse the potential for learning through its application. The testing procedure and practice was informed by the literature in serious games analysis such as Catalano and importantly Mitgutsch's use of Bateson's work to analyse learning 'in, through and beyond serious games'. Testing was focused on the gathering and analysis of qualitative data from the players/participants, with quantitative measures used as a baseline source of data to support general usability.

## Participants

This study focuses on the qualitative experience of ten participants aged between 19 and 30, four male participants and six female participants took part. There was various familiarity with meditation across the participants, but being of key importance to the study the participants have been broken down into 'meditation groups' to benefit qualitative analysis. Four categories were determined to help aid analysis. None: participants who had no experience with meditation or meditative practices (3 participants). Tried: one individual had a unique relationship with meditation, having tried it but not had a positive experience, this individual was placed in their own group to reflect this. Fair: participants who had practiced meditation, experienced it through activities like yoga or group meditation and had practiced it on occasion (3 participants). Practiced: participants who regularly practiced meditation or had done so for long periods of time (3 participants).

## Procedure

1. Participants were briefed generally on the study, the BCI system and the game experience.
2. Participants were asked to give consent and read through instructions.
3. Participants were asked to fill out a pre-test survey and reflect on their relationship with meditation and their practice of it if applicable and what current tools, if any, the used to engage with meditation. They were asked what might lead them to engage with meditation.
4. The experience was described and outlined to the player, as was the EEG headset they were asked to wear.
5. They were encouraged to play for around five to ten minutes, changing difficulties and reflecting on their experience.
6. Participants then filled out a post-test questionnaire. This includes a system usability scale questionnaire, to consider the general usability and playability of the experience. Additionally they were asked to reflect on the strategies that helped them interact with the game.
7. Participants were interviewed on their experience to gather further qualitative data.

## Usability Testing as a Basic Metric

Bateson's framework as reimagined for serious games provides the foundation for this approach to testing, looking to find learning 'in, through and beyond' serious games. To gain 'level zero' the player must be able to respond with ease to the experience and be able to learn its fundamental components. In terms of game design this means the player must feel comfortable to play the game as it was intended, to make sure that this low level of learning was achieved participants were asked fill out a 'system usability scale' (SUS) questionnaire. This was to measure generally for usability to make sure the experience was engaging enough to facilitate the further levels of learning. This SUS scale, created by Brooke (1986) (Usability.gov) is intended to measure the 'appropriateness to a purpose of any given artefact'. Though with only a small number of participants collectively this quantitative data is not particularly useful, within a more qualitative approach to evaluating the developed experience it can provide a baseline for usefulness to each participant and a value of how easy the system was to use. Confirming that 'level zero' could be achieved in the context of the experience with no hindrance.

## Qualitative Assessment of Exploration

Participants were observed while playing the game, observations were made on level of apparent relaxation, interest in the game, eagerness to explore the experience and adjust levels of difficulty. The process of engaging with the game and exploring its mechanic through gameplay allowed the players to understand the context of the experience, experimenting and achieve the first level of learning following Bateson's framework. Focusing on observing gameplay and listening to participant accounts provide a means of accessing this learning 'through serious games', allowing us to then consider the next and most important level of learning.

## Qualitative Analysis of Learning

The second and final level of learning as considered by Bateson supports the idea of 'deep learning' as described by Gee (2005). It is the level where through relating the learning achieved in previous levels to themselves and their existing knowledge and beliefs they can experience transformative learning. Taking the learning 'beyond' the game and into real world contexts. To monitor and look for traces of this kind of learning player's strategies towards and beliefs around meditation where compared before and after the experience. If the experience could facilitate adequate reflection for the player to reconsider their approach to meditation in a broader sense the game could be suggested to have had a successful, meaningful and individual impact on the player. By separating participants into individual categories based on their own relationship with meditation we can attempt to see this kind of shift in their thoughts and approaches, with reference to their existing knowledge and feelings before using the neurofeedback experience. This explorative approach aims to try to access the usefulness of the experience as a tool for advancing learning and engagement with meditation and potentially realizing how it may be practiced by that individual. Evaluating the overall usefulness of EEG BCI based neurofeedback experiences within the given context of serious games and educational experiences.

## Results

Using a SUS questionnaire to get a rough baseline for participant usability was originally intended to support the basic interactions required for 'level zero' learning. However when comparing the perceived usability on average between groups created around experience with meditation practice (no practice: 3, fair practice: 3 and well-practiced: 3) interesting differences appeared.

The questions are separated between agreeing on positive (5) and negative (5) aspects of the experience. With 0 being strongly disagree and 5 to strongly agree when represented below.

### Positive Question Agreement

- **I would use this frequently:** On average users agreed that they would like to use the system frequently (4.1/5). Fair (4.3) and well-practiced (4.7) participants were more enthusiastic about using the system when compared to those with no practice (3), who, on average, neither agreed nor disagreed to wanting to use the system again.
- **I thought it was easy to use:** On average participants found the system easy to use (4.6/5). Fair (4.7) and well-practiced (4.7) players found the systems slightly easier than average. While players with no experience still agreed the system was easy to use (4.3) but to a lesser extent when compared to the average and other groups.
- **I found the functions well integrated:** On average players agreed the experience's functions and features were well integrated (4). In this instance no practice and fair practice groups agreed (3.7) to a lesser extent than those well-practiced (4.3).
- **I imagine people would learn to use this quickly:** On average participants agreed that learning to use this system could be done quickly (4.1). Those well-practiced in meditation perceived the system to be easier to learn for others (4.7) when compared to no practice (4) and fair practice (3.3).
- **I felt confident using this:** On average players agreed to feeling confident using the experience (3.6). Well-practiced players (4.3) agreed more strongly than fair practice players (3.3). On average players with no experience leant more towards not being confident using the system (2.7).

#### *Findings*

On average players were positive about the experience, however when comparing those that practice meditation frequently with those who have no practice clear differences appear. Regarding agreeing to positive statements regarding the experience found in the SUS questionnaire; those well-practiced were consistently above average. Well-practiced players felt more confident using the system, found it easier to use and learn and they were enthusiastic about using such an experience frequently. Those with no practice where less positive about the experience, with averages consistently falling below the participant average. They were less enthusiastic about using the experience again and found the system less easy to use and more difficult to learn than well-practiced players. These findings could indicate a correlation between experience with meditation and perceived usability of the experience, suggesting that even though participants generally were positive about the experience when answering, players with more experience engaged with the experience more positively overall.

### Negative Question Agreement

- **I found this too complex:** On average players disagreed with the experience being too complex (1.3/5). The players with no experience disagreed less than the other two groups (1.7)
- **I feel I would need technical support:** On average players disagreed (2.3/5). However experienced meditators felt they would be less likely to need support (1.6), in comparison those without experience actually agreed that they would need technical support on average (3.3).
- **I thought the experience was inconsistent:** On average players disagreed (2/5). Again comparing well-practiced and no practice players, well-practiced felt there was less inconsistency (1.3), while those without practice felt there was more (2.3).
- **I found it cumbersome:** In general players disagreed (1.9). Well-practiced players actually found slightly more cumbersome than the average (2) and unexperienced players found it significantly more cumbersome when compared (2.3).
- **I need to learn a lot before I get going:** On average players mostly disagreed (2.4). However though well-practiced (2.3) and fair practiced (1.6) felt they did not need to learn a lot, non-practiced players actually agreed to need to learn a lot (3.7).

#### *Findings*

Players on average disagreed with the negative questions in the SUS questionnaire. However when examining meditation groups this is not true. Those without practice in meditation actually agreed to feeling a lot of learning was required and that they needed additional support. Again across questions non practiced players felt less positive compared to the average, while those with lots of practice were found to be more positive on average across questions, other than finding the system more cumbersome than participant average.

### Qualitative Data

'Meditation groups' are used again when analysing the qualitative reports and interviews provided by participants. This allows a focus on each participant's reflections and potential learning within the context of their current understanding.

## EVALUATION

This study has no usefulness if it is not aware of its own scope, this is a small study and though the findings are interesting, an area of research as broad as neurofeedback for educational purposes merits more scrutiny. Though conclusions and relationship can be discussed relating to the results of the study further research must be carried out, with greater numbers of participants, to draw conclusions. What the study may suggest will be the topic of the next chapter. This study can be scrutinized not only for its number of participants but also for elements of game design, development and testing.

## Game Design

Originally the contrast between the irritating office environment and the relaxing outdoor environment was intended to add to the narrative and differentiate the environments. It became clear that the soundscape used in the first environment was distracting and not conducive of meditation, though some players seemed to enjoy the challenge, many found it made the experience more difficult. A revised game would have a more peaceful starting environment so not to distract players. Furthermore players, especially those with no experience, felt there needed to be more explanation of the workings of the game. From a game design perspective this can be attributed to the failings of the user interface and the games heuristics. Additionally, as no explanation or description of mediation was given to players before the play session, information in-game could have helped address difficulty understanding the game and its premise. Particularly for players with less experience. Some players also questioned a lack of narrative, especially in the 'relaxing' environment as they felt this would motivate them to play. Overall a revised game would have to address many areas to support a better and more inclusive experience.

## Game Development

Problems are also present at a deeper development level. The value sent from the NeuroSky headset is between 0 and 100, that value becomes 0 to 10 by the time it reaches Unity. This results in a 10x reduction of resolution in the system. More important is the nature of that reduced signal, in code it is reduced using simple if statements. A value greater than 0 equals 1, a value greater or equal to 20 equals 2 and so on. This use of general if statements when reducing information to be sent across Arduino microprocessors results in a kind of stepping of the signal drastically from 1 to 2 (and so on) because of the way the signal is processed. This could add to the erratic nature the system sometimes takes, especially with unexperienced players. To address this the headset could send the value (0 to 100) that represents meditation directly to Unity via Bluetooth. This is possible and would remove the degradation of the signal. Resulting in a smoother experience with a greater resolution.

## Testing

Testing procedure can also be criticized, the participant group was small, only 10 people. There was an equal number of well, fair and non-practiced players. Though efforts were made to minimize noise players were sometimes distracted by students and other sounds when trying to relax using the experience. Some questions were unclear and had to be further explained to participants during pre and post questionnaires. Reference in questions should have been made to 'the experience' or 'the game' not 'the Aurora Experience' which confused participants, additionally the use of the word 'cumbersome' in the SUS caused difficulty for some participants, some whom did not have English as a first language. A more universal word should have been used for inclusivity.

## FUTURE RESEARCH DIRECTIONS

Basic user testing using the SUS questionnaire questions supports that generally players found the system easy to use and interact with. However when looking at result averages with relation to user experience well-practiced players found the system easier to use than those with no practice in meditation. This could suggest that the system was in fact able to measure meditation, with more experienced users having an easier time and perceiving the system to be more useable. It is important to note that no description of meditation practice was given to any of the participants, perhaps if a similar experience was supported by additional learning materials, a workshop or a professional practitioner, engagement could be improved for novice meditators. These findings are in stark contrast to the finding of Sas and Chopra (2015) who found neurofeedback experiences particularly useful for 'novice meditators'. Though the experiential learning tool developed seemed to be usable, and so support Bateson's 'level zero' of learning, it is felt further research into usability with regards to level of experience is needed. Additionally further research to identify the value additional learning materials can add when helping unexperienced players engage with experiential neurofeedback experiences would be valuable. Further studies should aim to record participant EEG levels during gameplay, this could provide quantitative data to define whether or not well-practiced players are better at the game than those with little or no practice. Fair practiced players seemed to have more 'deep' meditation strategies before playing the game, during play they often changed their strategies to a more 'mindful' approach. They were surprised by how little they had to close their eyes and by how much breathing techniques and the kind of calm awareness associated with mindfulness, helped control the experience. Well-practiced players on the other hand seemed to have ideas closer to mindfulness when approaching the experience, instead they used 'deep' meditation strategies such as relaxing the body and closing the eyes while playing the game. These changes in strategy from both fair and well-practiced players could represent a kind of learning or reassessment of their own meditation practices. However, it is felt that a longer study to try and map changes in practice over time would give a greater insight into the potential for 'transformational' learning. Though this study shows what may be traces of learning of this kind and a general usability to support the legitimacy of the system in monitoring meditation, further work must be carried out to create best practice in this emerging field. It is believed that BCI and neurofeedback have great potential for reflective experiential learning and serious games. The responses of practiced players were far more positive than that of those with no practice, this could reflect the accuracy of the system and the closeness of the meditation mechanic in the experience and the practice of meditation in real life. Alternatively those that regularly practice meditation may just have had more enthusiasm and interest in this kind of experience. It is felt the results would suggest the success of this approach, however user testing also highlighted several failings of the experience; from irritating sound design to lack of in-game information. Therefor this study is better seen as a 'toe in the water', an early look at how this kind of experience may benefit the world of serious games. As a heavily experiential method there is much that can benefit neurofeedback games in the experiential learning approaches found within serious game literature. Furthermore by adhering to serious game literature when considering design and development games can be assessed with greater accuracy with regards to their potential for learning. Importantly this study used consumer grade EEG hardware and was still successful in creating working and usable systems. This approach could provide low cost and accessible means for game developers and researchers to explore brain-computer interfacing.

## CONCLUSION

Brain-computer interfacing and neurofeedback provide an exciting new area for exploration in serious games. BCI offers a new frontier for learning and importantly learning about ourselves. Experiential neurofeedback games could provide engaging and novel new ways for us to learn about tacit and beneficial practices like meditation, answering age old questions about the human mind, its functions and how we can master them. Consumer facing solutions to brain-monitoring can allow greater access and experimentation in this field and as the fields of neurology and psychology advance serious games can benefit from attempting to frame the growing knowledge and approaches of these disciplines within its own literature and pedagogical theory. Importantly these kinds of solutions and approaches could help engage players with practices that can help them overcome real problems. How to relax when feeling stressed or how to focus when they have to, systems that can help players master these skills as they would master a skill in a game. Serious games often address external problems and knowledge, but through neurofeedback and BCI serious games can empower us to understand the mind.

## REFERENCES

Badcock, N. A., Mousikou, P., Mahajan, Y., De Lissa, P., Thie, J., & McArthur, G. (2013). Validation of the Emotiv EPOC® EEG gaming system for measuring research quality auditory ERPs. *PeerJ*, *1*, e38. doi:10.7717/peerj.38 PMID:23638374

Bateson, G. (1972). Steps to an ecology of mind: Collected essays. In *Anthropology, Psychiatry, Evolution, and Epistemology*. University of Chicago Press.

Bonnet, L., Lotte, F., & Lecuyer, A. (2013). Two brains, one game: Design and evaluation of a multiuser BCI video game based on motor imagery. *IEEE Transactions on Computational Intelligence and AI in Games*, *5*(2), 185–198.

Bos, D. P. O., Reuderink, B., Van De Laar, B., Gurkok, H., Muhl, C., Poel, M., . . . Nijholt, A. (2010). Human-computer interaction for bci games: Usability and user experience. In *Cyberworlds (CW), 2010 International Conference on* (pp. 277-281). IEEE.

Chen, Z., Hood, R. W., Jr., Yang, L., & Watson, P. J. (2011). Mystical experience among Tibetan Buddhists: The common core thesis revisited. *Journal for the Scientific Study of Religion*, *50*(2), 328-338.

Coffey, A. L., Leamy, D. J., & Ward, T. E. (2014). A novel BCI-controlled pneumatic glove system for home-based neurorehabilitation. In *Engineering in Medicine and Biology Society (EMBC), 2014 36th Annual International Conference of the IEEE* (pp. 3622-3625). IEEE. 10.1109/EMBC.2014.6944407

Djaouti, D., Alvarez, J., Jessel, J. P., Methel, G., & Molinier, P. (2007). Towards a classification of video games. In *Artificial and Ambient Intelligence convention*. Artificial Societies for Ambient Intelligence.

Duric, N. S., Assmus, J., Gundersen, D., & Elgen, I. B. (2012). Neurofeedback for the treatment of children and adolescents with ADHD: A randomized and controlled clinical trial using parental reports. *BMC Psychiatry*, *12*(1), 107. doi:10.1186/1471-244X-12-107 PMID:22877086

Friedrich, E. V., Sivanathan, A., Lim, T., Suttie, N., Louchart, S., Pillen, S., & Pineda, J. A. (2015). An effective neurofeedback intervention to improve social interactions in children with autism spectrum disorder. *Journal of Autism and Developmental Disorders*, *45*(12), 4084–4100. doi:10.100710803-015-2523-5 PMID:26210513

Gee, J. P. (2005). Learning by design: Good video games as learning machines. *E-Learning and Digital Media*, *2*(1), 5–16. doi:10.2304/elea.2005.2.1.5

Heinz, B. R. (1981). *The origins of meditation: Perspectives beyond the scientific research* (Unpublished doctoral dissertation). Loyola University Chicago. Retrieved July 10, 2018 from https://ecommons.luc.edu/luc_diss/2065

Hinterberger, T. (2011). The sensorium: A multimodal neurofeedback environment. *Advances in Human-Computer Interaction*, 3.

Hjelm, S. I., & Browall, C. (2000). Brainball: Using Brain Activity for Cool Competition. *Proceedings of the First Nordic Conference on Computer-Human Interaction (NordiCHI 2000).*

Huang-Storms, L. (2008). *Efficacy of neurofeedback for children with histories of abuse and neglect: Pilot study and meta-analytic comparison to other treatments*. University of North Texas.

Huster, R. J., Mokom, Z. N., Enriquez-Geppert, S., & Herrmann, C. S. (2014). Brain-computer interfaces for EEG neurofeedback: Peculiarities and solutions. *International Journal of Psychophysiology: Official Journal of the International Organization of Psychophysiology*, *91*(1), 36–45. doi:10.1016/j.ijpsycho.2013.08.011 PMID:24012908

IEEE Spectrum: Technology, Engineering, and Science News. (2017). *Silicon Valley's Latest Craze: Brain Tech.* Retrieved August, 10, 2017 from http://spectrum.ieee.org/biomedical/devices/silicon-valleys-latest-craze-brain-tech

Kennedy, J. F. (1962). *Moon Speech.* Rice Stadium. Retrieved July 10, 2018 from https://er.jsc.nasa.gov/seh/ricetalk.htm

Kim, S. G., & Uĝurbil, K. (1997). Comparison of blood oxygenattion and cerebral blood flow effect in fMRI: Estimation of relative oxygen consumption change. *Magnetic Resonance in Medicine*, *38*(1), 59–65. doi:10.1002/mrm.1910380110 PMID:9211380

Krepki, R., Blankertz, B., Curio, G., & Müller, K.-R. (2007). The Berlin Brain-Computer Interface (BBCI) – Towards a new communication channel for online control in gaming Applications. *Multimedia Tools and Applications*, *33*(1), 73–90. doi:10.100711042-006-0094-3

Lim, T., Louchart, S., Suttie, N., Hauge, J. B., Stanescu, I. A., Ortiz, I. M., ... Ott, M. (2014). Narrative serious game mechanics (NSGM)–insights into the narrative-pedagogical mechanism. In *International Conference on Serious Games* (pp. 23-34). Springer. 10.1007/978-3-319-05972-3_4

Miranda, E., & Brouse, A. (2005). Toward direct brain-computer musical interfaces. In *Proceedings of the 2005 Conference on New Interfaces for Musical Expression* (pp. 216-219). National University of Singapore.

Mitgutsch, K. (2011). Serious learning in serious games. In M. Ma, A. Oikonomou, & L. C. Jain (Eds.), *Serious Games and Edutainment Applications* (pp. 45–58). Springer London. doi:10.1007/978-1-4471-2161-9_4

Otten, L. J. & Rugg, M. D. (2005). Interpreting event-related brain potentials. *Event-Related Potentials: A Methods Handbook,* 3-16.

Sas, C., & Chopra, R. (2015). MeditAid: A wearable adaptive neurofeedback-based system for training mindfulness state. *Personal and Ubiquitous Computing, 19*(7), 1169–1182. doi:10.100700779-015-0870-z

Selwyn, N. (2009). The digital native–myth and reality. *Aslib Proceedings, 61*(4), 364–379. doi:10.1108/00012530910973776

Shields. (2016). Aristotle's Psychology. *The Stanford Encyclopedia of Philosophy (Winter 2016 Edition).* Retrieved July 10, 2018 from https://plato.stanford.edu/archives/win2016/entries/aristotle-psychology/

Sterman, M. B., & Egner, T. (2006). Foundation and practice of neurofeedback for the treatment of epilepsy. *Applied Psychophysiology and Biofeedback, 31*(1), 21–35. doi:10.100710484-006-9002-x PMID:16614940

Usability (Improving the User Experience). (2018). Retrieved July 10, 2018 from https://www.usability.gov/

Vidal, J. J. (1973). Toward direct brain-computer communication. *Annual Review of Biophysics and Bioengineering, 2*(1), 157–180. doi:10.1146/annurev.bb.02.060173.001105 PMID:4583653

Woodman, G. F. (2010). A brief introduction to the use of event-related potentials in studies of perception and attention. *Attention, Perception & Psychophysics, 72*(8), 2031–2046. doi:10.3758/BF03196680 PMID:21097848

## KEY TERMS AND DEFINITIONS

**Brain-Computer Interfacing (BCI):** The ability to interact with software and technology with our thoughts and feelings; it presents an exciting new frontier for serious games and learning.

**EEG or Electroencephalogram:** Is a method of using electrodes placed on the scalp to measure electrical brain activity, pioneered by Hans Berger in 1924.

**ERP or Event-Related Potential:** It uses EEG to monitor the brains response to specific stimulus. Using this technique specific internal or external events can be measured.

**Functional Magnetic Resonance Imaging or fMRI:** It is a neuroimaging approach that uses magnetic resonance imaging to monitor the change in blood as it flows around the brain. This nonintrusive approach causes the subject no harm and does not require direct contact with the scalp.

**Meditation:** It is the practice of focusing or drawing attention to one's thoughts in order to relax, clear the mind, or find peaceful or mindful states.

**Mixed Approaches:** Emerging approaches hope to address the failings of existing brain monitoring techniques. They are a combination of fMRI and EEG approaches that can allow for high spatial and temporal resolutions when gathering data.

**Serious Games:** They are games that have scope beyond recreation. They can be for training, teaching and propagating information, in fact games create uniquely customizable environments that excel in all of these areas.

**System Usability Scale (SUS):** It provides a reliable tool for measuring the usability. It consists of a ten-item questionnaire with five response options for respondents from “strongly agree” to “strongly disagree.” It was originally created by John Brooke in 1986.

# Chapter 4
# Virtual Reality Therapeutic Environments in Autism Spectrum Disorder (ASD) and Alzheimer's:
## Treatment, Diagnosis, and Refinement

**David W. Sime**
*Online Corporate Video Production Ltd., UK*

## ABSTRACT

*This chapter is devoted to observing and analyzing the role of virtual reality environments in the therapeutic treatment, analysis, and ongoing treatment planning of autistic spectrum disorders (ASD), Alzheimer's, and dementia. Using live real-world examples of the above activities in action and a literature review, the chapter will examine the level of empirical data and pre-existing qualitative and quantitative research to support these ongoing approaches. Critical analysis will also be made of the current level of empirical research available highlighting areas that should be focused on for future research.*

## INTRODUCTION

This researcher has been working in the field of virtual reality and digital interaction with both Google, the Chartered Institute of Marketing (LinkedIn, 2018) and the immersive VR agency Oncor Digital (Fair, 2015). Primarily with an approach focused on applied user psychology and marketing communications, the foci of the last decades' immersion in this field has nevertheless created links with many producers of Virtual Reality (VR) and Augmented Reality (AR) content across a wide range of other applications. These span entertainment, educational and promotional applications, all of which have significant realised and unrealised potential as fledgling VR/AR technology establishes itself as a mainstream technology. However, perhaps, the most affecting application of VR is in the field of healthcare – specifically mental healthcare. A great many aspects of mental health have been approached with VR treatments

DOI: 10.4018/978-1-5225-7168-1.ch004

and diagnostics. However, although much anecdotal evidence of benefits has been shared in online and offline media, perhaps because of the widely (and therefore thinly) dispersed activities, there has been a distinct lack of collected empirical research data in these fields. (Mikropuolos & Natsis, 2011). Although not an academic researcher, this author's two decades in the field of marketing (where arguably 70% of activities are research, testing, measuring, recording and adapting to qualitative and quantitative analysis of research – Jain, 1989) has generated a strong interest in capturing reliable and comparable data which can be usefully applied across the ongoing and collective progression of VR in all of its applications – particularly healthcare where the sharing of information has always been a lynchpin of the disciplines' development. (Walker et al., 2005). Similarly, the rapid progressions of the field of offline and online marketing media consumption, from primarily text and image based media through to audio, video and most recently immersive/interactive communications, has seen technological, behavioural and even sociological parallels that span all areas of human behaviour (Napoli, 2011) – not least healthcare. Finally, coming from an ongoing perspective based around psychology and sociology (stemming from regular study and application of consumer psychology) have highlighted the strong bidirectional link between media consumption/interaction and the psychological (even psychophysiological) condition of the participant (Shrum, 2009). It is the bidirectional and interactive nature of VR communication that provides the three specific foci for this chapter on its application to mental healthcare – namely not only treatment, but observation and recording of progress, and the resultant diagnostic potential of live and ongoing observation to continuously assess progress and accordingly adapt treatment plans. This chapter will examine precedents for these abilities across Autistic Spectrum Disorders (ASDs) and Alzheimer's/Dementia.

## ASD Virtual Environment Therapy

A recurrent issue in both lower and higher functioning Autistic Spectrum Disorders (ASD), most notably in younger sufferers, are the difficulties created by the breaking of routines (Schaaf et al., 2011). This is frequently an issue when coming into new and unfamiliar environments where ASD sufferers can be particularly prone to incidences of sensory overload and extreme resultant discomfort – but perhaps the most life restricting aspect of this is the avoidance behaviours which can result, restricting mobility, social interaction and even employment prospects in later life (Gustafsson & Papliński, 2004). Craig French Hendry (2018), a colleague working in the field of commercial and industrial immersive 360 walkthrough technology, was aware of this issue through a family connection with ASD. As a means of helping to prepare, and therefore alleviate, sufferers' symptoms, Hendry volunteered his services to a number of entertainment, historic and educational venues near his home base in Perth, Australia (Hendry, 2018). These services included capturing these areas using a combined infrared ranging and photogrammetry scanner. The output from this device is freely accessible via a cloud based online distribution network, viewable on devices from basic smartphones, tablets and computers through to VR Head Mounted Display (VR-HMD). To varying degrees, Hendry (2018) felt that, within a familiar home environment, and with the ability to pull out whenever the participant required, this approach would allow ASD sufferers and their carers to virtually 'pre-visit' the planned destination, familiarising themselves with the features and layouts of this new environment and beginning to form a more familiar pattern of awareness of the space. Although even a full VR walkthrough can only prepare the proposed visitor for a small section of the sensory stimulus likely to be encountered during a live visit - for instance, failing to replicate the noise and movement created by other visitors In-text: (Smith et al., 2014) – it was hoped that this would still go some way to alleviating symptoms caused by the unfamiliarity of environmental cues. Although responses to this and similar provisions elsewhere in the world have generated consistently positive anecdotal feedback from both sufferers, carers and hosts, as ad-hoc and not formally assessed activities, the empirical and quantifiable results of these have been extremely limited. Fortunately, a more structured application and assessment of this approach has been conducted by Cobb and Parsons (2011) conducting a comprehensive literature review of all similar applications of VR technology to ASD over a ten-year period. Their choice of VR in particular as a therapeutic medium was inspired by Parsons and Mitchel's (2002) assertion that virtual environments 'could be particularly helpful for people on the autism spectrum because: 1. The user has active control over their participation; 2. Interaction can take many forms and does not necessitate face-to-face communication (users may communicate via their avatars) which many people with autism might find particularly threatening; 3. The level and number of non-verbal and verbal features of communication can be directly controlled and manipulated; 4. Behaviours and responses can be practiced and built-upon in a context that shares some similarities with the real world, thereby offering greater potential for generalization; and 5. A more realistic representation of a situation on a computer-screen could, in theory at least, assist with the mental simulation of events, thereby improving social problem-solving'. Although Cobb and Parsons (2011) commented that there was (and still is) a surprising lack of large scale empirical studies on the topic, those studies included in their literature review still highlighted some very interesting findings. One set of studies in particular (Moore et al., 2005; Fabri & Moore, 2005; Fabri et al., 2007) were able to not only demonstrate far better real world participation in environments previously 'visited' in VR (in this case a café where they were asked to navigate to the counter, order a drink and take a seat), they were also able to demonstrate 'off target' behaviour in some of the participants, where they explored other areas of the café and even went behind the counter. What was particularly useful about this was that it allowed assessors to diagnose participants who might require extra support and preparation to be able to navigate the real world equivalent environment and task. Although the sample sizes on each of these studies were small (three sets of 12 ASD children, each grouped into a different age range from 4-5 up to 14-15), the results were consistent and borne out by subsequent qualitative monitoring. Familiarisation with environment was not the only application of VR examined in the context of young ASD sufferers – virtual environments were used to demonstrate safety procedures such as fire and tornado drills and even crossing a busy street. Not only were the vast majority (11 out of 12 and 5 out of 6 respectively) able to successfully complete these procedures in virtual reality, a lower but still significant proportion were also able to transfer this procedural learning to real world equivalent scenarios (Josman et al., 2008). To reiterate however, none of these studies were of a size which could be considered statistically significant enough for the results to be reliably repeatable, merely pointing towards the need for repetition amongst a larger sample size. As Cobb and Parsons (2011) themselves stated; 'Most of the studies tend to be fairly small-scale in nature, with limited extension beyond one or two preliminary investigations, which can present equivocal results. Although these do offer some positive support for the earlier arguments regarding potential of VR, there is still a considerable challenge in translating this into workable, useful tools that offer realistic applications'.

## Dementia Virtual Environmental Therapy

There has been a great deal of promising research into the beneficial effects of environmental therapies on sufferers of dementia; with changes to surroundings, furniture and even music to reflect that of the sufferer's pre-onset life experiences being shown to dramatically and consistently alleviate some of the most severe symptoms (Day et al., 2000). However the appropriate era of surroundings is very much dependent upon the age of each patient and the time of life when their symptoms came on, thus making an already complex and expensive process of recreation still more difficult to achieve across the range of sufferers, with the result that very few dementia patients are lucky enough to benefit from this type of immersion – referred to as 'Reminiscence Therapy' (Siriaraya & Ang, 2014). Suzanne Lee (2018) - at the time digital content communications specialist for Lloyds Banking Group - was very interested in VR technology and, having encountered dementia symptoms in two late members of her own family, began to explore if VR had ever been used for the condition. Initially encountering very promising video evidence of the application of immersive video for calming dementia patients by UK VR company TribeMix (2017). Lee (2018) was inspired to further this research directly. Undertaking bi-monthly visits to various care homes in collaboration with the Forget Me Not dementia training group (Elsley, 2018) Lee (2018) tested a variety of 360-degree videos on dementia patients depicting tranquil, calming environments. Not only did she notice consistent benefits in participants in terms of reduced agitation and increased post therapeutic engagement levels, she also noted that social interaction *between* these participants (limited or even absent beforehand) was dramatically increased – seemingly by their shared experience of the therapy. (Finkelstein et al., 2011). Based on this, Lee (2018) started to plan content which might be more meaningful to the specific patients, filming familiar local environments in 360 degrees which she was able to utilise with success in subsequent visits. Also, by observing online Alzheimers forums such as Twitter's "Alzchat" (Twitter.com, 2018), Lee (2008) observed and created content to address recurrent themes and threads based on their commonness, their impact etc. For example, in planning a virtual garden scene for the environment, Lee (2008) had learned that because of limitations to spatial navigation and decision making, and the confusion issues these could create, her interactive environments would need to avoid the incorporation of halting or forking paths, replacing these with continuous, looping pathways to facilitate smoother navigation. (Cushman, Stein & Duffy, 2008). Similarly, upon learning of the vision loss and depth perception issues common to many dementia sufferers, Lee (2008) was taught to avoid dark coloured areas, as these could be perceived as holes and therefore threatening obstacles. (Lewis & Griffin, 1997). For the same reasons, contrasts between different types of flooring could potentially be misinterpreted as changes in floor level or steps, so these were eliminated to avoid patients overcompensating in their step height. Conversely similarly coloured objects in relation to the floor, such as a blue bedspread over a blue carpet, cannot be easily differentiated as being at different heights, making identifying the object as a bed (if at all) very difficult. (Wallace et al., 2012). To illustrate these visual and spatial limitations and create greater understanding amongst to non-sufferers, a 3D modelling company - Wireframe Immersive in Glasgow – created a dementia simulation visor which showed first-hand how hard it is to differentiate colour and level changes in floors and walls, creating a need for extra definition of lines and outlines within VR environments to delineate, in particular, flat objects such as doors against the walls they were placed in (Mairs, 2018). Similarly, Alzheimer's research UK have created a 360 video of a dementia sufferer someone being lost, once again demonstrating the darkness/floor level colour misperception problems whilst seeking to generate empathy and understanding amongst non-sufferers. All these considerations had to be applied to Lee's next step – a connected series of virtual environments suitable for dementia sufferers to create benefits including memory recall, calming of agitation and building of real world community and communication in care homes and residential environments. A step beyond Reminiscence Therapy, Lee has titled this approach 'immersive reminiscence' (Lee, 2018). With a several year precedent of many of these sought after benefits having been achieved (albeit on a patient by patient basis) by a related system - Aloha VR based in San Francisco (Tsukayama, 2018), the observing physician concerned – Sonja Kim MD – stated that it over the two-year period of delivery it had proved more effective than any drug she might have been able to prescribe. It became apparent to Lee (2018) that, although there was real potential in this approach, there was also a wider audience for the content than she, or the likes of Dr Kim, could reach in person. Therefore, in order to reach a broader cross section of sufferers, carers and therapists, some form of hosting and platform would have to be created. Another precedent for this type of technology however – Rendever VR in Boston – applied a simultaneous multi user VR approach to focus on the social and communications benefits of VR. Allowing up to 4 people to participate in the same VR environment (which might include an Antarctic expedition or a canoeing excursion). These shared experiences appeared to generate some profound effects, with anecdotal results including one very withdrawn and incoherent patient being able to communicate clearly and continuing to do so for three months after a single exposure to the technology. More significantly however, sustained empirical research into the approach over the many sites using it reported quantitative feedback from participants of a 40% increase in stated happiness levels over the 12 month delivery period. (Zinck & Zinck, 2018). Like the ASD VR solutions mentioned earlier in this chapter – precedents for this type of technology have applications not only in treatment, but in research and diagnosis of Alzheimer's, in order to create more effective and bespoke treatment plans (Flynn et al., 2003). A freely available VR app – Sea Hero Quest – utilises a gaming format to monitoring spatial navigation abilities of people of any age, generating a huge dataset of comparative results across age ranges from its 2.5 million strong user-base. It's developers Alzheimers Research UK and University College London report that just 2 minutes of gameplay provides them with the equivalent of 5 hours of conventional research data, allowing them to leverage 'the collection, aggregation, and predictive analysis of large data volumes enabling timelier diagnosis and prevention strategies, and possibly overcoming current therapeutic limitations' (Ienca et al., 2018). There are a number of other virtual reality-based Alzheimer's diagnosis and data aggregation tools extant within the UK alone, including VITAE VR and Dorset NHS's 'VStore' gamified dementia diagnostic tool. This uses a realistic supermarket environment to assess the cognitive, spatial and decision making abilities of its users, allowing for remote diagnosis without the lack of real world application or observational bias inherent in most diagnostic procedures (McWilliam, 2018). These are just two of a growing number of VR diagnostic tools which include CogniSense and ACEmobile.

## CONCLUSION

Ienca et al. (2018) state that although these tools provide an unprecedented level and range of big data, which can be used for everything from broader trend analysis and prediction to the creation of personalised treatment regimes, these distinct datasets could become far more than the sum of their respective parts if they can be shared and used together – something which intellectual property and attempts by the developers to leverage value out of their own ring-fenced aggregated data sets seems unlikely to allow. Conversely the risk of too open a disclosure of personal data could include discrimination from health insurance companies. It is difficult to predict the long term outcome of this combination of VR therapy, diagnosis and treatment planning – or to what extent data might be shared between applications. In the meantime, Lee is leveraging her knowledge of the developing field to develop a multi therapeutic environment including a Garden area, a period living room with a turntable selection of period appropriate music potentially involving the Playlist for Life Initiative (2018), a cinema screening area and 360 videos for both sufferers and carers of people with dementia. The VR environment is multi user, with no upper limit to user numbers, but for the purposes of social familiarity is likely to be kept to smaller groups and even families. Recording and sharing of both data and development plans aim to get medical professionals, carers, family and academia involved with the development of the virtual environment, with the hope that this cross discipline approach will leverage the best possible outcomes for all stakeholders (García-Betances et al., 2015).

## REFERENCES

Cushman, L., Stein, K., & Duffy, C. (2008). Detecting navigational deficits in cognitive aging and Alzheimer disease using virtual reality. *Neurology*, *71*(12), 888–895. doi:10.1212/01.wnl.0000326262.67613.fe PMID:18794491

Day, K., Carreon, D., & Stump, C. (2000). The therapeutic design of environments for people with dementia: A review of the empirical research. *The Gerontologist*, *40*(4), 397–416. doi:10.1093/geront/40.4.397 PMID:10961029

Elsley, C. (2018). *About - Dementia Training from Forget Me Not - Dementia Training | Forget Me Not Dementia Training*. Retrieved July 10, 2018 from http://www.forgetmenotdementia.co.uk/about/

Fabri, M., Elzouki, S., & Moore, D. (2007). Emotionally expressive avatars for chatting, learning and therapeutic intervention. *Proceedings of the 12th International Conference on Human-Computer Interaction (HCI International)*, *4552*(3), 275–285.

Fabri, M., & Moore, D. J. (2005). The use of emotionally expressive avatars in Collaborative Virtual Environments. In *Proceedings of Symposium on Empathic Interaction with Synthetic Characters, held at Artificial Intelligence and Social Behaviour Convention 2005*. University of Hertfordshire.

Fair, A. (2015). *3D Scanning - OnCorVid*. Oncor Digital. Retrieved July 10, 2018 from https://oncorvideo.co.uk/3d-scanning/

Finkelstein, S., Nickel, A., Lipps, Z., Barnes, T., Wartell, Z., & Suma, E. (2011). Astrojumper: Motivating exercise with an immersive virtual reality exergame. *Presence (Cambridge, Mass.)*, *20*(1), 78–92. doi:10.1162/pres_a_00036

Flynn, D., Schaik, P., Blackman, T., Femcott, C., Hobbs, B., & Calderon, C. (2003). Developing a virtual reality–based methodology for people with dementia: A feasibility study. *Cyberpsychology & Behavior*, *6*(6), 591–611. doi:10.1089/109493103322725379 PMID:14756925

García-Betances, R., Waldmeyer, M., Fico, G., & Cabrera-Umpiérrez, M. (2015). A succinct overview of virtual reality technology use in Alzheimer's disease. *Frontiers in Aging Neuroscience*, 7.

Gustafsson, L., & Papliński, A. P. (2004). Self-Organization of an Artificial Neural Network Subjected to Attention Shift Impairments and Familiarity Preference, Characteristics Studied in Autism. *Journal of Autism and Developmental Disorders*, *34*(2), 189–198. doi:10.1023/B:JADD.0000022609.31371.4d PMID:15162937

Hendry, C. (2018). *Creative Aero – Craig French Hendry*. Retrieved July 10, 2018 from https://creative.aero/

Ienca, M., Vayena, E., & Blasimme, A. (2018). Big data and dementia: Charting the route ahead for research, ethics, and policy. *Frontiers in Medicine*, *5*, 13. doi:10.3389/fmed.2018.00013 PMID:29468161

Jain, S. C. (1989). Standardization of international marketing strategy: Some research hypotheses. *Journal of Marketing*, *53*(1), 70–79. doi:10.2307/1251525

Josman, N., Ben-Chaim, H. M., Friedrich, S., & Weiss, P. L. (2008). Effectiveness of virtual reality for teaching street-crossing skills to children and adolescents with autism. *International Journal on Disability and Human Development*, *7*(1), 49–56. doi:10.1515/IJDHD.2008.7.1.49

Lee, S. (2018). Suzanne Lee - Professional History. *LinkedIn*. Retrieved July 10, 2018 from https://www.linkedin.com/in/suzanne-lee/

Lewis, C., & Griffin, M. (1997). Human factors consideration in clinical applications of virtual reality. *Studies in Health Technology and Informatics*, 35–58. PMID:10175342

Mairs, J. (2018). New virtual reality tool helps architects create dementia-friendly environments. *Dezeen*. Retrieved July 10, 2018 from https://www.dezeen.com/2017/02/22/virtual-reality-empathy-platform-tool-help-architects-create-dementia-friendly-environments-david-burgher-aitken-turnbull-wireframe-immersive/

McWilliam, D. (2018). *The Product. V Store*. Retrieved July 10, 2018 from http://www.vitaevr.com/the-product/

Mikropoulos, T. A., & Natsis, A. (2011). Educational virtual environments: A ten-year review of empirical research (1999–2009). *Computers & Education*, *56*(3), 769–780. doi:10.1016/j.compedu.2010.10.020

Moore, D., Cheng, Y., McGrath, P., & Powell, N. (2005). Collaborative virtual environment technology for people with autism. *Focus on Autism and Other Developmental Disabilities*, *20*(4), 231–243. doi:10.1177/10883576050200040501

Napoli, P. M. (2011). *Audience evolution: New technologies and the transformation of media audiences*. Columbia University Press.

Parsons, S., & Cobb, S. (2011). State-of-the-art of virtual reality technologies for children on the autism spectrum. *European Journal of Special Needs Education*, *26*(3), 355–366. doi:10.1080/08856257.2011.593831

Parsons, S., & Mitchell, P. (2002). The potential of virtual reality in social skills training for people with autistic spectrum disorders. *Journal of Intellectual Disability Research*, *46*(5), 430–443. doi:10.1046/j.1365-2788.2002.00425.x PMID:12031025

Schaaf, R. C., Toth-Cohen, S., Johnson, S. L., Outten, G., & Benevides, T. W. (2011). The everyday routines of families of children with autism: Examining the impact of sensory processing difficulties on the family. *Autism, 15*(3), 373–389. doi:10.1177/1362361310386505 PMID:21430016

Shrum, L. (2009). Media consumption and perceptions of social reality: Effects and underlying processes. *Media Effects*, 66-89.

Sime, D. (2018). David Sime - Professional History. *LinkedIn*. Retrieved July 10, 2018 from https://www.linkedin.com/in/davidsime/

Siriaraya, P., & Ang, C. (2014). Recreating living experiences from past memories through virtual worlds for people with dementia. In *Proceedings of the SIGCHI Conference on Human Factors in Computing Systems (CHI '14)*. ACM. 10.1145/2556288.2557035

Smith, M. J., Ginger, E. J., Wright, K., Wright, M. A., Taylor, J. L., Humm, L. B., ... Fleming, M. F. (2014). Virtual reality job interview training in adults with autism spectrum disorder. *Journal of Autism and Developmental Disorders, 44*(10), 2450–2463. doi:10.100710803-014-2113-y PMID:24803366

Tribemix. (2017). *Commercial immersive virtual reality for people with dementia*. Retrieved August 10, 2017 from http://www.tribemix.co.uk/

Walker, J., Pan, E., Johnston, D., Adler-Milstein, J., Bates, D. W., & Middleton, B. (2005). The Value of Health Care Information Exchange and Interoperability: There is a business case to be made for spending money on a fully standardized nationwide system. *Health Affairs*, 24–1.

Wallace, J., Thieme, A., Wood, G., Schofield, G., & Olivier, P. (2012). Enabling self, intimacy and a sense of home in dementia: an enquiry into design in a hospital setting. In *Proceedings of the SIGCHI Conference on Human Factors in Computing Systems (CHI '12)*. ACM. 10.1145/2207676.2208654

Zinck, S., & Zinck, S. (2018). Virtual Reality: Not for Millennials only - Age and ability. *Age and Ability*. Retrieved July 10, 2018 from https://www.ibm.com/blogs/age-and-ability/2017/08/18/virtual-reality-not-millennials/

## KEY TERMS AND DEFINITIONS

**Augmented Reality (AR):** It is a technology that uses real world environment and enhances it by overlaying digital information on top of it.

**Head-Mounted Display:** A device worn over a user's head, providing a visual display in front of one or both of the user's eyes.

**Immersive Interactive Simulation System:** It is a system that provides state-of-the-art interactive environment that blurs the line between the real and virtual world.

**Immersive Reminiscence:** A connected series of virtual environments suitable for dementia sufferers to create benefits including memory recall, calming of agitation and building of real world community and communication in care homes and residential environments.

**Mixed Reality (MR):** It merges the real and digital environments that co-exist and interact with each other to produce new environment for the user to explore and manipulate.

**Virtual Reality Exposure Therapy (VRET):** The goal of VRET is to expose the patient to stimuli by combining advanced computer graphics, 3D visual displays, and body-tracking technologies to create realistic virtual non-threatening environment so that their mind and body can learn not to become alerted when they are exposed to similar stimuli in real life.

**Virtual Reality (VR):** It provides the user with computer-generated simulation of a real-life environment or situation. The headset gives the user a fully immersive experience, where what a user sees is a generated or an artificial environment and nothing of it is in the real world. Example of VR is gaming consoles.

# Chapter 5
# Virtual Reality (VR) as Medical Prevention of Adverse Childhood Experiences (ACEs)

**Anastasia Miron**
*Child Proof Yourself, USA*

## ABSTRACT

*This chapter identifies numerous cases on adverse childhood experiences (ACEs) and their link with post-traumatic stress disorders (PTSD). It explores the use of virtual reality (VR) as a clinical tool in diagnosis, prevention and treatment of ACEs. The emotional, physical, psychological and cognitive demands of a child going through ACEs are discussed using scientific researchers. The purpose of this chapter is to introduce the beneficial uses of virtual reality (VR) in the prevention, diagnosis, and treatment of ACEs.*

## INTRODUCTION

The chapter introduces the use of VR as a clinical instrument to address the appraisal, counteractive action, and treatment of ACEs. A concise discourse of the definition and method of reasoning for clinical utilization of VR is trailed by a depiction of VR application intended for the conveyance of prolonged exposure (PE). The clinical utilization of VR is discussed, especially in regard to its ability to break down barriers.

### VR's Role in Treating ACEs

Child maltreatment is a serious and general public health concern in the United States. Studies (Zimmerman & Merci, 2010), revealed that the public child protective services agencies received in 2007 reports of alleged maltreatment involving 5.8 million children. Sixty-two percent of reports to child protective services, involving 3.5 million children, were screened for further investigation; 794,000 were determined to be victims of abuse or neglect. In 86% of these cases, parents or other relatives were responsible for the maltreatment. Neglect was the problem in 60% of the cases. Young children, under

DOI: 10.4018/978-1-5225-7168-1.ch005

7 years old, constitute the majority of child abuse/neglect cases (55.7%) and suffer the greatest harm. Infants less than 1 year old have the highest rates of child victimization at 22 victims per 1,000 children (Zimmerman & Merci, 2010). The Economic Burden of Child Maltreatment in the United States and Implications for Prevention (Fang et al., 2012), found the aggregate lifetime monetary expenses related to only one year of affirmed instances of child abuse such as sexual abuse, physical abuse, neglect and physiological abuse to be about $124 billion. VR plays an important role in treating ACEs because it has a variety of uses. A study (Slater et al., 2010) presented by researchers of the University of Barcelona showed that VR experiences may improve empathy in violent people having lack of emotional recognition. According to Slater et al. (2010), virtual bodies can be radically not quite the same and the involved individual goes under a subjective illusion of owning the virtual body. The illusions participants are subjected have a strong impact altering perceptions, behavior, and attitudes of the participants (Slater et al., 2008, 2009). The results of the research (Slater et al., 2010) revealed that bottom-up perceptual mechanisms can temporarily override top down knowledge resulting in a radical illusion of transfer of body ownership. Moreover, immersive virtual reality is a powerful tool in the study of body representation and experience (Slater et al., 2010).

## CHILD MALTREATMENT (CM): A SERIOUS HEALTH PROBLEM

Childhood experiences have a great impact on the future of a person. Researchers refer to such experiences as Adverse Childhood Experiences (ACEs) (Foege, 1998; Hardt & Rutter, 2004). ACEs Include:

- Sexual abuse
- Physical abuse
- Emotional abuse
- Physical neglect
- Emotional neglect
- Household substance abuse
- Mother treated violently
- Parental divorce and separation
- Mental household illness
- Poisoned household member

ACEs have been linked to chronic health conditions, risky health behaviors, early death and low life potential. These events can be single, acute or sustained over time. These conditions may include the detrimental effect of the community, parents' death, poverty and violence. Most children aged between 0 to 18 have one or more ACEs. Childhood stress may become toxic with time if prolonged, leading towards activation of the body's stress-response system. The biological reaction to toxic stress can drastically affect the health of a person and last a lifetime. Most common life-threatening conditions that researchers have studied include heart disease, obesity, drug use and alcoholism. A child who suffers from ACEs can have behavioral and learning issues. These effects move on through generations if these traumatic conditions are not resolved. The financial loss to society and the individual is also significant (Herman et al., 1997; Foege, 1998; Hardt & Rutter, 2004; Zimmerman & Merci, 2010). Technology that helps diagnosing the health of an individual from infancy to adulthood is now available. It allows us to have a look at the life of an individual, not as disconnected stages, but as integrated. Studies issued from distinct disciplines (e.g. Behavioral science, neuroscience, medicine, sociology) enables child healthcare professionals the chance to diagnose what care is required to maximize the child's lifelong health. Extensive research showing effects of traumatic stress on brain development are now available. Prolonged pathologic stress disrupts or impairs healthy brain development, leading to lifelong implications of health, behavior and adult functioning. The Centers for Disease Control and Prevention promote well-being and lifelong health regarding essentials for childhood, making stable, safe, nurturing relationships and environments for kids (Centers for Disease Control and Prevention, n.d.). Basic childhood experiences have a long-term impact on a wide range of developmental and health problems, and on skills that will lead children to reach their potential. In a report of the Centre for Youth Wellness, a data analysis was done on ACEs in California (Centre for Youth Wellness, n.d.). Over 60% of the population suffered from at least one of the mentioned ACEs, and 16.7% suffered from four or more experiences. The 16.7% population was more likely to suffer from different psychological diseases. There is a misconception that early life difficulties are always linked to low income communities and/or the discrimination they may face. The data collected in California shows, that this is the problem of every income level household and neighborhood (Centre for Youth Wellness, n.d.). Pediatrician Nadine Burke Harris, founder of the Center for Youth Wellness, explains that 'childhood trauma is not a thing you get over as you continue to grow up'. She further elaborated that neglect, repeated stress of abuse, parents struggling with mental health or drug abuse all have a drastic effect on brain development. Children who go through high levels of trauma in their life are 3 times more likely to have lung cancer and heart diseases. The pediatrician said: 'I was observing health outcomes of ACEs and also toxic stress every day in my clinic, after observing I realized some people are aware of them, I wanted to wake people up. ACEs are something that parents, teachers, and grandparents should know about' (Centre for Youth Wellness, n.d.; Gross, 2018). ACEs lead towards adulthood physical illnesses. The conditions of stress vary from child to child, depending on the child's sensitivity level and how he reacts to things. Some serious conditions may not affect a child, while some minor stress conditions can be greatly traumatic. Toxic stress responses occur when a child feels frequent, strong and long-term stress in the form of emotional and physical abuse, chronic neglect, caregiver abuse or mental illness, violence exposure situations, or burden related to the family's poor economic situation, and an absence of a parent or adult support (Centre for Youth Wellness, n.d.; Gross, 2018; Baglivio et al., 2014; Foege, 1998). According to The National Child Traumatic Stress Network (NCTSN, n.d.), traumatic stress is defined as - the emotional and physical responses of a child to actions that threaten the life or physical reliability of the child or of someone most important to the child (e.g., parent, sibling). It is this uncontrolled physiological stimulation that is the cause of stress that becomes traumatic and can provoke what is initially an adaptive response to the stressor that ultimately becomes destructive and maladapted (National Child Traumatic Stress Network, n.d.). While an occurrence of a natural disaster or physical attack by a stranger may cause toxic stress, the effects increase and get worse when the trauma continues, whether by repetition of (e.g., Domestic violence or parental drug abuse) or gathering of disparate ones (e.g., Hurricane, parental illness) (National Child Traumatic Stress Network, n.d.). The effect of toxic stress resulting from trauma may not be soon visible or appear as expected. In addition, some traumatic sources of toxic stress may not be apparent to the physician. Psychological mismanaged treatment can be stressful and traumatic as well (National Child Traumatic Stress Network, n.d.; Gross, 2018; Baglivio et al., 2014; Foege, 1998). Children who are neglected in certain ways can also be traumatized. Neglect is always in a chronic state and can include basic life needs such as shelter, food, or emotional security (Herman et al., 1997; Foege, 1998; Hardt & Rutter, 2004).

Current advancements in research have given amazing opportunities to understand how healthy brain development is done. The human body is designed in such a way that it is influenced by behavioral, social, genetic and even neuroendocrine factors. The brain continues to develop under these influences and the capability of an individual to recover from trauma relies on these factors. Environmental cues guide the structural development of the brain. A newborn brain is capable of adapting what it hears, sees and feels. Researchers have shown critical periods for good development of the brain's systems. Proper brain development requires a stimulating and loving environment (Herman et al., 1997; Foege, 1998; Hardt & Rutter, 2004; Butler et al., 2006; Baglivio et al., 2014). Interaction with other people also helps in development of the brain. Children may not be able to interact with people due to their age limiting factors, but they learn from their surroundings. People, especially caregivers and educators must give the child a positive learning environment (National Child Traumatic Stress Network, n.d.; Foege, 1998; Butler et al., 2006).

## Why Is the Prevention of ACEs Important?

Child abuse is a genuine and predominant public health issue in the United States. In 2008, Child Protective Specialists (CPS) received over 3 million reports of youngsters being abused or facing an adverse condition. An expected 772,000 kids were characterized by CPS specialists as being abused and 1,740 children aged between 0 to 17 died from such instances. The evaluated normal lifetime cost of a child facing abuse was $210,012 in 2010, incorporating $32,648 in youth medicinal services costs; $10,530 in grown-up therapeutic expenses; $144,360 in efficiency misfortunes; $7,728 in child welfare costs; $6,747 in criminal equity costs; and $7,999 in specialized curriculum costs (Fang et al., 2012).

## Studies About VR as a Behavioral Change Tool

There's a growing body of research on how VR can be utilized to develop empathy (Benyoucef et al., 2017; Freeman & Freeman, 2017; Rizzo et al., 2010). The United Nations is applying VR experiences to enable watchers to feel for Syrian displaced people, or a family in Gaza, dividers burned and stippled by gunfire and bombs (United Nations Virtual Reality, n.d.). Different tasks from the University of Southern California's Institute for Creative Technologies embed clients in a sensible battle reenactment to enable them to better comprehend the encounters of friends and family members who are experiencing Post-Traumatic Stress Disorder (PTSD) subsequent to serving in the military. VR is also utilized as a part of police training, to recreate situations that require split-second basic decision making (Rizzo et al., 2010; Rizzo & Kim, 2005). A new project, directed by scientists from the University of Georgia, Stanford and the University of Connecticut, intended to see whether VR could enable users to sympathize with animal experiences. In the first trial, the associates requested that participants embark on a cow's journey to the slaughterhouse. The second trial reproduced the vibe of coral kicking the bucket in an acidifying sea. To make the experience immersive, members felt vibrations in the floor and heard splitting sounds as the coral's branches broke off. The scientist found that the VR members felt for the situations in excess of a controlling bunch viewing a comparative experience on video only (Ahn et al., 2016). It has been proposed that VR experiences may help fill up the gap between intention and action by enabling members to react in a way that is more authentic. The proliferation of accessible VR tools has seen expanded use in test psychological research settings in the course of the most recent years. VR has developed as an interesting tool to help in various distinctive issues, especially to treat patients with mental disorders. One in five individuals in the U.S. have a diagnosable mental disorder, even individuals who don't experience much stress and anxiety (Senson, 2016). Mental conditions and psychological wellness influences people's lives and costs an expected $467 billion to the U.S. in medical expenses. For some disorders, there are very effective treatments that don't require drugs. However, many specialists still tend to over-endorse prescriptions that have irritating reactions or are totally superfluous. Some part of the issue is an absence of emotional well-being, joined with the trouble to discover and get to qualified mental health professionals. While serious disorders may, in any case, require cognitive behavioral treatment (CBT) and exposure therapy (ET) (Senson, 2016; Rizzo et al., 2010; Rizzo & Kim, 2005). VR has been utilized for quite a long time as a tool for the therapists to oversee virtual reality exposure treatment (VRET) in a controlled way. Because of cost and innovation limitations, it has not been generally accessible. A challenge today is the absence of clinical proof and information to help if and how VR can be utilized to control successful treatment both in the clinic and remotely. Organizations wishing to infiltrate this market should lead all around outlined, randomized, controlled, legitimately clinical examinations keeping in mind the end goal to change or influence treatment standards.

## Cognitive Behavioral Therapy (CBT) and Exposure Therapy (ET)

CBT is a psychotherapeutic treatment directed by a professional of mental wellness. Patients normally go to a predetermined number of sessions that emphasize on a particular issue, helping the patient distinguish, perceive and change irritating emotions that are prompting negative or dangerous convictions and practices. CBT can be used to overcome mental restrictions. CBT and ET are not separable. After some sessions, this therapy adequately brings down the peak of anxiety the individual encounters when he/she is presented with whatever causes the anxiety (Senson, 2016). In addition to this, there are numerous other mental conditions, for example, childhood developmental disorders and extreme autism, where VR assume a crucial role (Benyoucef et al., 2017; Bellani et al., 2011).

## VR Used for Prolonged Exposure Therapy (PET)

VR has been utilized extensively to convey prolonged exposure therapy (PET) for PTSD since the 1990s, for the most part for the treatment of warriors and war veterans (Senson, 2016). A recently published study (Senson, 2016; Rizzo et al., 2010; Rizzo & Kim, 2005) found that the VR treatment alone was a combination of medication treatment and VR treatment. Military funding has enabled thorough studies to be conducted. Be that as it may, less privately-owned businesses creating VR treatment applications with restricted spending plans should even now show clinical adequacy in the event that they want to enter this market. Beyond Care (Senson, 2016), for instance, is working on a VR programming solution for PTSD utilizing Eye Movement Desensitization and Reprocessing (EMDR). EMDR works by having a patient review a horrible memory while following a moving object with their eyes. The dual task of memory review in addition to eye development affects the working memory, making the horrible memory turn out to be less clear and distinctive. After sufficient repetition, the memory forever loses its capacity to trigger such extraordinary emotional reactions. After an effective review of the pilot, Beyond Care is currently working with the Dutch University to organize a patient trial to offer specific mental treatment over the Internet. The outcome of this investigation will decide whether the new VR desensitization and reprocessing treatment, called Beyond Care PTSD works and whether it can be effectively practiced under the semi-supervision of a therapist. Military PTSD isn't the main kind of PTSD. There are around 7.7

million individuals in the U.S. with PTSD, most of them have endured assault or sexual abuse in their past. It is likely that a significant number of these cases go unreported and untreated (Senson, 2016).

## VR for Phobias, Anxiety Disorders and Stress Relief

VR has for a long time been utilized for the treatment of anxiety disorders, phobias and stress relief (Rus-Calafell et al., 2018; Senson, 2016). Anxiety disorders influence more than 40 million individuals in the U.S. Due to the tremendous number of patients distressed by some type of tension issue, decentralization of treatment through telemedicine or independently directed treatment could have a significant effect (Senson, 2016). Particular fears influence around 19 million people in the U.S. A recently published meta-examination of 14 clinical trials demonstrated that VRET was comparatively successful in regard to particular phobias as a genuine presentation therapy (Senson, 2016). The Virtual Reality Medical Center has a system for treating those with a fear of flying. It incorporates programming and equipment, complete with plane seats and a subwoofer system to imitate the sights, sounds, and feelings of flying. An organization from Sweden called Immerse is creating gasified psychological treatment apparatuses for VR for the mass market in association with the Swedish Government and Stockholm University. Their first VR application, 'Tiny' is centered on treating arachnophobia without supervision of a live therapist. Along with the VR application's release on the Gear VR application store, a randomized controlled investigation is being led comparing VRET with genuine presentation treatment (Senson, 2016). Regardless of whether a man experiences a particular diagnosable mental health condition or not, most people experience fluctuating levels of stress, pressure and nervousness. Reflection and meditation have long been known to be useful methods for relaxation and unwinding. As an example, Pious and Virtual Ret VR offer VR based solutions for relaxation. DEEP is another VR application where the user explores an immersive submerged world generated by biofeedback. DEEP uses guided breathing techniques to navigate the VR environment, and with the custom DEEP controller, the user's breathing harmonizes with what is found in the virtual world and controls how the user travels through it (Senson, 2016).

## VR as a Teaching Tool

Over the last couple of years, VR has moved from being mostly used in the military and aviation industry to mainstream professional development of managers, instructors, coaches as well as therapists who have claimed increasing benefits. Many researchers (Oigara, 2018; Wu et al., 2013; Winn, 1993) have investigated the viability of virtual environments (VEs), digital simulations that involve representations of teachers, students, and/or content for learning applications. VEs enable transformed social interaction (TSI), the ability of teachers and students to use digital technology to strategically alter their online representations and contexts in order to improve learning (Bailenson et al., 2004). A series of empirical studies demonstrate how breaking social physics of traditional learning environments can increase learning in VEs. Of course, immersive VR currently is not yet an easily acquired technology in classroom settings. Nevertheless, VEs are becoming more common place, and it is important to understand how this digital technology will aid the basic learning process. Application of VR in training and education seems to give excellent promise in providing an alternative and virtual environment in situations where it is impossible for students to experience in person (Oigara, 2018; Wu et al., 2013; Winn, 1993).

## VR as Prevention

Social scientists have long pointed out that a human being's social environment has a profound and sustained impact on his emotional and physical health. Neuroscientists have extended this work to propose that the brain is responsible for regulating behavioral, autonomic, and immune responses to the social environment, particularly for perceptions of relative safety and threat. The National Institute of Mental Health (NIMH, n.d.) suggested that there may be discrete brain circuits associated with both acute and chronic stressors. The brain's response to threats can vary greatly by an individual's developmental status and beliefs about the causes of the threat and ability to survive or overcome them. When threats are interpreted as significantly life-threatening or negatively life-changing, we often refer to them as traumatic and become concerned about their short and long-term impact on health (National Institute of Mental Health, n.d.). The National Child Traumatic Stress Network (NCTSN) separates serious threats into two main categories: acute and chronic. Acute traumatic events include witnessing violence, facing imminent threats of injury, or experiencing violation of personal physical integrity (e.g., School shootings, sudden or violent loss of a loved one, sexual assault etc.). Chronic traumatic situations occur repeatedly over long periods of time (e.g., Living with abusive parents or in poverty etc.). Using these and similar definitions, general population studies have found that more than two-thirds of children and adolescents report past or present exposure to at least one form of trauma (National Child Traumatic Stress Network, n.d.). Response to stressors is highly variable and can be immediate or delayed. Predictors include both personal characteristics such as temperament and environmental characteristics such as social support. There is evidence supporting that specific psychological interventions can help prevent or ameliorate the development of long-term consequences including PTSD, which is associated with a myriad of mental and physical problems in adults (National Child Traumatic Stress Network, n.d.). The American Academy of Pediatrics (AAP, n.d.) advocates that pediatricians do more to address trauma, not only because of the developmental and behavioral support offered by primary care providers (PCPs), but also because of their ability to identify and treat early physiologic markers that may be associated with adverse physiologic responses (e.g., Abnormal weight, blood pressure, glucose and lipid metabolism) (American Academy of Pediatrics, n.d.). By building longitudinal and broadly-based relationships with families, PCPs can become part of an ongoing support system and serve as a point of entry and coordination for additional services. Primary care practices have long made referrals for emotional and behavioral problems, but it is only recently that PCPs have begun to consider the extent to which they can help identify and address trauma-related physical and psychological problems (American Academy of Pediatrics, n.d.). Given that the 2010 Patient Protection and Affordable Care Act requires coverage of screening for depression and that Medicaid's Early and Periodic Screening, Diagnosis, and Testing requires children to be screened for mental health problems, the use of screening interventions within the pediatric medical home is likely to increase over time (Patient Protection and Affordable Care Act, 2010). The challenge lies in determining which interventions are feasible, sustainable, and effective for use in the pediatric primary care setting. Pediatric providers face a number of challenges in providing mental health services such as limited training on how to address the psychosocial concerns of their patients. The goal of this systematic review was to examine the existing evidence base on preventing and addressing traumatic stress exposure in pediatric primary care to better understand what is effective in this setting. Specifically, it is aimed to identify the types of interventions that have been implemented and assess their impact on a variety of outcomes including provider behavior and, where studied, clinical outcomes (Patient Protection and Affordable Care Act, 2010). There is a growing interest in integrating the prevention and management of trauma-related problems into pediatric primary care visits, yet very little is known about effective approaches to address trauma in this setting. According to an American Academy of Pediatrics policy statement 'the reduction of toxic stress in young children ought to be a high priority for medicine as a whole and for pediatrics in particular' (American Academy of Pediatrics, n.d.). Studies concluded that the interventions studied had a positive impact on their intended outcomes. The findings suggest that training/education and screening interventions in primary care settings can enhance a range of provider skills and increase provider knowledge and perceived competence (American Academy of Pediatrics, n.d.). Reductions in adverse child outcomes such as child physical abuse and maltreatment (as assessed by Parent's Guide to Child Protective Services Report, n.d.), domestic violence exposure, delinquent behavior, aggression, and injury were achieved by a majority of the interventions that measured these outcomes (Parent's Guide to Child Protective Services Report, n.d.). The current evidence suggests that primary care may be well suited to implementing interventions related to prevention, detection, and early intervention of trauma-related problems. The review highlights the impact and effectiveness of primary care-based trauma interventions. Issues of cost-effectiveness and sustainability of the interventions reviewed remain to be studied in depth (Parent's Guide to Child Protective Services Report, n.d.). Samsung Electronics introduced mental health diagnosis programs that utilize portable VR headsets (Swaney, 2018). The tech industry consented to a collaboration agreement with Gangnam Severance Hospital and VR content creator FNI for the projects, with the objective to popularize them in 2018 in dementia focused clinics, and schools, before being extending to homes at a later date. The three firms will utilize Samsung's Gear VR headset, FNI's VR substance improvement innovation, and the clinic's medicinal information to make the projects. Organizations around the globe are progressively utilizing VR for healthcare services (Swaney, 2018). In 2016 Build VR revealed their Solis VR unit for Australian care homes. Their Gear VR handset highlights audio-visual simulations that attempt to trigger positive feelings for dementia patients (Singletary, 2016). There are many other VR apps that are focusing on end of life positive experiences, but not that many that focus on preventing a bad experience from happening. The United States has made noteworthy progress in reducing the devastating effects of ACEs. This has in turn resulted in millions of dollars in investments to the state budget. The US has seen a significant decline in high school dropout rates, teenage pregnancy, youth and teenage suicide, and in community ACEs scores over the past 10 years. This is just one example of how important it is to allocate resources for the prevention of ACEs (Herman et al., 1997; Foege, 1998; Hardt & Rutter, 2004; Zimmerman & Merci, 2010).

## VR as a Training Tool for Parents to Prevent ACEs

There is a lot of research that indicates how a person is going to perform as a parent - by making sense of his/her own past. However, one's childhood may be the last place a person might look into when he/she becomes a parent (Foege, 1998; Anda et al., 2002; Hardt & Rutter, 2004). Although most of what has happened during childhood is going to show up in the parenting style, this does not mean same parenthood style will always be simulated, but often it does happen. In fact, no matter how much distress or trauma is endured during the early years, what actually matters most is one's ability to reflect and understand the pain from one's childhood to create a coherent narrative of personal experiences. It ultimately brings in the realization that the 'instinctive' reactions are not always representative of the desired parenting style. Only after accepting this fact it is possible to begin to understand why children trigger us in the manner they do (Anda et al., 2002; Hardt & Rutter, 2004; Baviglio et al., 2014). The following are ways in which past ACEs can affect how future behavior unfolds:

- **Imitating:** During parenthood, parents often repeat the maladaptive treatments of 'their' parents. One of the most extreme examples of this is physical punishment. Numerous parents justify physically abusing their children by simply stating that: 'This is how I was disciplined!'
- **Overreacting:** Instead of deciding on the various qualities that matter to the parent, the parent is actually only reacting to the things that happened to them in the past.
- **Recreating:** A parent might internalize 'their' parents' point of views and generate a family environment similar to the one the parent lived in, exposing the children to the negative atmosphere of 'their' own childhood.
- **Projecting:** Attempt to overcompensate for parents' mistakes by projecting 'ourselves' or the feelings 'we' felt onto our children.

It can be a vicious cycle, but it doesn't have to be. Parents who have experienced ACEs are more likely to recreate environments where ACEs can occur for the next generations. These intergenerational ACEs include depression, suicide, alcohol and drug abuse, substance abuse, and relationship problems. While many parents do not repeat the violence they experienced or were exposed to as children, the mental health consequences and unhealthy coping behaviors associated with childhood victimization can compromise the parenting skills (Anda et al., 2002; Hardt & Rutter, 2004; Felitti & Anda, 2010; Baviglio et al., 2014). By introducing VR in this parenthood formula and by using VR as a teaching tool, it is possible to create what is long asked for throughout history, an operating manual for how to be a connected parent- a how to guide for the everyday experiences of the hard yet rewarding challenges of preventing ACEs and raising an authentic child. Through simulating experience like a toddler throwing a tantrum, talking to a 12 year old about sex or effectively disciplining a teenager, VR is able to wire paths in the brain that creates deep empathy and understanding, connecting the user deeper to the child and in turn providing the user with strategies to more effectively and consciously handle 'yours' and 'their' needs and emotions (Rus-Calafell et al., 2018; Oigara, 2018; Freeman & Freeman, 2017; Slater et al., 2010; Rizzo & Kim, 2005). It would move the experience from the drama and trauma of disconnection to the ease and stability of awareness and connection. By creating mobile VR apps, that are easily accessible and highly customizable by immediate feedback, the parent is empowered to learn new paths much faster and implement them more effectively. Teaching parents and actually showing in VR how children react to emotional and psychological trauma is helpful and long lasting (Rus-Calafell et al., 2018; Oigara, 2018; Freeman & Freeman, 2017; Slater et al., 2010; Rizzo & Kim, 2005). By showcasing some normal responses to injury and approaches to enable the child to manage them we empower the parents with the following knowledge to recognize three early symptoms of trauma:

- **Relapse:** Numerous children need to come back to a prior perception of self when they felt more secure. Younger children may return to bed wetting or needing a pacifier or bottle; more children may fear to be alone. It's imperative to comprehend and console your child if he/she reacts this way.

- **Thinking the Occasion Is Their Fault:** Children younger than 8 tend to think that if something turns out badly, it is their fault. Parents should assure their child they are not at fault.
- **Rest Issue:** Some children experience issues trouble falling and staying asleep.

## VR as a Training Tool for Children to Prevent ACEs as a Part of Self-Care

VR can be used as detection tool to enable children to identify ACEs and then learn how to act in their own interest in order to stop the process of stress, abuse and discomfort and undertake beneficial steps towards healing (Rus-Calafell et al., 2018; Freeman & Freeman, 2017). A mobile VR app can be used by the teenagers/children in a homelike, de-institutionalized environment supportive of patient autonomy and control over a personal environment with noise control, privacy, and personal safety/security. Intimacy is not typically a term utilized when describing healthcare settings. However, an individual's health and well-being are extremely personal. When the VR app design is approached from an intimate level—looking at each personal human interaction using the biofeedback, the stress level is lower and the delivered information is best assimilated. Results suggest that design features in which patients have choice and control offer greater perceptions of calm during the immersive VR experience and after the use of it (Rus-Calafell et al., 2018; Oigara, 2018; Freeman & Freeman, 2017; Slater et al., 2010; Rizzo & Kim, 2005).

## Teaching About Emotional Symptoms of Trauma

Emotional Trauma is characterized by the American Psychological Association (APA) as the emotional response when someone is subjected to a negative event. While it is an ordinary response to an appalling occasion, the impacts can be severe to the point that they interfere with a person's ability to carry on with normal, everyday life (American Psychological Association, n.d.). Emotion is the most common way by which trauma is felt. Some basic emotional side effects of trauma incorporate disavowal, outrage, trouble, and outburst. A victim of trauma may divert the mind-boggling feelings that are encountered toward different sources, for example, friends or relatives. This is one reason why trauma is also a problem for friends and family (American Psychological Association, n.d.; Glasers, 2002). It is difficult to help someone who does not welcome it, however, understanding the passionate side effects that come after a traumatic event can help facilitate the process.

## Teaching About Physical Symptoms of Trauma

Trauma frequently shows physically and not just emotionally. Some normal physical indications of trauma are fatigue, lethargy, poor focus and racing heartbeat. The victim may have uneasiness or fits of anxiety and be not able to adapt to specific conditions. The physical side effects of a psychological injury can be as genuine and disturbing as those of physical illness or sickness, and care must be taken to overcome stress levels after a traumatic event (American Psychological Association, n.d.; Glasers, 2002). Teaching through VR how to recognize the first signs of ACEs, such as disbelieve, denial and shock will help children recognize they are experiencing an ACE. Once initial signs die down, the individual may appear distant when requested to talk about the ACE or attempt to avoid the topic. This disengagement is a technique for adapting to the trauma and a sign that the individual needs assistance.

## Explaining Aggression and Empowering Self-Diagnosis in VR

Individuals who have endured physiological trauma will often experience aggression. Sometimes, it might be express outrage or blame towards themselves or others. The Reconnect Integrative Trauma Treatment Center (2018) says it's 'vital to perceive that this individual isn't to be faulted, as their upheavals are frequently a cry for help'. VR helps explain and visualize how sleep plays a fundamental role in mental well-being and highlights that after encountering a traumatic event, a person may encounter disturbances in their sleeping patterns. These can include occasional insomnia, bad dreams, or night terrors. Chronic sleep issues reduces one's ability to concentrate and leaves one feeling continually tired and exhausted (Freeman & Freeman, 2017; Rus-Calafell et al., 2018; Wiederhold & Wiederhold, 2005; Rizzo & Kim, 2005). Using VR to simulate the relationship between physiological trauma and anxiety helps individuals to recognize the link between anxiety and the causing trauma. VR can also be used in explaining and making the concept of dissociation clear and unthreatening and stating that dissociation is another basic indication of psychological trauma. These changes in the cerebrum can cause memory loss, and also separation or withdrawal from others. Such social isolation can add to the sentiments of sadness, depression, and hopelessness. Through VR it is possible to draw attention to the many signs of psychological trauma (emotional or behavioral). Humans react in different ways to trauma, experiencing a wide range of emotional and physical reactions (Freeman & Freeman, 2017; Rus-Calafell et al., 2018; Wiederhold & Wiederhold, 2005; Rizzo & Kim, 2005). In Summary, VR can be used to simulate the following emotional, psychological and physical symptoms:

- Disbelief, denial or shock
- Difficulty concentrating, confusion
- Mood swings, irritability, anger
- Fear and anxiety
- Self-blame, guilt, and shame
- Withdrawing from others
- Feeling hopeless or sad
- Feeling numb or disconnected
- Insomnia or nightmares
- Aches and pains
- Fatigue
- Being startled easily
- Difficulty concentrating
- Racing heartbeat
- Edginess and agitation
- Muscle tension

Based on the biofeedback of a patient, a healthcare provider can assess whether to recommend a VR or not VR experience as a treatment. Considering well known facts such as working out, staying social and not isolating, visualizing how to self-regulate the nervous system, can mitigated the tension. By staying physically active and bringing to rescue the sensory input the irritation is reduced and helps to cope with the trauma in a less stressful way. Some small tips as murmuring a favorite song, smelling a calming aroma, touching some silky or soft materials can go along way (Freeman & Freeman, 2017;

Rus-Calafell et al., 2018; Wiederhold & Wiederhold, 2005; Rizzo & Kim, 2005). For children, ACE evaluations might arise in the setting of child care visits or other health care encounters like hospitalizations. For children, such experiences can also include an evaluation of current (vs historic/past) experiences. This raises vital questions as to the procedure for doing so in a manner that ensures trust with the parents and family. As suggested in procedures related with several ACE tools, evaluation of ACEs might be effective in a larger setting where health elevation discussions proactively encourage constructive health and resilience for families and children. Such settings might also involve simultaneous evaluation of:

1. Resilience
2. Biological indicators of stress or trauma
3. Mental and physical functioning and symptoms
4. Protective factors like family connection
5. Positive functioning and well-being

By combining VR with prevention techniques, the effects of childhood trauma can be mitigated by offering him/her educational courses, self-management lectures, and other critical teachings which reduce the feeling of actually being in the scenario. Within any given context or purpose for measurement, identifying a standardized method to assess ACEs is important to accurately evaluate the effect of ACEs on children's outcomes as well as to understand how ACE assessments might inform or improve a child's well-being. Also essential is establishing the feasibility, validity, and specific implementation approach for ACE assessment methods. Considering the known data about the short and long-term negative effects of ACEs and VR's powerful effects on human brains, there is enough evidence to say that a VR application can be an efficient tool for self-diagnosis and prevention of traumas (Freeman & Freeman, 2017; Rus-Calafell et al., 2018; Wiederhold & Wiederhold, 2005; Rizzo & Kim, 2005).

## VR Displays for Children

ACEs are associated with children who are in the early years of their childhood. Researchers suggest that VR is not suitable to be use by children under the age of 12. Most VR viewers manufacturers say their VR displays are not suitable for children under age 12 or 13 (Mukamal, 2017). Although there are no long-term studies, and ophthalmologists agree there is no reason to be concerned that VR headsets will damage eye development. In fact, age limitations for VR technology is for the content accessible online without adult supervision. Moreover, any digital device used for a protracted period may cause eye fatigue (Mukamal, 2017). However, the problem also lies in the fact that the age limits are set by the VR headset manufacturers. The Oculus Rift and Samsung Gear VR headset have an age limit of 13+. Sony PlayStation VR cannot be used by children younger than 12 years of age. However, HTC has not specified an age limit and does not warn children against the use of Vive. There is not enough evidence to conclude whether VR is safe for children or not. VR's safety varies from device to device, time spent on using it as well as the child using it. Ethical regulations should be planned to enhance the benefits and minimize the potential harm of VR technology (Darvasi, 2016).

## USING VR AS A TRAINING TOOL FOR PARENTS TO PREVENT ACEs

Parents should be interested in reprogramming the status quo of parenting. VR technology is a promising tool for education and for children's cognitive and emotional development, but parents have some concerns about potential side effects (Common Sense Report Highlights Potential Impact of Virtual Reality on Children's Development, 2018). By using VR techniques, parents are able to learn how to emotionally, neurologically and bio-chemically fulfill the needs of their children and their own. Prevention of trauma early on leads to the well-being of the parent and child. Using VR as a detection tool to enable children to identify ACEs and act in their own interest in order to stop the process of stress, abuse and discomfort and undertake beneficial steps towards healing.

## THE FUTURE OF VR USE FOR ACEs

VR can be exceptionally successful in treating ACEs. VR appears to offer an approach to help close the gap between humans' conduct and the more extensive outcomes. There should be proper training systems for physicians and awareness programs for parents to know what conditions children are going through and what will be the long-term effects (Freeman & Freeman, 2017; Rus-Calafell et al., 2018; Wiederhold & Wiederhold, 2005; Rizzo & Kim, 2005).

## CONCLUSION

VR outcomes are promising and it appears that it can be used in treating PTSD in people who have had ACEs. Preventive medicine for mental health care is being underestimated and not enough public funds are being dedicated to it, meanwhile the private sector is running trials and studies by using cutting edge technologies such as VR and machine learning. One of the most important pillars for mental health is to feel understood, included and accepted. It can be achieved through empathic communication. VR as preventive and prescriptive medicine for ACEs aims to equip the parents with the tools they need to prevent the pain of exclusion or traumas. VR does this by helping the parent empathize with the child's experience. For the child, VR can be used to train themselves how to identify and self-diagnose ACEs and take corrective actions. Used in this capacity, VR can be seen as a sort of empathy machine. Parents have the power to teach their kids almost anything; love, hate, respect, creativity, resilience and much more. Today's adults have the moral responsibility to teach the future generation how to stay prepared for the unknown that lies in front of them (Freeman & Freeman, 2017; Rus-Calafell et al., 2018; Wiederhold & Wiederhold, 2005; Rizzo & Kim, 2005). The children of tomorrow have to be empowered for a more self-sovereign life and self-diagnose and identifying ACEs is one way of preparing themselves for a better future. VR may soon become one of the most widely prescribed treatments for people who are suffering from phobias, PTSD, anxiety and ACEs. Hopefully prevention through VR will be taken more seriously and become a bigger share of the mental health space.

## REFERENCES

Ahn, S. J., Bostick, J., Ogle, E., Nowak, K. L., McGillicuddy, K. T., & Bailenson, J. N. (2016). Experiencing nature: Embodying animals in immersive virtual environments increases inclusion of nature in self and involvement with nature. *Journal of Computer-Mediated Communication*, *21*(6), 399–419. doi:10.1111/jcc4.12173

American Academy of Pediatrics (AAP). (n.d.). Retrieved from https://www.aap.org/

American Psychological Association (APA). (n.d.). Retrieved from http://www.apa.org/

Anda, R. F., Whitfield, C. L., Felitti, V. J., Chapman, D., Edwards, V. J., Dube, S. R., & Williamson, D. F. (2002). Adverse childhood experiences, alcoholic parents, and later risk of alcoholism and depression. *Psychiatric Services (Washington, D.C.)*, *53*(8), 1001–1009. doi:10.1176/appi.ps.53.8.1001 PMID:12161676

Baglivio, M. T., Epps, N., Swartz, K., Huq, M. S., Sheer, A., & Hardt, N. S. (2014). The prevalence of adverse childhood experiences (ACE) in the lives of juvenile offenders. *Journal of Juvenile Justice*, *3*(2), 1.

Bailenson, J. N., Beall, A. C., Loomis, J., Blascovich, J., & Turk, M. (2004). Transformed social interaction: Decoupling representation from behavior and form in collaborative virtual environments. *Presence (Cambridge, Mass.)*, *13*(4), 428–441. doi:10.1162/1054746041944803

Bellani, M., Fornasari, L., Chittaro, L., & Brambilla, P. (2011). Virtual reality in autism: State of the art. *Epidemiology and Psychiatric Sciences*, *20*(3), 235–238. doi:10.1017/S2045796011000448 PMID:21922965

Benyoucef, Y., Lesport, P., & Chassagneux, A. (2017). The emergent role of virtual reality in the treatment of neuropsychiatric disease. *NCBI*. Retrieved May 10, 2018 from https://www.ncbi.nlm.nih.gov/pmc/articles/PMC5591848/

Butler, A. C., Chapman, J. E., Forman, E. M., & Beck, A. T. (2006). The empirical status of cognitive-behavioral therapy: A review of meta-analyses. *Clinical Psychology Review*, *26*(1), 17–31. doi:10.1016/j.cpr.2005.07.003 PMID:16199119

Centers for Disease Control and Prevention. (n.d.). Adverse Childhood Experiences (ACE's). Retrieved from https://www.cdc.gov/violenceprevention/acestudy/index.html

Centre for Youth Wellness. (n.d.). Children can thrive: Report. Retrieved July 18, 2018 from https://centerforyouthwellness.org/wp-content/themes/cyw/build/img/building-a-movement/children-can-thrive.pdf

Common Sense Report Highlights Potential Impact of Virtual Reality on Children's Development, (2018). Common Sense Media. Retrieved from https://www.commonsensemedia.org/about-us/news/press-releases/common-sense-report-highlights-potential-impact-of-virtual-reality-on

Darvasi, P. (2016). Five ethical considerations for using virtual reality with children and adolescents. *KQED*. Retrieved July 3, 2018 from https://www.kqed.org/mindshift/46103/five-ethical-considerations-for-using-virtual-reality-with-children-and-adolescents

Fang, X., Brown, D. S., Florence, C. S., & Mercy, J. A. (2012). The economic burden of child maltreatment in the United States and implications for prevention. *Child Abuse & Neglect*, *36*(2), 156–165. doi:10.1016/j.chiabu.2011.10.006 PMID:22300910

Felitti, V. J., & Anda, R. F. (2010). The relationship of adverse childhood experiences to adult medical disease, psychiatric disorders, and sexual behavior: Implications for healthcare. In The impact of early life trauma on health and disease: The hidden epidemic (pp. 77-87).

Foege, W. H. (1998). Adverse childhood experiences. A public health perspective. *American Journal of Preventive Medicine*, *14*(4), 354–355. PMID:9635083

Freeman, D., & Freeman, J. (2017). Why virtual reality could be a mental health gamechanger. *The Guardian*. Retrieved July 10, 2018 from https://www.theguardian.com/science/blog/2017/mar/22/all. AnesthAnalg

Glaser, D. (2002). Emotional abuse and neglect (psychological maltreatment): A conceptual framework. *Child Abuse & Neglect*, *26*(6-7), 697–714. doi:10.1016/S0145-2134(02)00342-3 PMID:12201163

Gross, A. (2018). Pediatrician Nadine Burke Harris explains how childhood trauma can have lasting health impacts. *KNKX*. Retrieved July 18, 2018 from http://knkx.org/post/pediatrician-nadine-burke-harris-explains-how-childhood-trauma-can-have-lasting-health-impacts

Hardt, J., & Rutter, M. (2004). Validity of adult retrospective reports of adverse childhood experiences: Review of the evidence. *Journal of Child Psychology and Psychiatry, and Allied Disciplines*, *45*(2), 260–273. doi:10.1111/j.1469-7610.2004.00218.x PMID:14982240

Herman, D. B., Susser, E. S., Struening, E. L., & Link, B. L. (1997). Adverse childhood experiences: Are they risk factors for adult homelessness? *American Journal of Public Health*, *87*(2), 249–255. doi:10.2105/AJPH.87.2.249 PMID:9103105

Mukamal, R. (2017). Are virtual reality headsets safe for eyes? Retrieved July 10, 2018 from https://www.aao.org/eye-health/tips-prevention/are-virtual-reality-headsets-safe-eyes

National Child Traumatic Stress Network (NCTSN). (n.d.) Retrieved from https://www.nctsn.org/

National Institute of Mental Health (NIMH). (n.d.) Retrieved from https://www.nimh.nih.gov/

Oigara, J. N. (2018). Integrating virtual reality tools into classroom instruction. In J. Keengwe (Ed.), *Handbook of Research on Mobile Technology, Constructivism, and Meaningful Learning* (pp. 147–159). Hershey, PA: IGI Global. doi:10.4018/978-1-5225-3949-0.ch008

Parent's Guide to Child Protective Services. (n.d.) Retrieved from https://www.dshs.wa.gov/sites/default/files/SESA/publications/documents/22-484.pdf

Patient Protection and Affordable Care Act. (2010). Retrieved from https://www.healthcare.gov/glossary/patient-protection-and-affordable-care-act/

Reconnect Integrative Trauma Treatment Center. (2018). Retrieved from http://www.reconnectcenter.com/

Rizzo, A., & Kim, J. G. (2005). A SWOT analysis of the field of virtual reality rehabilitation and therapy. *Presence (Cambridge, Mass.)*, *14*(2), 119–146.

Rizzo, A. S., Difede, J., Rothbaum, B. O., Reger, G., Spitalnick, J., Cukor, J., & McLay, R. (2010). Development and early evaluation of the Virtual Iraq/Afghanistan exposure therapy system for combat-related PTSD. *Annals of the New York Academy of Sciences*, *1208*(1), 114–125. doi:10.1111/j.1749-6632.2010.05755.x PMID:20955333

Rus-Calafell, M., Garety, P., Sason, E., Craig, T. J. K., & Valmaggia, L. R. (2018). Virtual reality in the assessment and treatment of psychosis: A systematic review of its utility, acceptability and effectiveness. *Psychological Medicine*, *48*(3), 362–391. doi:10.1017/S0033291717001945 PMID:28735593

Senson, A. (2016). Virtual reality therapy: Treating the global mental health crisis. *Tech Crunch*. Retrieved January 10, 2018 from https://techcrunch.com/2016/01/06/virtual-reality-therapy-treating-the-global-mental-health-crisis/

Singletary, C. (2016). Solis VR takes elderly patients to places long thought out of reach. Retrieved July 10, 2018 from https://uploadvr.com/patients-solis-vr-edlerly/

Slater, M., Perez-Marcos, D., Ehrsson, H. H., & Sanchez-Vives, M. (2008). Towards a digital body: The virtual arm illusion. *Frontiers in Human Neuroscience*, *2*(8). PMID:18958207

Slater, M., Perez-Marcos, D., Ehrsson, H. H., & Sanchez-Vives, M. V. (2009). Inducing illusory ownership of a virtual body. *Frontiers in Neuroscience*, *3*(2), 214–220. doi:10.3389/neuro.01.029.2009 PMID:20011144

Slater, M., Spanlang, B., Sanchez-Vives, M. V., & Blanke, O. (2010). First person experience of body transfer in virtual reality. *PLoS One*, *5*(5), e10564. doi:10.1371/journal.pone.0010564 PMID:20485681

Swaney, R. (2018). Virtual reality delivers real-world benefits to dementia patients. *Samsung*. Retrieved from https://insights.samsung.com/2018/03/13/virtual-reality-delivers-real-world-benefits-to-dementia-patients/

United Nations. (n.d.). Virtual Reality. Retrieved from http://unvr.sdgactioncampaign.org/

Wiederhold, B. K., & Wiederhold, M. D. (2005). *Virtual reality therapy for anxiety disorders: Advances in evaluation and treatment*. American Psychological Association. doi:10.1037/10858-000

Winn, W. (1993). A conceptual basis for educational applications of virtual reality. Human Interface Technology Laboratory, Washington Technology Center, University of Washington, USA.

Wu, H. K., Lee, S. W.-L., Chang, H. Y., & Liang, J. C. (2013). Current status, opportunities and challenges of augmented reality in education. *Computers & Education*, *62*, 41–49. doi:10.1016/j.compedu.2012.10.024

Zimmerman, F., & Merci, J. A. (2010). A better start. Child maltreatment prevention as a public health priority. Retrieved July 18, 2018 from https://vetoviolence.cdc.gov/apps/phl/docs/A_Better_Start.pdf

## ADDITIONAL READING

Anda, R. F., Croft, J. B., Felitti, V. J., Nordenberg, D., Giles, W. H., Williamson, D. F., & Giovino, G. A. (1999). Adverse childhood experiences and smoking during adolescence and adulthood. *Journal of the American Medical Association*, *282*(17), 1652–1658. doi:10.1001/jama.282.17.1652 PMID:10553792

Beitchman, J. H., Zucker, K. J., & Hood, J. E., daCosta, G. AAkman, D. (1991). A review of the short-term effects of child sexual abuse. *Child Abuse & Neglect*, *15*(4), 537–556. doi:10.1016/0145-2134(91)90038-F PMID:1959086

Chartier, M. J., Walker, J. R., & Naimark, B. (2010). Separate and cumulative effects of adverse childhood experiences in predicting adult health and health care utilization. *Child Abuse & Neglect*, *34*(6), 454–464. doi:10.1016/j.chiabu.2009.09.020 PMID:20409586

Danese, A., & McEwen, B. S. (2012). Adverse childhood experiences, allostasis, allostatic load, and age-related disease. *Physiology & Behavior*, *106*(1), 29–39. doi:10.1016/j.physbeh.2011.08.019 PMID:21888923

Dube, S. R., Anda, R. F., Felitti, V. J., Chapman, D. P., Williamson, D. F., & Giles, W. H. (2001). Childhood abuse, household dysfunction, and the risk of attempted suicide throughout the life span: Findings from the Adverse Childhood Experiences Study. *Journal of the American Medical Association*, *286*(24), 3089–3096. doi:10.1001/jama.286.24.3089 PMID:11754674

Herman, D. B., Susser, E. S., Struening, E. L., & Link, B. L. (1997). Adverse childhood experiences: Are they risk factors for adult homelessness? *American Journal of Public Health*, *87*(2), 249–255.

Jiang, J. Y., Xu, W., Li, W. P., Gao, G. Y., Bao, Y. H., Liang, Y. M., & Luo, Q. Z. (2006). Effect of long-term mild hypothermia or short-term mild hypothermia on outcome of patients with severe traumatic brain injury. *Journal of Cerebral Blood Flow and Metabolism*, *26*(6), 771–776. doi:10.1038j.jcbfm.9600253 PMID:16306933

Larkin, H., & Park, J. (2012). Adverse childhood experiences (ACEs), service use, and service helpfulness among people experiencing homelessness. *Families in Society*, *93*(2), 85–93.

Prandoni, P., Lensing, A. W., Cogo, A., Cuppini, S., Villalta, S., Carta, M., ... Prins, M. H. (1996). The Long-term Clinical Course of Acute Deep Venous Thrombosis. *Annals of Internal Medicine*, *125*(1), 1–7. doi:10.7326/0003-4819-125-1-199607010-00001 PMID:8644983

Schilling, E. A., Aseltine, R. H., & Gore, S. (2007). Adverse childhood experiences and mental health in young adults: A longitudinal survey. *BMC Public Health*, *7*(1), 30. doi:10.1186/1471-2458-7-30 PMID:17343754

Trzpuc, S. J., Wendt, K. A., Heitzman, S. C., Skemp, S., Thomas, D., & Dahl, R. (2016). Does space matter? An exploratory study for a child–adolescent mental health inpatient unit. *HERD: Health Environments Research & Design Journal*, *10*(1), 23–44. doi:10.1177/1937586716634017 PMID:27081193

Wantland, D. J., Portillo, C. J., Holzemer, W. L., Slaughter, R., & McGhee, E. M. (2004). The effectiveness of Web-based vs. non-Web-based interventions: A meta-analysis of behavioral change outcomes. *Journal of Medical Internet Research*, *6*(4), e40. doi:10.2196/jmir.6.4.e40 PMID:15631964

Whitfield, C. L., Dube, S. R., Felitti, V. J., & Anda, R. F. (2005). Adverse childhood experiences and hallucinations. *Child Abuse & Neglect*, *29*(7), 797–810. doi:10.1016/j.chiabu.2005.01.004 PMID:16051353

## KEY TERMS AND DEFINITIONS

**Augmented Reality (AR):** It is a technology that uses real world environment and enhances it by overlaying digital information on top of it.

**Avatar:** A computer-generated representation of an individual in a virtual environment.

**Cybersickness:** A form of motion or simulator sickness related to sensory mismatch or conflict; symptoms include dizziness, nausea, eye strain and fatigue.

**Head-Mounted Display:** A device worn over a user's head, providing a visual display in front of one or both of the user's eyes.

**Mixed Reality (MR):** It merges the real and digital environments that co-exist and interact with each other to produce new environment for the user to explore and manipulate.

**Traumatic Stress:** The emotional and physical responses of a child to actions that threaten the life or physical reliability of the child or of someone important for the child (e.g. parent, sibling). It is this uncontrolled physiological stimulation that is the cause of stress that becomes traumatic and can provoke what is initially an adaptive response to the stressor that ultimately becomes destructive and maladapted.

**Virtual Reality (VR):** It provides the user with computer-generated simulation of a real life environment or situation. The headset gives the user a fully immersive experience, where what a user sees is a generated or an artificial environment and nothing of it is in the real world. Example of VR is gaming consoles

**Virtual Reality Exposure Therapy (VRET):** It is a virtual reality-based exposure therapy for treating Post Traumatic Stress Disorder (PTSD) as well as severe phobias. The goal of VRET is to expose the patient to stimuli by combining advanced computer graphics, 3D visual displays, and body-tracking technologies to create realistic virtual non-threatening environment so that their mind and body can learn not to become alerted when they are exposed to similar stimuli in real life.

# Chapter 6
# A SWOT Analysis of Virtual Reality for Seniors

**Pooya Soltani**
*Aix Marseille University, France*

## ABSTRACT

*The population of older people is increasing. In this book chapter, the author reviewed some of the applications of virtual reality (VR) for seniors in form of a strengths, weaknesses, opportunities, and threats (SWOT) analysis. This approach is commonly used to assess and guide internal and external parameters to accomplish a mission. Some of the challenges that the elderly are facing were reviewed and the way VR can help in overcoming those challenges were discussed. A comparison of VR technologies was also presented. The results show that VR's feasibility and concept are linked to existing technologies and the characteristics of each system control immersion, interaction, and stimulation. VR interventions might have the potential to be used as ecologically valid e-health screening systems. Systems should be specifically designed and adapted for seniors and usability issues should be addressed. Ideally, VR interventions work best in addition to traditional methods. Future studies should use more subjects to ensure the efficacy of such interventions for seniors.*

## INTRODUCTION

Human life expectancy and the population of elderly people over 60 years old are increasing. People might be less available to properly support older family members. Costs of hospitalization and nursery homes, as well as physical barriers, loneliness, and isolation, are among challenges that elderly are facing (Marcelino et al., 2018). Research has shown that regular physical activity (PA) is important for good health. It could also prevent various diseases and lower the risk of fall (Ofstedal, Zimmer, & Lin, 1999). Additionally, PA could improve memory and executive functions in the short and long term. However, aging is usually accompanied by deterioration of muscular strength, sensory sensitivity, and functional capacities (Park & Yim, 2016). These physiological changes affect the seniors' willingness to participate in regular PA (Lin et al., 2018). The physical decline also affects the elderly's quality of life, falls, admission to the healthcare centers, and mortality. Cognitive impairments also affect the

DOI: 10.4018/978-1-5225-7168-1.ch006

elderly's functional autonomy and result in a decline in physical performance and unsafe decisions and behaviors (Dommès et al., 2015).

By means of computers interfaces, virtual reality (VR) allows users to enter a virtual world. It uses various audiovisual technologies to provide high interaction leading to a feeling of immersion (Lin, Jeng, and Yeh, 2018). VR simulates environments and activities by using real-time stimulation of one or more sensory channels. Its feasibility and concept have been linked to the existing technologies for simulation and interaction. VR settings provide immediate feedback that could be necessary for all forms of learning (Manera et al., 2016). They also offer personalized environments according to the needs of the different participants.

Although seniors shape a considerable portion of our population, they are often overlooked when it comes to newly introduced technologies. They may not always be willing to accept new technologies, in fear of not being able to use them (Lin et al., 2018). Despite the functional loss, seniors still have the abilities to acquire and re-learn performance skills (Skjæret et al., 2016). Technology might be used to promote better performance for them. Jeng, Pai, and Yeh (2017) suggested that to encourage the elderly to use technology, psychological barriers should be broken. Teaching and providing hands-on experience and assistance, increase their willingness to experience new things. VR may have the advantage to control the type and amount of experience each patient receives and may boost learning transfer to the identified targets (Maillot et al., 2017). VR also has the ability to change the existing scenarios by modifying physics and other aspects of reality. Virtual tasks might be designed according to the elderly's needs for acquiring and practicing new skills repeatedly. The immersive nature of these interventions may also offer implicit learning processes without the patient's awareness (Rand et al., 2017).

Telerehabilitation uses information and communication technology and offers accessible and affordable services to people in their homes (Kizony et al., 2017). The use of VR and serious games for older adults are generally categorized in improving upper and lower limbs movements, balance, mobility training, daily living, neglect, and cognition (cf. Deutsch and Westcott, 2017). The challenge is to provide enough amount and intensity and therefore, various technological approaches have been proposed. VR could also be used as an add-on to robotic devices for execution of movement or to be used as standalone systems using visual stimulation and interaction (Hoermann et al., 2017; Cameirão, Bermudez, & Verschure, 2008).

Considering these issues, this book chapter will present a SWOT analysis of using VR for seniors. SWOT stands for strengths, weaknesses, opportunities, and threats, and is usually used in business to analyze the parameters that affect the company's competitive position in the market. A strength is a positive capacity that allows an entity reaching to its defined goals. A weakness is a limitation that slows the progress towards the defined goals. An opportunity is an internal or external force in favor of that entity. A threat is an unfavorable situation that could present a barrier or limitation in achieving goals. SWOT analysis is done to reveal the optimal match between strengths, weaknesses, opportunities, and threats that the company is facing. SWOT framework could also be applied outside of the business domain (Rizzo & Kim, 2005). Based on a SWOT analysis, strategies could take advantage of opportunities by using their strengths and by actively addressing threats by correcting the weaknesses.

## BACKGROUND

In this part, some of the challenges that elderly people might face are explained:

Falls affect approximately one-third of older adults per year and could significantly reduce their independent functionality (Talamo et al., 2017). Injuries and fall-related costs are high and their prevention are important public health challenges. Fall risks can be attributed to both motor and cognitive deficits. Multimodal interventions that target both motor and cognitive functions may contribute to fall reduction (Mirelman et al., 2013). Surveys and physical tests are used to measure both intrinsic and extrinsic risk factors. Physical tests are easy to administer but they lack ecological validity or the degree of similarity between the training environment and the real-world. Moreover, traditional tests may not have the ability to isolate specific sensory defects (Saldana et al., 2017). This is important as ecologically valid tests add value for predicting improvements in everyday functioning.

Static and dynamic balance training are usually prescribed to overcome day to day tasks in the older population. Biofeedback systems could also be beneficial for building new motor skills. They allow motor-cognitive systems integration and self-perception of treatment effectiveness (Montero-Alia et al., 2016). However, these systems are expensive, are not highly accessible, and require an expert to operate them. Other existing proactive interventions for fall prevention may also produce mixed success results because these exercises do not specifically target the neuromuscular skills required for fall prevention (Parijat et al., 2015).

Stroke is the main cause of long-term disability, and the majority of stroke patients are over 65. It creates many problems such as difficulties in completing daily living activities. Neuroplasticity and recovery after strokes are improved by repetitive, task-oriented, and intensive training. However, general barriers of cost, transport, information (on how and where to exercise), and time exist. Moreover, it seems that motivation is a major challenge for rehabilitation adherence (Paquin et al., 2016). Other parameters such as the number of exercises, their effectiveness, and their complexities might also contribute to the adherence (Pallazo et al., 2016). Stroke patients may also experience visual neglect as a result of brain dysfunction. In clinical practice, these patients are often observed for far and near space sight check.

Personally lived events are called episodic memories and they shape our identity and connect us the past and future. Changes in this type of memory (e.g. due to age) could predict the evolution towards neurodegenerative disorders (Abichou, La Corte, & Piolino, 2017). Alzheimer's disease (AD) is a common form of dementia and results in a decline in cognition and daily living activities. Mild cognitive impairment (MCI) is the limited declination of cognitive abilities in the AD. Patients with MCI have problems remembering the relationship between objects or between objects and their contexts. Spatial disorientation is another early manifestation of AD and MCI in which patients have problems in unfamiliar places.

Cognitive and functional tools are usually used to detect early manifestation of the disease. Assessing instrumental activities of daily living (e.g. using a bus or a telephone) is important for choosing better interventions for AD patients. Traditional neuropsychological tools use simple situations and are able to partially measure the characteristics of episodic memory. Ecological tasks might be more beneficial compared to subjective questionnaire-based assessments (Vallejo et al., 2017). Novel screening tests use new technologies and game principles and focus on the immersion of the users in various scenarios to mislead and deceive patients' minds (Fernandez & Argyriou, 2017). Assessing patients with VR application seems legitimate because they could recreate conditions similar to that of the real world. In the next section, the differences between different forms of VR are discussed and after, a SWOT analysis of how VR could address the mentioned challenges is presented.

## MAIN FOCUS OF THE CHAPTER

### Differences Between Exergames and the VR

Early studies have characterized active video games (exergames) as forms of VR. In fact, these two terms are usually used interchangeably. We have heard research findings like these: Elderly may have higher interests in participation in exergame sport activities than real-world activities (Wollersheim et al., 2010); When exergames are used for rehabilitation, elderly are more motivated and rarely drop out (Pigford & Andrews, 2010). There are also demented pieces of evidence on better control over posture stability and balance when using exergames (Chiang et al., 2011). So, what are the differences between exergames and VR?

For a system to create the illusion of interacting with a virtual world, it should offer presence, immersion, and flow. The presence or the realness of the world is partly created by the system's ability to deliver an illusion or degree of immersion. This is where the differences of exergames and other types of hardware is more visible. Exergame platforms detect your movements with their sensors and transfer them to computerized avatars inside the games. Nintendo Wii also comes with a balance board, a small portable force platform that could be coupled with various Wii Fit games. It adds enhanced immersion by monitoring center of gravity while the participants interact with the on-screen characters (Rendon et al., 2012). More immersive virtual environments include cave automatic virtual environments (CAVE) which are basically a video theater within a room. The walls of the cave are made up of rear-projection screens. Users enter the cave while wearing 3D glasses and their movements are monitored to continuously adjust viewers' perspective. Newer technologies such as head-mounted displays (HMD) use participant-centric perspective. They have a larger field of view (FOV) and stereoscopic visual fields that are constantly modified by head position and rotation. The recent HMDs have higher FOV, display resolution, and tracking latency resulting in a better creation of the visual illusion of real objects and scenarios.

One reason to consider exergames as VR might be that exergame platforms provide immediate feedback to players' movements, offering immersive feelings. Therefore, VR's feasibility and concept are linked to the existing technologies for immersion, interaction, and stimulation. The characteristics of each concept are responsible for delivering an illusion of reality (immersion). These characteristics later affect presence or the sense of being in the VR (Borrego et al., 2018). For example, one might argue that HMDs and CAVEs are more immersive than exergames because they provide higher visual stimulation. However, this degree of immersion is not necessarily related to the effectiveness of the system (Deutsch & Westcott, 2017), and both VR and video games create a state of flow, the optimal performance zone of the players.

Lee, Chen, and Chang (2016) argued that tasks presented on LCD displays are in fact presented in 2D. In a 2D virtual environment, there is no stereo vision and subjects see one planar view. Other cognitive and sensory cues may be used to indicate depth; for example, an avatar walking in a jungle. As patients need to imagine 3D patterns, a huge cognitive load is created when the information is presented in a 2D format (Sweller et al., 1998). It has been suggested that augmented reality (AR) provides better 3D stimuli and manual spatial manipulation (Sweller et al., 1998). On the other hand, by using AR, users might change their behavior when they are aware of being observed (Sweller et al., 1998). Liebermann et al. (2012) also compared arm reaching movements made in 2D video VR environment with the real-world environment. They showed that movements patterns were affected by viewing angle and were slower, shorter, and less accurate compared to the real condition. They also suggested that a

2D VR environment may be perceptually and cognitively challenging for the participants because the intended 3D illusion presented by their VR was likely based on previous memories and experiences. They concluded that caution needs to be taken when using these environments for improving the quality of movement for rehabilitation of upper limb.

Another issue to consider is that visual systems contribute to balance and visual perturbation cause instability. Exergames do not completely encompass the viewer's FOV, and visual information from surroundings of the VR environment (e.g. TV or screen) can still provide stability cues (Menzies et al., 2016). HMDs obscure unwanted additional visual cues and add ecological validity through the addition of depth perception (Saldana et al., 2017). However, it may cause simulator sickness and if not properly designed or performed without supervision, may lead to falls.

## Strength

Riva et al. (2004) used a VR-based multidimensional approach to treat body image (perception of the aesthetics or sexual attractiveness of one's body) attitudes. Their results showed positive short-term results in improving the overall psychological state of the participants compared to the traditional cognitive-behavioral training. Chang et al. (2014) compared the effects of a VR gaming system on sleep quality of elderly people with a disability. They showed that regular VR exercise significantly reduces stress among the older patients, confirming that it can improve their sleep quality. In his meta-analysis, Cardinale (2018) suggested that VR balance training using Nintendo Wii improves Borg balance scale score compared to no balance training, and helps people to multi-task during balance training. Parijat et al. (2015) used VR as a perturbation-based training tool for older adults. They found that their VR environment could induce perturbations similar to a slip. It could also reduce the incidence of balance loss during the actual experiment on a slippery surface. Mirelman et al. (2016) targeted the interplay between cognitive and mobility deficits and combined non-immersive VR gaming with treadmill training. After 6 months of training, those who trained on the treadmill using VR had a significantly lower fall incident rate compared to the treadmill only group.

Yasuda et al. (2017) examined the immediate effects of an immersive VR rehabilitation program (a reaching task and a visual searching task) using HMD. They concluded that this program might be beneficial for the visual searching task in far spatial neglect. Self-training compliance using video games for post-stroke rehabilitation is shown to be higher compared to traditional methods in elderly patients (Rand et al., 2017). Parsons and Barnett (2017) developed a VR measure of memory and validated it with traditional methods in older adults. Not only the VR measure was similar to traditional methods for memory measures, it provided objective measurements of individual memory components. Their subjects also preferred the VR task over the pen-and-paper measures. Vallejo et al. (2017) developed a VR serious game to assess cognitive function in healthy and AD patients using an ecological approach of daily living activities. Differences were expected between healthy and AD patients in terms of percentage of achievements and the time needed to achieve those tasks. However, the additional qualitative information regarding the errors in the achievement of the tasks provided information about cognitive functions.

Nir-Hadad et al. (2017) also validate their VR shopping task for the assessment of executive function in stroke elderly population. Maillot et al. (2017) developed an affordable and transportable VR system to help older pedestrians make safer street crossing decisions. They also measured whether training with the small-scale simulator transfers to a full-size simulator where they could actually walk. They showed that the small-scale simulator triggers more unsafe decisions compared to full-scale. It also allowed learning new skills and modify behavior to use in the large-scale simulator (learning transfer).

## Weakness

Manera et al. (2016) argued that their VR task needs to be improved to fix usability issues. They attributed the lower performance of elderly in VR to the difficulties elderly have with using the mouse and possibly to eye strain from wearing the 3D glasses. In general, the senior population suffers from technological illiteracy. For maximum efficacy, VR systems should promote a user-centered design and their primary focus should be on inclusive design, usability, and accessibility. Different sensors might demand higher body performances. For example, to use Kinect, it is necessary to move the whole body. Some sensors might require players to have better coordination and in elderly it might cause lower levels of performance. Other technologies like touch screens may not require high levels of body movement but may demand higher mental agility (Palacio et al., 2017).

Bezerra et al. (2018) showed that VR environments provide improvements of performance in healthy older adults. However, there is no transfer of performance from VR to the real task and vice versa. Rand et al. (2017) compared video game and traditional self-training for upper limb rehabilitation in older adults after a stroke. Although improvements were observed in the two methods, they showed that the differences were not significant. Zygouris et al. (2015) used a virtual supermarket task for MCI screening. Although the task displayed a high correct classification rate between MCI and healthy elderly, it was unable to differentiate between MCI subtypes. Dommes et al. (2012) assessed the effectiveness of a VR training program for elderly on the street crossing decision making. Although they showed that immediately after the training, the intervention group and the control group differed significantly, these differences were not significant after 6 months. However, a clear shift to making more safe decisions was observed for all participants. In general, due to the lower number of subjects in different studies, the generalization of the results are somewhat restricted (Yeşilyaprak et al., 2016).

## Opportunities

Mattan et al. (2017) discussed that age is associated with reduced perspective-taking capacity. They showed that compared to younger adults, older people are relatively more egocentric and more accurate when they are in the first person perspective compared to the third person perspective. Mohammadi et al. (2018) also used two VR navigation tasks (allocentric and egocentric virtual neighborhoods) in different AD patients. They showed that patients needed more time to find the goal in egocentric tasks. It might be possible to properly distinguish specific types of AD patients from others. Sobral Monteiro-Junior et al. (2017) showed that exergaming could offer improvements in short-term memory, working memory, and semantic memory/executive function over time. Valladares-Rodriguez et al. (2017) used a digital game to assess episodic memory, which is used to evaluate potential cognitive impairments in the elderly. Using the new ecological, non-intrusive, and better administrable tool, they conducted the test in a shorter time. They could also introduce scenarios that are closer to real life while being more engaging and highly acceptable compared to the classical pen-and-paper based method.

Fernandes and Argyriou (2017) used VR as an affordable approach for creating e-health screening AD diagnostic systems. They proposed VR tests that could evaluate memory loss related to common objects, recent events, expressing and understanding languages, and the ability to recognize abnormalities accurately and similarly for the presence of AD. From their research, Plancher et al. (2012) concluded that VR is better adapted for early diagnosis of AD compared to traditional verbal memory tools. Manera et al. (2016) tested the feasibility of an image-based VR system in MCI and dementia. Their patients reported high feelings of security and low discomfort, anxiety, and fatigue. Although the VR task was more difficult, they were also more satisfied with the VR condition and preferred it to the paper condition.

Lin et al. (2018) used means-end chain techniques to examine elderly's awareness and personal values regarding VR activities. Elderly population mentioned leisure VR activities to be fun, safe, easy, and physically and mentally healthy. While playing with VR, they were also seeking enjoyment, improved quality of life, and a sense of belonging. Goršič et al. (2017) explored the role of competition while using VR. They concluded that stroke patients (including elderly) who exercise with a peer in an unsupervised situation (e.g. home) exhibit higher enjoyment and exercise intensity compared to those who exercise alone. Brunner et al. (2017) explored the effectiveness of their upper extremity VR rehabilitation system and showed that the improvements were similar to the conventional therapy. They also suggested that the motivating nature of VR could be a supplement to standard rehabilitation.

Saldana et al. (2017) used HMD in VR to objectively assess balance by using visual-vestibular conflict and by comparing the results of postural sway with a force plate. Their preliminary results showed that the HMD is a valid, reliable, and comparable to traditional mechanical perturbation approaches for measuring balance. Popular HMDs allow easy navigation in life-size virtual environments and provide required spatial requirements of non-immersive serious games, exergames, and motor rehabilitation applications (Borrego et al., 2018). Such interaction allows natural navigation and exploration and therefore, the improved ecological validity of the task while facilitating skill transfer. Albiol-Pérez et al. (2017) designed a low-cost active balance rehabilitation system and measured the performance of balance control during 15 sessions of virtual rehabilitation. Although there were no statistically significant differences between the left, central, and right positions, their results indicated a trend of improvement, especially in the left and right sway which are important in avoiding risks of falls. Tsang and Fu (2016) compared the efficacy of their VR balance system with traditional balance training. They attributed the improvements in VR system to the real-time performance feedback and cuing stimuli that supports error-free learning.

Paquin et al. (2016) used a VR rehabilitation program for fine motor recovery of stroke patients. All of their subjects experienced a perceived increase in hand function and that they would recommend the program to other stroke survivors. McDonald et al. (2013) used a VR pain coach for the effects on the communication of pain by older adults. They measured pain and depressive symptoms before and one month after the intervention. Older adults shared a significant amount of clinically important pain information with the pain coach than the pain communication-only group. Pain intensity and depressive symptoms reduction showed a non-significant trend one month after the intervention. The VR pain coach shows a possible strategy for pain management discussions between practitioners and older adults.

### Threats

Previous research has suggested side effects of display characteristics, obstacles, cost/benefit of the technology as weaknesses for the adoption of VR in rehabilitation (Rizo & Kim, 2005). Dizziness and imbalance might occur after using VR applications. Chairovano et al. (2018) perturbed visual inputs and measured their effects on self-report (complaint) vs. balance measurement (posturography). As they found no correlation between these two methods, it is important not to only rely on subjective measurement of dizziness, but also to objectively measure the imbalance; especially because questionnaires could be influenced by age, sex, motivation, and cognitive and emotional parameters (Yardley & Redfern, 2001). Eggenberger et al. (2015) also compared long-term multi-component cognitive-physical tasks: one was treadmill walking with simultaneous verbal memory training and the other VR video game dancing. Both types of training resulted in significant advantages in improving gait parameters compared to physical training only. However, these two interventions resulted in different training-specific adaptations in the gait. Cardinale (2018) suggests that VR balance training should be used in supplement with other interventions. With multi-component processes such as balance, there might be the possibility of errors leading to falls. The lower number of patients, especially in different types of AD might limit the generalization of the results (Mohammadi et al., 2018).

## SOLUTIONS AND RECOMMENDATIONS

Technology is constantly evolving, and it has the potential to be applied to various domains. However, it needs to be adapted to meet the seniors' needs. Lee et al. (2016) designed a VR based rehabilitation and explored patients' perceived difficulty and enjoyment. They suggested that the level of enjoyment could be an indicator of the appropriateness of the difficulty levels. They identified five parameters that could affect this relationship: ease of following the directions, the experience of pain, achieved scores, novelty and immediate feedback, and self-perceived effectiveness. Participants' physical, cognitive, proprioceptive differences should also be considered while tailoring the VR systems. As mentioned by Lin et al. (2018), elderly people's decision-making processes are restricted to certain leisure activities. Different platforms should identify their feature and consider elderly's physiological functions to establish a marketing focus.

From their systematic review, Molina et al. (2014) concluded that most of the studies on the efficacy of inclusion of exergames for elderly have methodological problems. The duration of gameplay varies widely and therefore, it is hard to be conclusive about the physical benefits. Miller et al. (2014) also mentioned that although VR/gaming systems are effective and feasible, there is a high risk of bias for addressing impairments and participation. Booth et al. (2014) also systematically reviewed 251 articles on the effects of VR gaming systems on improving balance in older adults. The pooled results showed no significant differences. What is important is that video games for older people could help them to be more socially active. However, several parameters such as simplicity, social enjoyability, and entertaining new games should be considered. Video game controller should allow adequate time for the elderly to make decisions in order to achieve the games' objectives (Palacio et al., 2017).

## FUTURE RESEARCH DIRECTIONS

As mentioned before, most of the studies lack an adequate number of participants which makes it hard to generalize the efficacy of results. Future studies should use a larger sample size and consider culture and gender-oriented tasks (Vallejo et al., 2017; Yeşilyaprak et al., 2016). Future studies should also have appropriate dosages of use to improve the validity of treatment prescription and safe functioning levels of the seniors (Cardinale, 2018). Follow-up and longitudinal studies with normalized baseline levels are required to identify the consistency of the beneficial effects of VR (Maillot et al., 2017; Nawaz et al., 2016; Mirelman et al., 2016). Feasibility studies are important in enhancing performance and other cognitive tasks in the target population. However, randomized controlled trial (RCT) efficacy studies should be conducted with control groups of healthy elderly participants, while creating more complex versions of the task (Kizony et al., 2017; Marena et al., 2016). Control groups and blinding participants and the tests also help in avoiding bias and learning effects (Yasuda et al., 2017). Similar VR and real tasks could also help in better understanding the transferability of the intervention (Bezerra et al., 2018). It is also important to assess psychosocial and cognitive emotion improvements after VR interventions (Cardinale, 2018). As suggested before, it is also important to consider the VR training as part of a holistic platform and not the sole effects (Cardinale, 2018).

## CONCLUSION

VR is a rapidly developing subject and in this book chapter, the author discussed how VR could help in overcoming various struggles of the seniors. Both exergames and newer VR technologies have the ability to immerse players and their effectiveness may not be related to the levels of immersion they offer. However, each technology might address specific needs. As shown in Table 1, it seems that VR interventions have the potential to offer ecologically valid scenarios for screening various diseases. It is suggested that these interventions are used in addition to traditional interventions. More subjects and longer duration of use are needed to validate the efficacy of VR for seniors.

*Table 1. Summary of SWOT analysis of using VR for seniors*

<table>
<tr><th>Strengths</th><th>Weaknesses</th></tr>
<tr><td>1. Short term overall psychosocial state improvements<br>2. Improved balance and decreased risks of falls<br>3. Improved visual searching<br>4. Higher compliance to self-training<br>5. Similar validity to traditional memory tests<br>6. Enhanced ecological validity</td><td>1. Adaptation issues (usability, display technologies, platforms)<br>2. Limitations in skill transfer<br>3. Limitation is differentiating between subtypes of cognitive tests<br>4. Short lasting results<br>5. Restricted generalization of the results</td></tr>
<tr><th>Opportunities</th><th>Threats</th></tr>
<tr><td>1. Ability to modify physics and scenarios according to the needs<br>2. Efficiency<br>3. Affordable<br>4. Possible similar results to traditional interventions</td><td>1. Mixed positive and negative results<br>2. Low number of subjects<br>3. Little cost/benefit proofs for VR adoption</td></tr>
</table>

## ACKNOWLEDGMENT

This research was supported by Institut Carnot STAR and Collège de France.

## REFERENCES

Abichou, K., La Corte, V., & Piolino, P. (2017). Does virtual reality have a future for the study of episodic memory in aging? *Gériatrie et Psychologie Neuropsychiatrie du Vieillissement*, *15*(1), 65–74. doi:10.1684/pnv.2016.0648 PMID:28266343

Albiol-Pérez, S., Gil-Gómez, J. A., Muñoz-Tomás, M. T., Gil-Gómez, H., Vial-Escolano, R., & Lozano-Quilis, J.-A. (2017). The effect of balance training on postural control in patients with Parkinson's disease using a virtual rehabilitation system. *Methods of Information in Medicine*, *56*(2), 138–144. doi:10.3414/ME16-02-0004 PMID:28244545

Bezerra, Í. M. P., Crocetta, T. B., Massetti, T., Silva, T. D. D., Guarnieri, R., Meira, C. M. Jr, ... Monteiro, C. B. M. (2018). Functional performance comparison between real and virtual tasks in older adults: A cross-sectional study. *Medicine*, *97*(4), e9612–e9612. doi:10.1097/MD.0000000000009612 PMID:29369177

Booth, V., Masud, T., Connell, L., & Bath-Hextall, F. (2014). The effectiveness of virtual reality interventions in improving balance in adults with impaired balance compared with standard or no treatment: A systematic review and meta-analysis. *Clinical Rehabilitation*, *28*(5), 419–431. doi:10.1177/0269215513509389 PMID:24188913

Borrego, A., Latorre, J., Alcaniz, M., & Llorens, R. (2018). Comparison of Oculus Rift and HTC Vive: Feasibility for Virtual Reality-Based Exploration, Navigation, Exergaming, and Rehabilitation. *Games for Health Journal*, *7*(3), 151–156. doi:10.1089/g4h.2017.0114 PMID:29293369

Brunner, I., Skouen, J. S., Hofstad, H., Aßmus, J., Becker, F., Sanders, A. M., ... Verheyden, G. (2017). Virtual reality training for upper extremity in subacute stroke (VIRTUES): A multicenter RCT. *Neurology*, *89*(24), 2413–2421. doi:10.1212/WNL.0000000000004744 PMID:29142090

Cameirão, M. S., Bermúdez, S., & Verschure, P. F. M. J. (2008). Virtual reality based upper extremity rehabilitation following stroke: A review. *Journal of Cyber Therapy and Rehabilitation*, *1*(1), 63–74.

Cardinale, J. (2018). *Does Virtual Reality Balance Training Utilizing the Wii Balance Board Improve Balance in Community Dwelling Older Adults: A Meta-Analysis* [Doctoral dissertation]. California State University, Fresno, CA.

Chang, L. C., Wang, C. Y., & Yu, P. (2014). Virtual reality improves sleep quality amongst older adults with disabilities. *International Journal of Geriatric Psychiatry*, *29*(12), 1312–1313. doi:10.1002/gps.4172 PMID:25394270

Chiang, I. T., Chen, M. L., Chang, P. S., & Lee, J. Y. (2011). Effects of a video game-based intervention on balance learning for institution-dwelling elderly in veterans home. In *The 2011 International Educational Technology Conference Proceedings Book* (Vol. 1, pp. 393-398).

Chiarovano, E., Wang, W., Reynolds, P., & MacDougall, H. G. (2018). Imbalance: Objective measures versus subjective self-report in clinical practice. *Gait & Posture*, *59*, 217–221. doi:10.1016/j.gaitpost.2017.10.019 PMID:29080510

Deutsch, J. E., & Westcott McCoy, S. (2017). Virtual reality and serious games in neurorehabilitation of children and adults: Prevention, plasticity, and participation. *Pediatric Physical Therapy: The Official Publication of The Section on Pediatrics of the American Physical Therapy Association*, *29*(Suppl. 3), S23–S36. doi:10.1097/PEP.0000000000000387 PMID:28654475

Dommes, A., & Cavallo, V. (2012). Can simulator-based training improve street-crossing safety for elderly pedestrians? *Transportation Research Part F: Psychology and Behaviour*, *15*(2), 206–218. doi:10.1016/j.trf.2011.12.004

Dommès, A., Le Lay, T., Vienne, F., Dang, N. T., Beaudoin, A. P., & Do, M. C. (2015). Towards an explanation of age-related difficulties in crossing a two-way street. *Accident; Analysis and Prevention*, *85*, 229–238. doi:10.1016/j.aap.2015.09.022 PMID:26476193

Eggenberger, P., Theill, N., Holenstein, S., Schumacher, V., & de Bruin, E. D. (2015). Multicomponent physical exercise with simultaneous cognitive training to enhance dual-task walking of older adults: A secondary analysis of a 6-month randomized controlled trial with 1-year follow-up. *Clinical Interventions in Aging*, *10*, 1711–1732. doi:10.2147/CIA.S91997 PMID:26604719

Fernandez Montenegro, J. M., & Argyriou, V. (2017). Cognitive evaluation for the diagnosis of Alzheimer's disease based on Turing Test and Virtual Environments. *Physiology & Behavior*, *173*, 42–51. doi:10.1016/j.physbeh.2017.01.034 PMID:28137425

Goršič, M., Cikajlo, I., Goljar, N., & Novak, D. (2017). A multisession evaluation of an adaptive competitive arm rehabilitation game. *Journal of Neuroengineering and Rehabilitation*, *14*(1), 128–128. doi:10.118612984-017-0336-9 PMID:29208017

Hoermann, S., Ferreira Dos Santos, L., Morkisch, N., Jettkowski, K., Sillis, M., Devan, H., ... Cutfield, N. J. (2017). Computerised mirror therapy with augmented reflection technology for early stroke rehabilitation: Clinical feasibility and integration as an adjunct therapy. *Disability and Rehabilitation*, *39*(15), 1503–1514. doi:10.1080/09638288.2017.1291765 PMID:28478736

Jeng, M.-Y., Pai, F.-Y., & Yeh, T.-M. (2017). The virtual reality leisure activities experience on elderly people. *Applied Research in Quality of Life*, *12*(1), 49–65. doi:10.100711482-016-9452-0

Kizony, R., Weiss, P. L., Harel, S., Feldman, Y., Obuhov, A., Zeilig, G., & Shani, M. (2017). Tele-rehabilitation service delivery journey from prototype to robust in-home use. *Disability and Rehabilitation*, *39*(15), 1532–1540. doi:10.1080/09638288.2016.1250827 PMID:28004980

Lee, I. J., Chen, C. H., & Chang, K. P. (2016). Augmented reality technology combined with three-dimensional holography to train the mental rotation ability of older adults. *Computers in Human Behavior*, *65*, 488–500. doi:10.1016/j.chb.2016.09.014

Lee, M., Pyun, S. B., Chung, J., Kim, J., Eun, S. D., & Yoon, B. (2016). A further step to develop patient-friendly implementation strategies for virtual reality-based rehabilitation in patients with acute stroke. *Physical Therapy*, *96*(10), 1554–1564. doi:10.2522/ptj.20150271 PMID:27149961

Liebermann, D. G., Berman, S., Weiss, P. L. T., & Levin, M. F. (2012). Kinematics of reaching movements in a 2-D virtual environment in adults with and without stroke. *IEEE Transactions on Neural Systems and Rehabilitation Engineering: A Publication of the IEEE Engineering in Medicine and Biology Society, 20*(6), 778-787. doi:10.1109/TNSRE.2012.2206117

Lin, C. S., Jeng, M. Y., & Yeh, T. M. (2018). The elderly perceived meanings and values of virtual reality leisure activities: A means-end chain approach. *International Journal of Environmental Research and Public Health, 15*(4), 663. doi:10.3390/ijerph15040663 PMID:29614012

Maillot, P., Dommes, A., Dang, N. T., & Vienne, F. (2017). Training the elderly in pedestrian safety: Transfer effect between two virtual reality simulation devices. *Accident; Analysis and Prevention, 99*, 161–170. doi:10.1016/j.aap.2016.11.017 PMID:27898369

Manera, V., Chapoulie, E., Bourgeois, J., Guerchouche, R., David, R., Ondrej, J., ... Robert, P. (2016). A feasibility study with image-based rendered virtual reality in patients with mild cognitive impairment and dementia. *PLoS One, 11*(3), e0151487–e0151487. doi:10.1371/journal.pone.0151487 PMID:26990298

Marcelino, I., Laza, R., Domingues, P., Gómez-Meire, S., Fdez-Riverola, F., & Pereira, A. (2018). Active and assisted living ecosystem for the elderly. *Sensors (Basel), 18*(4), 1246. doi:10.339018041246 PMID:29673234

Mattan, B. D., Quinn, K. A., Acaster, S. L., Jennings, R. M., & Rotshtein, P. (2017). Prioritization of self-relevant perspectives in ageing. *Quarterly Journal of Experimental Psychology, 70*(6), 1033–1052. doi:10.1080/17470218.2015.1127399 PMID:26652616

McDonald, D. D., Walsh, S., Vergara, C., & Gifford, T. (2013). Effect of a virtual pain coach on pain management discussions: A pilot study. *Pain Management Nursing: Official Journal of The American Society of Pain Management Nurses, 14*(4), 200–209. doi:10.1016/j.pmn.2011.03.004 PMID:24315243

Menzies, R. J., Rogers, S. J., Phillips, A. M., Chiarovano, E., de Waele, C., Verstraten, F. A., & MacDougall, H. (2016). An objective measure for the visual fidelity of virtual reality and the risks of falls in a virtual environment. *Virtual Reality (Waltham Cross), 20*(3), 173–181. doi:10.100710055-016-0288-6

Miller, K. J., Adair, B. S., Pearce, A. J., Said, C. M., Ozanne, E., & Morris, M. M. (2014). Effectiveness and feasibility of virtual reality and gaming system use at home by older adults for enabling physical activity to improve health-related domains: A systematic review. *Age and Ageing, 43*(2), 188–195. doi:10.1093/ageing/aft194 PMID:24351549

Mirelman, A., Rochester, L., Maidan, I., Del Din, S., Alcock, L., Nieuwhof, F., ... Hausdorff, J. M. (2016). Addition of a non-immersive virtual reality component to treadmill training to reduce fall risk in older adults (V-TIME): A randomised controlled trial. *Lancet, 388*(10050), 1170–1182. doi:10.1016/S0140-6736(16)31325-3 PMID:27524393

Mirelman, A., Rochester, L., Reelick, M., Nieuwhof, F., Pelosin, E., Abbruzzese, G., ... Hausdorff, J. M. (2013). V-TIME: A treadmill training program augmented by virtual reality to decrease fall risk in older adults: Study design of a randomized controlled trial. *BMC Neurology*, *13*(1), 15–15. doi:10.1186/1471-2377-13-15 PMID:23388087

Mohammadi, A., Kargar, M., & Hesami, E. (2018). Using virtual reality to distinguish subjects with multiple- but not single-domain amnestic mild cognitive impairment from normal elderly subjects. *Psychogeriatrics: The Official Journal of the Japanese Psychogeriatric Society*, *18*(2), 132–142. doi:10.1111/psyg.12301 PMID:29409155

Molina, K. I., Ricci, N. A., de Moraes, S. A., & Perracini, M. R. (2014). Virtual reality using games for improving physical functioning in older adults: A systematic review. *Journal of Neuroengineering and Rehabilitation*, *11*(1), 156–156. doi:10.1186/1743-0003-11-156 PMID:25399408

Monteiro-Junior, R. S., da Silva Figueiredo, L. F., Maciel-Pinheiro, P. T., Abud, E. L. R., Braga, A. E. M. M., Barca, M. L., ... Laks, J. (2017). Acute effects of exergames on cognitive function of institutionalized older persons: A single-blinded, randomized and controlled pilot study. *Aging Clinical and Experimental Research*, *29*(3), 387–394. doi:10.100740520-016-0595-5 PMID:27256080

Montero-Alia, P., Munoz-Ortiz, L., Jimenez-Gonzalez, M., Benedicto-Pañell, C., Altimir-Losada, S., López-Colomer, Y., ... Torán-Monserrat, P. (2016). Study protocol of a randomized clinical trial evaluating the effectiveness of a primary care intervention using the Nintendo Wii console to improve balance and decrease falls in the elderly. *BMC Geriatrics*, *16*(1), 8. doi:10.118612877-015-0178-x PMID:26796956

Nir-Hadad, S. Y., Weiss, P. L., Waizman, A., Schwartz, N., & Kizony, R. (2017). A virtual shopping task for the assessment of executive functions: Validity for people with stroke. *Neuropsychological Rehabilitation*, *27*(5), 808–833. doi:10.1080/09602011.2015.1109523 PMID:26558414

Ofstedal, M. B., Zimmer, Z. S., & Lin, H. S. (1999). A comparison of correlates of cognitive functioning in older persons in Taiwan and the United States. *The Journals of Gerontology. Series B, Psychological Sciences and Social Sciences*, *54*(5), S291–S301. doi:10.1093/geronb/54B.5.S291 PMID:10542831

Palacio, R. R., Acosta, C. O., Cortez, J., & Morán, A. L. (2017). Usability perception of different video game devices in elderly users. *Universal Access in the Information Society*, *16*(1), 103–113. doi:10.100710209-015-0435-y

Palacio, R. R., Acosta, C. O., Cortez, J., & Morán, A. L. (2017). Usability perception of different video game devices in elderly users. *Universal Access in the Information Society*, *16*(1), 103–113. doi:10.100710209-015-0435-y

Palazzo, C., Klinger, E., Dorner, V., Kadri, A., Thierry, O., Boumenir, Y., ... Ville, I. (2016). Barriers to home-based exercise program adherence with chronic low back pain: Patient expectations regarding new technologies. *Annals of Physical and Rehabilitation Medicine*, *59*(2), 107–113. doi:10.1016/j.rehab.2016.01.009 PMID:27050664

Paquin, K., Crawley, J., Harris, J. E., & Horton, S. (2016). Survivors of chronic stroke - participant evaluations of commercial gaming for rehabilitation. *Disability and Rehabilitation*, *38*(21), 2144–2152. doi:10.3109/09638288.2015.1114155 PMID:26728133

Parijat, P., Lockhart, T. E., & Liu, J. (2015). Effects of perturbation-based slip training using a virtual reality environment on slip-induced falls. *Annals of Biomedical Engineering*, *43*(4), 958–967. doi:10.100710439-014-1128-z PMID:25245221

Park, J., & Yim, J. (2016). A new approach to improve cognition, muscle strength, and postural balance in community-dwelling elderly with a 3-D virtual reality Kayak program. *The Tohoku Journal of Experimental Medicine*, *238*(1), 1–8. doi:10.1620/tjem.238.1 PMID:26656425

Park, Y. S., & Kim, H. J. (2005). Effects of a taping method on pain and ROM of the knee joint in the elderly. *Journal of Korean Academy of Nursing*, *35*(2), 372–381. doi:10.4040/jkan.2005.35.2.372 PMID:15860951

Parsons, T. D., & Barnett, M. (2017). Validity of a newly developed measure of memory: Feasibility study of the virtual environment grocery store. *Journal of Alzheimer's Disease*, *59*(4), 1227–1235. doi:10.3233/JAD-170295 PMID:28759971

Pigford, T., & Andrews, A. W. (2010). Feasibility and benefit of using the Nintendo Wii Fit for balance rehabilitation in an elderly patient experiencing recurrent falls. *Journal of Student Physical Therapy Research*, *2*(1), 12–20.

Plancher, G., Tirard, A., Gyselinck, V., Nicolas, S., & Piolino, P. (2012). Using virtual reality to characterize episodic memory profiles in amnestic mild cognitive impairment and Alzheimer's disease: Influence of active and passive encoding. *Neuropsychologia*, *50*(5), 592–602. doi:10.1016/j.neuropsychologia.2011.12.013 PMID:22261400

Rand, D., Weingarden, H., Weiss, R., Yacoby, A., Reif, S., Malka, R., ... Zeilig, G. (2017). Self-training to improve UE function at the chronic stage post-stroke: A pilot randomized controlled trial. *Disability and Rehabilitation*, *39*(15), 1541–1548. doi:10.1080/09638288.2016.1239766 PMID:27793071

Rendon, A. A., Lohman, E. B., Thorpe, D., Johnson, E. G., Medina, E., & Bradley, B. (2012). The effect of virtual reality gaming on dynamic balance in older adults. *Age and Ageing*, *41*(4), 549–552. doi:10.1093/ageing/afs053 PMID:22672915

Riva, G., Bacchetta, M., Baruffi, M., & Molinari, E. (2001). Virtual reality–based multidimensional therapy for the treatment of body image disturbances in obesity: A controlled study. *Cyberpsychology & Behavior*, *4*(4), 511–526. doi:10.1089/109493101750527079 PMID:11708731

Rizzo, A. S., & Kim, G. J. (2005). A SWOT analysis of the field of virtual reality rehabilitation and therapy. *Presence (Cambridge, Mass.)*, *14*(2), 119–146. doi:10.1162/1054746053967094

Saldana, S. J., Marsh, A. P., Rejeski, W. J., Haberl, J. K., Wu, P., Rosenthal, S., & Ip, E. H. (2017). Assessing balance through the use of a low-cost head-mounted display in older adults: A pilot study. *Clinical Interventions in Aging*, *12*, 1363–1370. doi:10.2147/CIA.S141251 PMID:28883717

Skjæret, N., Nawaz, A., Morat, T., Schoene, D., Helbostad, J. L., & Vereijken, B. (2016). Exercise and rehabilitation delivered through exergames in older adults: An integrative review of technologies, safety and efficacy. *International Journal of Medical Informatics*, *85*(1), 1–16. doi:10.1016/j.ijmedinf.2015.10.008 PMID:26559887

Sweller, J., Van Merrienboer, J. J., & Paas, F. G. (1998). Cognitive architecture and instructional design. *Educational Psychology Review*, *10*(3), 251–296. doi:10.1023/A:1022193728205

Talamo, A., Camilli, M., Di Lucchio, L., & Ventura, S. (2017). Information from the past: How elderly people orchestrate presences, memories and technologies at home. *Universal Access in the Information Society*, *16*(3), 739–753. doi:10.100710209-016-0508-6

Tsang, W. W. N., & Fu, A. S. N. (2016). Virtual reality exercise to improve balance control in older adults at risk of falling. *Hong Kong Medical Journal*, *22*(1 Suppl. 2), S19–S22. doi:10.12809/hkjr1615298 PMID:26908338

Valladares-Rodriguez, S., Perez-Rodriguez, R., Facal, D., Fernandez-Iglesias, M. J., Anido-Rifon, L., & Mourino-Garcia, M. (2017). Design process and preliminary psychometric study of a video game to detect cognitive impairment in senior adults. *PeerJ*, *5*, e3508. doi:10.7717/peerj.3508 PMID:28674661

Vallejo, V., Wyss, P., Rampa, L., Mitache, A. V., Müri, R. M., Mosimann, U. P., & Nef, T. (2017). Evaluation of a novel Serious Game based assessment tool for patients with Alzheimer's disease. *PLoS One*, *12*(5), e0175999. doi:10.1371/journal.pone.0175999 PMID:28472049

Wollersheim, D., Merkes, M., Shields, N., Liamputtong, P., Wallis, L., Reynolds, F., & Koh, L. (2010). Physical and psychosocial effects of Wii video game use among older women. *International Journal of Emerging Technologies and Society*, *8*(2), 85–98.

Yardley, L., & Redfern, M. S. (2001). Psychological factors influencing recovery from balance disorders. *Journal of Anxiety Disorders*, *15*(1-2), 107–119. doi:10.1016/S0887-6185(00)00045-1 PMID:11388354

Yasuda, K., Muroi, D., Ohira, M., & Iwata, H. (2017). Validation of an immersive virtual reality system for training near and far space neglect in individuals with stroke: A pilot study. *Topics in Stroke Rehabilitation*, *24*(7), 533–538. doi:10.1080/10749357.2017.1351069 PMID:28701101

Yeşilyaprak, S. S., Yıldırım, M. Ş., Tomruk, M., Ertekin, Ö., & Algun, Z. C. (2016). Comparison of the effects of virtual reality-based balance exercises and conventional exercises on balance and fall risk in older adults living in nursing homes in Turkey. *Physiotherapy Theory and Practice*, *32*(3), 191–201. do i:10.3109/09593985.2015.1138009 PMID:27049879

Zygouris, S., Giakoumis, D., Votis, K., Doumpoulakis, S., Ntovas, K., Segkouli, S., ... Tsolaki, M. (2015). Can a virtual reality cognitive training application fulfill a dual role? Using the virtual supermarket cognitive training application as a screening tool for mild cognitive impairment. *Journal of Alzheimer's Disease. JAD*, *44*(4), 1333–1347. doi:10.3233/JAD-141260 PMID:25428251

## KEY TERMS AND DEFINITIONS

**Alzheimer's Disease:** Is a neurodegenerative disease that involves short-term memory loss, language disorientation, and other behavioral issues.

**Ecological Validity:** Refers to the extent to which the results of a research could be generalized to the real-life settings.

**Exergame:** A combination of exercise and gaming, exergame are video games that are also a form of exercise.

**Mild Cognitive Impairment:** Is a neurological disorder that happens in older adults and involves cognitive and instrumental activities of daily living impairments.

**Serious Game:** A game that is designed for a primary purpose other than pure entertainment. The serious adjective refers to issues such as defense, education, health care, engineering, and politics.

**Skill Transfer:** Is the concept of exploring how individuals would transfer learning in one context to another one.

**Virtual Reality:** An interactive computer generate experience within a simulate environment and involves different types of sensory feedbacks.

Section 2

# Virtual and Augmented Reality in Mental Health Treatment:

## Pedagogy, Psychology, and Technology

# Chapter 7
# Virtual and Augmented Reality Mirrors for Mental Health Treatment:
## Analysis and Future Directions

**Sergio Casas**
*University of Valencia, Spain*

**Cristina Portalés**
*University of Valencia, Spain*

**Lucía Vera**
*University of Valencia, Spain*

**José Vicente Riera**
*University of Valencia, Spain*

## ABSTRACT

*Virtual and Augmented Reality are technologies widely used in a variety of areas, including the medical sector. On the other hand, regular mirrors have been traditionally used as tools to aid in mental health treatment for a variety of diseases and disorders. Although it is possible to build Virtual and Augmented Reality experiences based on mirror metaphors, there are very few contributions of this kind in the medical sector. In this chapter, the great benefits that regular mirrors have brought for mental health treatment are addressed. In addition, a review on the state of the art in mirror-based Virtual and Augmented Reality applications is given, highlighting the potential benefits that these enhanced mirrors could bring for the mental health treatment.*

DOI: 10.4018/978-1-5225-7168-1.ch007

## INTRODUCTION

A regular mirror can be defined as a special kind of object usually flat and made of polished metal or reflective glass that is capable of reflecting light in such a way that it provides a faithful representation of the objects reflected on it. Mirrors have a natural attraction for human beings since they allow people to see themselves in a third-person view, which is not the one we usually have of our own body, and have been referred to provide uncanny experiences (Rochat & Zahavi, 2011).

Although the daily use of mirrors is commonly associated with cosmetics and superficial activities, they have been used in medical therapy for a long time in order to treat several medical conditions, many of them related to mental health. Pain relief (such as in phantom limb pain (Desmond, O'neill, De Paor, McDarby, & MacLachlan, 2006)), rehabilitation (such as motor rehabilitation or the treatment of patients with cerebral palsy), psychological disorders (such as body dysmorphic disorder or anorexia nervosa) and neurological disorders (such as asomatognosia or mirror agnosia) are some of the areas where Mirror Therapy (MT) has been used in the past, to name a few.

One characteristic of regular mirrors is that they are constrained to reflect a real image of the environment where they are located (although some optical distortion can be applied using curved mirrors) and are thus limited by the physical space and vision angle that the specific set-up offers. Therefore, their potential uses are rather restricted to a set of certain conditions. However, the use of Information Technologies (IT), such as Virtual Reality (VR) or Augmented Reality (AR) can radically change the way mirrors are used in medical therapy, extending their use to other medical problems such as phobias, autism spectrum disorders (ASD) or even neurodegenerative diseases. VR and AR can be presented with many different set-ups, using different display devices and exploiting different interaction paradigms and metaphors. One of these paradigms is the mirror metaphor, by which a VR or AR system is designed to behave like a mirror, regardless of whether it is implemented using an actual mirror or not.

This chapter has three major goals. The first one is to clearly define and classify the different mirror-based IT solutions that are based on either VR or AR. As these enhanced mirrors are relatively new, the literature offers different terminologies for similar proposals, which can be confusing. The chapter will try to clarify the different options and methods that can supply mirror-like images using IT solutions. The second goal is to review the works that already exploit the use of VR and AR mirrors for mental health treatment, reviewing the state of the art. Since the technology is relatively new and the research area of this particular review is restricted to mental health applications, the number of works is relatively small. Nevertheless, they are enough to demonstrate the benefits of this technology and show its potential. Last, but not least, the chapter aims to discuss the possible benefits of these technologies for the treatment of other mental health illnesses, disorders, syndromes, problems and conditions, which are currently not explored with IT solutions. The chapter will try to identify opportunities, strengths, weaknesses and future research lines, so that readers and practitioners get a clearer picture about these devices.

This chapter is organized as follows. In a first place, a short review is given regarding to the use of regular mirrors in mental therapy. In this regard, several illnesses and mental disorders are addressed. Afterwards, the use and potential of VR and AR in mental therapy is discussed. First, the VR and AR mirror metaphors are given, and then a review on the state of the art is provided. The review also covers a few applications of enhanced mirrors to other (mind-related) medical fields, since the number of applications of this technology for mental health is still small. Finally, some conclusions and further directions are outlined.

## THE USE OF REGULAR MIRRORS IN MENTAL THERAPY

Regular mirrors have been traditionally used in a variety of medical therapy applications for a long time, which is referred as Mirror Therapy (MT). In this sense, mirrors have been mainly used in pain relief, rehabilitation, in the treatment of anxiety disorders or in the treatment of phantom limb pain (PLP), among others. Several works have dealt with the use of MT for PLP (Chimes, Bernstein, Cortazzo, & Huber, 2009) and it has been proven to be effective (Chan et al., 2007) in the treatment of this condition, although the amount of pain relief obtained is controversial. MT for PLP and other conditions causing limb impairment is used in patients with unilateral limb impairment (such as unilateral amputation). It consists in the use of a mirror so that the motion of the healthy limb is reflected and creates the illusion that the opposite (impaired or amputated) limb is present or healthy and moves appropriately.

MT in rehabilitation includes the treatment of patients with recovery from hemiparesis (Altschuler et al., 1999; Dohle et al., 2009; Stevens & Stoykov, 2003), cerebral palsy (Feltham, Ledebt, Deconinck, & Savelsbergh, 2010) and motor rehabilitation after a stroke (Rossiter, Borrelli, Borchert, Bradbury, & Ward, 2015; Thieme, Mehrholz, Pohl, Behrens, & Dohle, 2012, 2013), to name a few. For instance, in Harmsen, Bussmann, Selles, Hurkmans, and Ribbers, (2015) 37 participants in chronic stage after a stroke were instructed to perform an upper-arm reaching task as fast and as fluently as possible. In Colomer, Noe, and Rodríguez, (2016) 31 post-stroke chronic subjects with severely impaired upper limb function were evaluated. In Park, Chang, Kim, and Kim, (2015) a group of chronic stroke patients were tested to perform a comparison based in paretic upper-extremity function and hand coordination abilities. In Vural, Yuzer, Ozcan, Ozbudak, and Ozgirgin, (2016) the participants were 30 patients with first-time stroke and simultaneous complex regional pain syndrome type 1 of the upper extremity at the dystrophic stage. The huge amount of research in this topic is an indicator of the benefits that MT brings for patients needing rehabilitation.

Other uses of MT include the treatment of anxiety disorders, such as anorexia nervosa (Key et al., 2002) or body dysmorphic disorder (Windheim, Veale, & Anson, 2011), and other rarer conditions such as mirror agnosia, mirrored-self misidentification or asomatognosia (Connors & Coltheart, 2011; Fotopoulou et al., 2011; Paysant, Beis, Le Chapelain, & André, 2004). For instance, in Probst, (2015) patients with eating disorders, where the body image is a problem, were evaluated. The relationship between mirror exposure and body satisfaction has been widely studied. According to the literature, it has been proved that mirror exposure increases satisfaction in patients with normal weight eating disorder (Hildebrandt, Loeb, Troupe, & Delinsky, 2012), anorexia nervosa (Key et al., 2002), obese adolescents (Jansen et al., 2008), normal weight and overweight in binge eaters (Hilbert, Tuschen-Caffier, & Vögele, 2002) or in body unsatisfied students (Luethcke, McDaniel, & Becker, 2011). For instance, in Jansen et al., (2016) a study is presented that shows that the exposure to one's body using a mirror increases body satisfaction in body-dissatisfied young women. They proved it in two experiment conditions: focusing on attractive body parts and focusing on unattractive body parts. In both cases, mirror exposure led to increasing body satisfaction.

Another study about MT is the one presented in Deconinck et al., (2015), where a review on the effect of mirror visual feedback (MVF) on the brain is presented. This study concludes that MVF can exert a strong influence on the motor network, mainly through increased cognitive penetration in action control.

As it can be seen from the many examples given above, the use of regular mirrors has been proved beneficial for the treatment of a variety of medical conditions and disorders. It can be added that Mirror Therapy has been used for a long time with little economic impact, as mirrors are inexpensive devices.

The question now is if new technologies, such as VR and AR could bring additional benefits to Mirror Therapy, while keeping a simple setup and without increasing costs.

## USE AND POTENTIAL OF VR AND AR MIRRORS IN MENTAL THERAPY

Whereas the application of MT with regular mirrors for mental health treatment is limited to some particular applications due to the small amount of set-ups that can be considered, the combination of mirrors and Information Technologies (IT) provides the possibility of using MT for mental health treatment in many different ways and applications. Unlike a real mirror, which is constrained to its optical and physical properties, the image in a mirror-like IT-based application can be augmented by means of virtual objects (AR mirrors) or can be substituted by a virtual depiction (VR mirrors). Therefore, the possibilities are almost unlimited.

### VR and AR Interaction Paradigms and the Mirror Metaphor

The concept of VR was born around 1930. Already in 1929, E. Link created the Link Trainer, which is considered the first flight simulator, being completely electromechanical. During the same years, the science fiction writer S. G. Weinbaum writes a story (Pygmalion's Spectacles) that contains the idea of a pair of goggles that makes users experience a synthetic world through holograms, smell, taste and touch. He further describes uncanny experiences for those wearing the goggles, aligned with the modern concept of VR. Some years later, M. Heilig developed the Sensorama (patented in 1962), which resembled a kind of arcade-style theatre cabinet. That technology allowed a user seeing stereoscopic films enhanced with seat motion, vibration, stereo sound, wind, and aromas, which were triggered during the films (Heilig, 1962). Since then, many works have arisen that use VR as platforms that support a variety of fields, such as learning and training (Gavish et al., 2015; Gimeno, Fernández, Morillo, Coma, & Pérez, 2007; Pan, Cheok, Yang, Zhu, & Shi, 2006), entertainment (Díaz, Boj, & Portalés, 2016; Vargas González, Kapalo, Koh, & LaViola, 2017), driving and flight simulation (Casas, Coma, Portalés, & Fernández, 2016; Cox et al., 2010; Tudor, Carey, & Dubey, 2015), digital cultural heritage (Gaitatzes, Christopoulos, & Roussou, 2001; Portalés, Alonso-Monasterio, & Viñals, 2017; Richards-Rissetto et al., 2014), and scientific or medical visualizations (Cruz-Neira et al., 1993; Chirico et al., 2016; Moro, Stromberga, & Stirling, 2017), to name just a few.

Overall, VR can be defined as the technology by which one or several individuals experience the sensation of belonging to an alternative reality, which is not the one they are actually living in (outside the VR world). This alternative reality is generated by a computer or by a network of computers and it is important that the participants of this simulated experience accept this virtual synthetic world as a suitable deception of the real world. In this sense, it can be argued that VR is all about perception. For this reason, VR applications need to incorporate visual, aural, gravito-inertial, haptic, tactile, or even olfactive and gustatory perceptual cues (Anthes, García-Hernández, Wiedemann, & Kranzlmüller, 2016) in order to induce a feeling of immersion in the virtual world. However, as a complete recreation of the real world is usually impossible, it is often acceptable that the feeling of immersion and the perception of belonging to this new virtual world be only partial. Some of the characteristics of VR that makes it valuable as a medical tool are (Casas Yrurzum, 2014; Perpiñá, Botella, & Baños, 2003):

- The recreated VR experience is a 'safe environment', since none of the issues can harm patients.
- The fact that, within VR, 'protected' contexts are generated, makes it more feasible to persuade the patient to take the step and enter into action.
- Within VR, it is possible to graduate the situation, progressing from simple to complex settings.
- As events can be synthetically recreated, it is not necessary to wait for those events to take place in the real world.

On the other hand, AR is a technology by which a view of the real world (or even the world itself) is augmented using synthetic images that are superimposed or projected over this image of the real world. However, AR systems need to provide some other features to be considered as true AR applications. The definition currently accepted is that AR systems are those that simultaneously (Azuma, 1997): i) combine virtual and real objects; ii) are completely interactive in real time and iii) are registered in 3D. The interaction and 3D registration are essential features of an AR application since they allow a seamless blending of virtual and augmented objects. AR applications should provide virtual objects that fit in the real world regardless of the position from which the user observes them. AR is a fairly popular technology because it provides a number of advantages that other technologies cannot offer (Bimber & Raskar, 2005):

- *The ability to enhance/augment reality.* By using this technology, physical entities can be enhanced with additional elements, such as images, sounds, virtual models, etc. that are not present in the real scene.
- *Seamless interaction between virtual and real objects.* Interfaces are said to have seams (Ishii, Kobayashi, & Arita, 1994) if there is a functional, temporal, spatial or cognitive element that forces the user to change the way in which he/she interacts with the interface. When using properly designed AR applications, interaction is performed in a natural seamless way, since users can visualize and interact with virtual elements as if they belong to the real environment.
- *It supports a tangible interface.* In AR applications, there is a very intimate relationship between virtual objects and the physical world. Physical objects can be augmented through virtual elements, allowing the overlap of these elements dynamically. These objects can be accessible to all users (public use) or may be individualized for each user (private use), so that particular interactions can be defined for different users. Similarly, physical objects can be used to manipulate virtual elements in an intuitive manner.
- *The presence of spatial cues for face-to-face and remote collaboration.* Augmented Reality allows that the elements generated *in silico* (by a computer) be spatially distributed according to the physical environment.

Perhaps because of these benefits and the increasing capabilities of computers, AR is being widely used in a variety of scenarios such as medical treatment and rehabilitation (Casas, Herrera, Coma, & Fernández, 2012; Tang, Kwoh, Teo, Sing, & Ling, 1998), learning and training (Dunleavy & Dede, 2014; Wu, Lee, Chang, & Liang, 2013), engineering and construction (Boyer, 2009; Gimeno, Morillo, Casas, & Fernández, 2011), entertainment (Díaz et al., 2016), culture heritage (Galatis, Gavalas, Kasapakis, Pantziou, & Zaroliagis, 2016; Gimeno, Portalés, Coma, Fernández, & Martínez, 2017), etc.

The use of mirror metaphors in VR and AR systems leads to VR Mirrors (VRM) and AR Mirrors (ARM). A VRM can be defined as a VR application that displays a virtual depiction of the user's own image on a display device as if that device was a mirror. The virtual depiction can be based on previous photographs of the user or it can be an avatar acting as the person being "reflected" on the VRM, for instance. The fact that the virtual world replicates and communicates with the real world is something that makes VRMs be slightly different from most of the rest of VR applications, where the goal is to extract the user from the real world and teleport them to a different virtual world where there is no communication whatsoever with the real world. VRM are not typically built with actual mirrors, but with computer-based immersive displays that render a mirror-like image of the user.

Augmented Reality Mirrors (ARM) are AR applications in which a real mirror-like real-time image of the user is augmented by means of virtual objects registered in 3D and properly blended with the image of the real environment (Giner Martínez & Portalés Ricart, 2005; Portalés, Gimeno, Casas, Olanda, & Martínez, 2016). The image of the user can be captured by means of a video camera (video-based ARM, e.g. (Giner Martínez & Portalés Ricart, 2005)) or can be produced by a real mirror on which virtual objects are projected (optical-based ARM, e.g. (Alhamid, Eid, & El Saddik, 2012)). Video-based ARMs are more commonly used than optical-based ARMs, because optical setups usually require the use of semi-transparent mirror displays (to create virtual objects with a rear projection) where the blending of virtual and real objects could be difficult, whereas the setup of a video-based ARM typically requires a simple camera and occlusion problems are easier to handle. Education, entertainment and retail are the areas of application where ARMs are more frequently used, although medical therapy has also been explored.

In Figure 1, the mirror metaphors in VR and AR are depicted, in comparison to regular mirrors. As it can be seen, while in an ARM the user sees its own image merged with virtual objects, in a VRM the visual reference to the real environment disappears. Therefore, strictly speaking, face-to-face interaction of users is only possible with the ARM metaphor, although a VRM can eventually simulate that effect. Some works use different terms to refer to VRM or ARM, such as *magic mirror* (Bork et al., 2017; Kim, Lee, & Kim, 2004), *magic face* (Javornik, Rogers, Gander, & Moutinho, 2017), *mixed-reality (MR) mirror* (Sato, Kitahara, & Ohta, 2009) or *real-time mirror* (Gonzalez-Franco, Perez-Marcos, Spanlang, & Slater, 2010). The terms *virtual mirror* or *immersive mirror* are also sometimes used for either VRM or ARM, creating some additional confusion. For this reason, it is important to clarify and define these terms.

*Figure 1. The mirror metaphors in VR and AR: regular mirror, AR mirror and VR mirror*

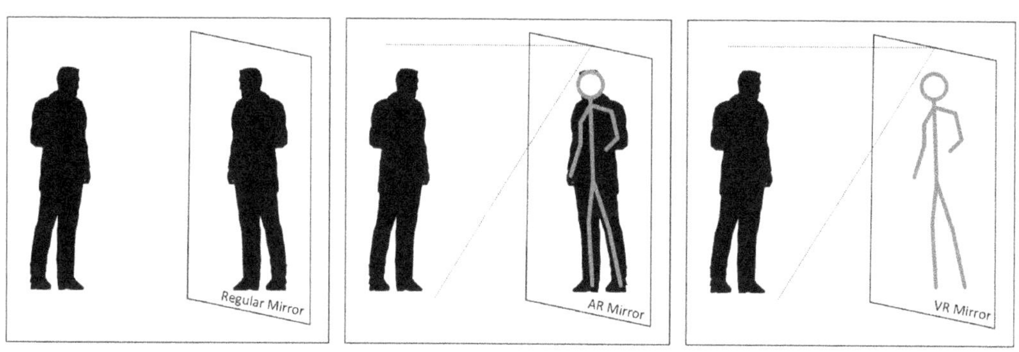

## VR and AR Mirrors in Medical and Mental Therapy

Medicine has been traditionally, and still is, one prominent application area of VR and AR. As computers have gradually invaded our societies with smarter and more computationally efficient devices, the application of IT solutions to medical procedures has become increasingly common. Examples of IT applications in medicine include computer vision and imaging (Doi, 2007), robotics (Taylor & Stoianovici, 2003), database and information systems (Müller, Michoux, Bandon, & Geissbuhler, 2004), and also VR (Krijn, Emmelkamp, Olafsson, & Biemond, 2004; Malloy & Milling, 2010; Rose, Brooks, & Rizzo, 2005) and AR (Chicchi Giglioli, Pallavicini, Pedroli, Serino, & Riva, 2015; Kilgus et al., 2015; Thomas, 2016), to name a few. On the other hand, VRMs and ARMs are typically used in applications for cosmetics, clothing and optical retail, since they provide a way for customers to see how products would look like if they wore them. These *virtual try-on* applications have become very popular for entertainment, commercial or even cultural applications (Javornik et al., 2017), but can be used also for medical purposes. For instance, AR has been used in the field of plastic surgery to depict the results before the intervention of the patient (Ilusio, 2016). This application can be considered as an ARM, since the potential patient is able to see how a particular breast augmentation surgery would result, simply looking at an augmented mirror. Nevertheless, the use of ARMs and VRMs can be extended to other medical areas of application, such as medical treatment for mental disorders, where only a few cases have been reported by the research community up to date, such as Perpiñá et al., (2003), where the VRM paradigm is employed to treat eating disorders (anorexia nervosa and bulimia nervosa) or Mölbert et al., (2018) where a VR mirror scenario is used to analyze desired body weights in patients with anorexia nervosa. Although enhanced mirrors (not only VRMs but also ARMs) could provide a very important role for treating eating disorders, in which the mirror image is usually problematic for patients, there is a clear lack of research in the use of mirrors with IT technologies for these applications.

Since the first X-Ray images were taken back in 1896, a great deal of effort was driven to create devices that allowed physicians to see inside the human body. After Computer Tomography was invented in the 1970s, and MRI became available in the 1980s (Sielhorst, Feuerstein, & Navab, 2008), research for innovative medical imaging procedures focused on the development of VR and AR tools that allowed physicians to obtain more information about the patient's body. In this regard, VR technology can be relevant to reconstruct the human body for educational and training purposes. On the other hand, other research focused on the X-Ray paradigm to obtain see-through images of the body in real time, without having to perform surgical incisions (or making small ones) in the patient's body. In this sense, AR is especially important in microsurgery where minimum invasive techniques are required (being spine and brain surgery the main reference in microsurgery). The smaller the incision the less the surgeon is able to actually see. Thus, the use of AR is fully justified in order to enhance the view of the surgeon. Examples of these ideas can be seen in Birkfellner et al., (2002); Fuchs et al., (1998); Marescaux, Rubino, Arenas, Mutter, and Soler, (2004). A short review can be looked up in Shuhaiber, (2004).

Regarding to VR in the medical sector, many works can be found. For instance, in Connelly et al., (2010) a pneumatic glove was developed for hand rehabilitative training after stroke, that can be used to train grasp-and-release movements either with real objects or with virtual objects. In Hoffman et al., (2011) VR was used as a non-pharmacologic analgesic for some medical procedures (VR used as distraction). In Rizzo, Hartholt, Grimani, Leeds, and Liewer, (2014) a flexible VR system was created that offers significantly enhanced prolonged exposure treatment possibilities to be used as therapy in post-traumatic stress disorders. In Gromala, Tong, Choo, Karamnejad, and Shaw, (2015) a system was developed that includes biofeedback sensors and a virtual environment, which can be used as a form of meditation in order to reduce stress. However, very few examples can be found that use the VRM metaphor in the medical sector, and usually they are not referred as such and/or cannot be considered as pure VRMs, but the described setup indicates that they use some kind of mirror metaphor. For instance, in Johnsen et al., (2005) a projector-based life-sized system was developed that allows medical students to experience the interaction between a patient and a medical doctor – though the student is not represented by an avatar, the setup is similar to a VRM and there is tracking of the student's head and hand movements. On the other hand, in Sucar et al., (2014) a VR-based platform for upper limb rehabilitation was presented. This work uses the rehabilitation exercises as actions within computer games – in this case, only the upper limb is represented in the VRM. Similarly, in Lozano et al., (2005) a VRM is employed for mental practice in post-stroke rehabilitation, where the mirror is also representing the arm and hand which are being rehabilitated, whereas Roosink et al., (2015) uses a virtual mirror to help in physical rehabilitation tasks. A different set-up is the one presented in Liao et al., (2015) where a Wii Fit device is used to improve obstacle-crossing performance and dynamic balance in patients with Parkinson's disease. This setup cannot be considered as a pure VRM, although it somehow acts like a mirror since the Wii Fit tracks the motion of the patient's center of mass, and this motion is then mirrored and shown with a virtual avatar.

Another interesting work is the research presented in Waltemate, Gall, Roth, Botsch, and Latoschik, (2018) where a VRM is utilized to study emotional responses and body ownership with respect to different avatars representing the body of several persons. Although this application is not currently used for the treatment of any particular mental health condition, it could be used in patients with visual agnosia, or for the study of the psychological and psychophysical factors in therapies relying on embodied virtual interfaces. VRMs can also be utilized to analyze or identify racial biases (Groom, Bailenson, & Nass, 2009). It is interesting that racial biases extend beyond digital spaces and these findings could be used to address racial identity problems and racial prejudices with VR applications.

Similarly to VR, there is a variety of AR applications in the medical sector, some built for the treatment of disorders such as phobias (Botella, Bretón-López, Quero, Baños, & García-Palacios, 2010; C. M. Botella et al., 2005; Juan et al., 2005) or cognitive problems (Richard, Billaudeau, Richard, & Gaudin, 2007). AR is being used also for the treatment of PLP, as in Carrino et al., (2014), for cerebral palsy rehabilitation (Correa, Ficheman, do Nascimento, & De Deus Lopes, 2009) or for the treatment of motor impairment (Alamri, Jongeun, & El Saddik, 2010). In summary, the capability of adding virtual objects to the real life environment seems to be a very useful tool for the treatment of a big variety of day-to-day difficulties related to the mind.

Immersive VR (IVR) applications represent another area where VR can be successfully applied in medicine, like in Mathur, (2015); and Won et al., (2017). IVR has many uses in the medical sector, and can be used as a pain distractor (burn wound cleaning, cancer, dental work, etc.) or as an educational tool for children (Bailey & Bailenson, 2018), to name a few. However, the powerful nature of IVR experiences may also pose some risks and should be utilized with caution in children (Won et al., 2017).

IVR can be used as well for the treatment of different specific mental conditions and disorders. For instance, IVR with a Head-Mounted-Display (HMD) has been repeatedly used for the treatment of PLP (Ambron, Miller, Kuchenbecker, Buxbaum, & Coslett, 2018; Bach et al., 2010; Henriksen et al., 2016; Murray et al., 2007; Rodriguez, Aruanno, Bordegoni, Rossini, & Molteni, 2017; Zanfir, Georgescu, Turturica, Eczedi, & Mironiuc, 2017). Although further studies are necessary, it seems that IVR can be effective in the treatment of PLP for some patients (Murray et al., 2009) or at least encourages patient's motivation leading to a potential analgesic effect (Osumi et al., 2017). A deeper study of the effectiveness of these approaches can be found in Herrador Colmenero et al., (2017).

These systems can be considered partial VRM applications, because they are based on the Mirror Therapy. Although the view of the patient is not a third-person view and therefore they do not see a complete mirror image of themselves, the VR application tracks the motion of the healthy limb and (virtually) mirrors these movements to the other limb, creating a mirror effect that enhances the traditional mirror-box therapy used for the treatment of PLP.

Eating disorders can also benefit from immersive VR mirrors (IVRM), such as the experiments described in Riva, Bacchetta, Baruffi, and Molinari, (2001) where virtual mirrors were utilized in patients with bulimia and anorexia nervosa.

There are also immersive ARM applications for the treatment of PLP, like Ortiz-Catalan, Sander, Kristoffersen, Håkansson, and Brånemark, (2014), where a video input is used to track a fiducial marker placed on the amputated arm and several electrodes provide myoelectric signals corresponding to some common movements. This particular application can be used for bilateral amputees since it does not mirror the other limb. However, it can display a mirror image of the patient and, therefore, it can be considered as a true ARM application.

Although some ARM works can be found in other related medical fields, such as anatomy education (Blum, Kleeberger, Bichlmeier, & Navab, 2012; Bork et al., 2017; Kugelmann et al., 2018), it is harder to find ARM systems for medical therapy use, such as Mouraux et al., (2017), where an augmented mirror is used to treat neuropathic pain. There are also some related works, such as Bach et al., (2010); Desmond, O'Neill, Paor, McDarby, & MacLachlan, (2006); Regenbrecht, Franz, McGregor, Dixon, and Hoermann, (2011); and Trojan et al., (2014), although they are partial ARM systems based on adaptations of the Mirror Therapy. They make use of the mirror paradigm but in a first-person fashion instead of allowing the users to see a complete reflected image of themselves. Also, the VirHab system introduced by Feintuch, Tuchner, Lorber-Haddad, Meiner, and Shiri, (2009), targeted at treating pain and impairment of upper extremities, is based on video processing rather than providing a 3D registration of virtual and real objects. An example in which a true ARM is used for medical therapy is the work presented in Lozano-Quilis et al., (2014); and Lozano-Quilis et al., (2013), where a Kinect-based ARM is used in patients with multiple sclerosis. This is one of the very few examples of the use of enhanced mirrors with neurodegenerative diseases, an area where enhanced mirrors are still not commonly used.

One of the most interesting contributions in which the use of both VRM and ARM technologies is combined for mental health therapy can be found in the Pictogram Room (Casas et al., 2012; Herrera, Jordan, & Gimeno, 2006; Orange, 2012). This system was designed to aid children with ASD to advance in basic aspects of the communication (such as joint attention), to improve knowledge about their corporal scheme and to achieve imitation skills. These critical skills can be addressed in an entertaining way, so that children with ASD can learn while playing (see Figure 2). In order to build the mirror methapor in both VR and AR, a back projection screen is present in front of users. The movement of the users is tracked with a Kinect (for both VRM and ARM setups), as well as the image of the real environment (only for the ARM setup). The Pictogram Room is nowadays installed in multiple schools and centres, being a successful case study. In fact, autism disorders are one of the few areas where enhanced mirrors (either VRM or ARM) have been repeatedly proposed for mental health. Several research works can be found in this regard (Bai, 2012; Bai, Blackwell, & Coulouris, 2013; Bhatt, De Leon, & Al-Jumaily, 2014; Chen, Lee, & Lin, 2015). These systems exploit the advantages that augmented or virtual objects can offer to autistic people, which have difficulties with imagination, communication, imitation and self-body recognition. Even the Diminished Reality (DR) paradigm in combination with the mirror metaphor - it could be called Diminished Reality Mirror (DRM) - has been explored (Yantaç, Çorlu, Fjeld, & Kunz, 2015). DR is useful for eliminating, rather than augmenting, elements of the real world that could be distractive for some patients, such as people with autism.

One of the main benefits of the use of VRM/ARM for people with ASD is in the improvement of self-recognition (Escribano, Herrera, Jordan, & Gimeno, 2010) and in the development of their body outline. People with autism and intellectual disabilities tend to show a lack of sense of self-recognition (Ferrari & Matthews, 1983). One of the most used experimental procedures to study the development of self-awareness in young children has been the use of mirrors and the "test of the mark" (Amsterdam, 1972). In this procedure, the child's nose is marked with some kind of mark and using a mirror it is possible to check if the child touches more times his/her own nose than the one in the mirror; in that case it is considered that they have self-recognition. Using VRM and ARM setups it is possible to develop activities to help users acquire these self-identification skills. In addition, with the incorporation of some kind of picture with the body outline in a virtual mirror (controlled and synchronized with the motion of the user in front of it), patients could improve the recognition of his/her body and the understanding and identification of each part of it. Another important aspect where VRMs and ARMs offer significant potential benefits is in the differentiation of oneself with respect to others, in which people with ASD show many difficulties. Using a virtual representation of the patient in the mirror, and integrating elements to facilitate the distinction of each user in the scene, it is possible to develop in the patient the awareness of himself/herself with respect to others. In addition, ARM technologies allow us to easily analyze the salience of the cause-effect reactions of patients with respect to environment changes (such as light intensity, sounds, colors, textures, a blur of the scene, etc.) without having to wait for them to happen.

As seen from the literature review shown above, very few examples exist where the VR and/or AR mirror metaphor is used in mental health therapy. However, successful examples exist, such as the Pictogram Room. In these setups, little has to be invested in hardware technology. Basically, a projector, a screen and a Kinect is enough for both setups. However, building AR and VR experiences is not always trivial, and usually an IT expert is required to deal with modelling, building the virtual environment and implementing the interaction. This fact might be the main reason that makes the use of VRM and ARM in mental therapy more complex than the use of regular mirrors. Therefore, the question is whether the benefits that VR and AR technologies might bring for the medical sector do compensate for the bigger efforts needed to build them.

*Figure 2. Dealing with autism with the ARM developed in Casas et al., (2012), where: in the left image the ARM setup is shown; in the right image, the VRM setup is shown.*

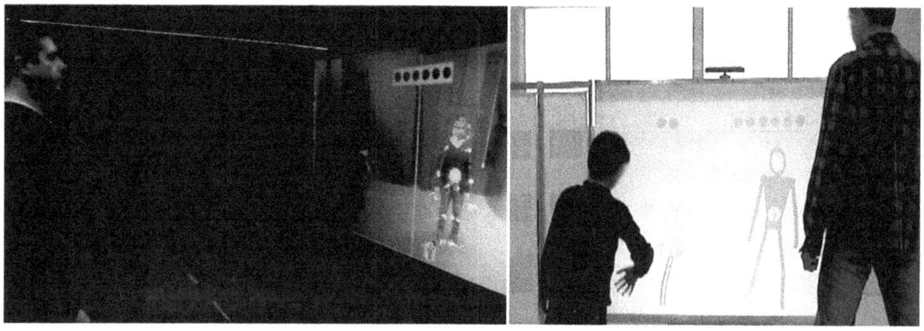

## CONCLUSION AND FUTURE DIRECTIONS

In this chapter, the topic of VR and AR mirrors is studied as an emerging but little explored solution to deal with mental health treatment. As it has been shown through the paper, there is an extensive literature related to the use of regular mirrors in medicine, though when referred to VR and AR mirrors the examples are just a few. From these examples, the Pictogram Room stands out as an application where both mirror metaphors are used (VRM and ARM) to successfully aid children with ASD. In fact, autism-related disorders are one of the few mental-health-related areas in which enhanced mirrors have been repeatedly proposed. Phantom limb pain has been also repeatedly treated with immersive VRM applications; although these latter applications are not complete mirrors but partial interactive mirrors, these systems represent the continuation of the Mirror Therapy through the use of IT technology.

As the VRM and ARM metaphors can bring enhanced experiences to regular mirrors, the authors argue that the combination of mirrors or mirror-like perspectives with the use of the VR and AR paradigms can bring a completely new set of applications and therapies, and can enhance and improve the traditional uses of medical therapy. However, because of the very few examples found in the literature, the authors believe that the potential of VRM and ARM systems for medical therapy is not being fully exploited, probably because not all the medical therapies require a mirror image, and simpler VR or AR systems are sufficient in most cases where IT solutions are employed, or maybe because the shortcomings of current technology prevent to achieve better results. Regarding to costs, the hardware technology needed to build VRMs or ARMs is not cumbersome. However, the need of an IT expert to build the experiences can increase costs. In this sense, one has to value the potential benefits that AR and VR might bring compared to regular mirrors, and decide if it is worth investing on that.

Besides, ARM and VRM can radically change the way mirrors are used in medical therapy, extending their use to other medical problems where Mirror Therapy is still not commonly used, such as phobias, eating disorders, or even neurodegenerative diseases. For instance, an ARM application could be used to depict an entire image of oneself but with other virtual elements that cause phobias, such as insects or animals – this purpose has been explored in AR, but not with the use of a mirror metaphor. In this case, an application could be built where the doctor could choose between different virtual elements (spiders, snakes, rats, etc.), select the number of elements (one, tens, hundreds, etc.), select the kind of followed path (around the user, on its head, on its hands, etc.), select the time, the speed, etc.

Another potential use would be to treat eating disorders. In this sense, the image of the patient could be easily distorted (enlarged, widen, etc.), only processing the video feed of a camera. In this way, an application could be built where doctors could choose the degree of distortion, and interactively modify it according to the patient's feedback. In this particular case, the IT application is extremely simple and it would be as having hundreds of regular mirrors embedded in a single application, so the cost/benefit ratio would be optimal compared to regular mirrors. More sophisticated applications with ARMs or VRMs (such as in Perpiñá et al., (2003) could be also built. A possible set-up could include an avatar with the face of the patient, which could gain or lose weight. In this case, the doctor could choose to show the avatar with a specific weight (50 Kg, 100 Kg, etc.).

Another possible use for mental therapy would be to reinforce the personality of patients by providing an enhanced image of themselves. The influence that a change of the perceived oneself image might bring in oneself behavior in AR experiences has been reported through artistic pieces (Giner Martínez & Portalés Ricart, 2005; Portalés Ricart, 2009), but not yet in the medical sector. For instance, with VR and/or AR technology one can be a superhero, a famous actor, a composer, etc. Even, a change in gender (for the treatment of gender dysphoria) and/or race (for racial identity disorders) can be explored. In the case of the VRM paradigm, a complete avatar would replace the user's body, whereas in an ARM the patients' body would be complimented with virtual elements that transform them in a new person. Therefore, imagine an application were the doctor could choose between different persons to infer in the way patients perceive themselves and thus modify certain aspects of their behavior.

On the other hand, it has to be pointed out that an additional reason on why these systems are not fully exploited might be that the medical community is not fully aware of the last advances in AR and VR, the benefits that they might bring, and the possibility to build a mirror metaphor within them. Therefore, it is in the aim of this chapter to serve as a catalyzer to boost new applications in this field.

## REFERENCES

Alamri, A., Jongeun, C., & El Saddik, A. (2010). AR-REHAB: An Augmented Reality Framework for Poststroke-Patient Rehabilitation. *IEEE Transactions on* Instrumentation and Measurement, *59*(10), 2554–2563. doi:10.1109/tim.2010.2057750

Alhamid, M. F., Eid, M., & El Saddik, A. (2012, May 18-19). A multi-modal intelligent system for biofeedback interactions. *Paper presented at the 2012 IEEE International Symposium on Medical Measurements and Applications Proceedings (MeMeA).*

Altschuler, E. L., Wisdom, S. B., Stone, L., Foster, C., Galasko, D., Llewellyn, D. M. E., & Ramachandran, V. S. (1999). Rehabilitation of hemiparesis after stroke with a mirror. *Lancet*, *353*(9169), 2035–2036. doi:10.1016/S0140-6736(99)00920-4 PMID:10376620

Ambron, E., Miller, A., Kuchenbecker, K. J., Buxbaum, L. J., & Coslett, H. (2018). Immersive low-cost Virtual reality Treatment for Phantom limb Pain: Evidence from Two cases. *Frontiers in Neurology*, *9*, 67. doi:10.3389/fneur.2018.00067 PMID:29515513

Amsterdam, B. (1972). Mirror self-image reactions before age two. *Developmental Psychobiology*, *5*(4), 297–305. doi:10.1002/dev.420050403 PMID:4679817

Anthes, C., García-Hernández, R. J., Wiedemann, M., & Kranzlmüller, D. (2016). State of the art of virtual reality technology. *Paper presented at the 2016 IEEE Aerospace Conference.* 10.1109/AERO.2016.7500674

Azuma, R. T. (1997). A Survey of Augmented Reality. *Presence (Cambridge, Mass.)*, *6*(4), 355–385. doi:10.1162/pres.1997.6.4.355

Bach, F., Schmitz, B., Maaß, H., Çakmak, H., & Diers, M., B-Bodmann, R. … Flor, H. (2010). Using interactive immersive VR/AR for the therapy of phantom limb pain. *Paper presented at the 13th International Conference on Humans and Computers.*

Bai, Z. (2012). Augmenting imagination for children with autism. *Paper presented at the 11th International Conference on Interaction Design and Children.*

Bai, Z., Blackwell, A. F., & Coulouris, G. (2013). Through the looking glass: Pretend play for children with autism. *Paper presented at the 2013 IEEE International Symposium on Mixed and augmented reality (ISMAR).* 10.1109/ISMAR.2013.6671763

Bailey, J. O., & Bailenson, J. N. (2018). *Immersive Virtual Reality and the Developing Child. In Cognitive Development in Digital Contexts* (pp. 181–200). Elsevier.

Bhatt, S., De Leon, N., & Al-Jumaily, A. (2014). Augmented reality game therapy for children with autism spectrum disorder. *International Journal on Smart Sensing and Intelligent Systems*, *7*(2), 519–536. doi:10.21307/ijssis-2017-668

Bimber, O., & Raskar, R. (2005). *Spatial Augmented Reality: Merging Real and Virtual Worlds*. A. K. Peters, Ltd. doi:10.1201/b10624

Birkfellner, W., Figl, M., Huber, K., Watzinger, F., Wanschitz, F., Hummel, J., ... Bergmann, H. (2002). A head-mounted operating binocular for augmented reality visualization in medicine--design and initial evaluation. *IEEE Transactions on Medical Imaging*, *21*(8), 991–997. doi:10.1109/TMI.2002.803099 PMID:12472271

Blum, T., Kleeberger, V., Bichlmeier, C., & Navab, N. (2012). mirracle: An augmented reality magic mirror system for anatomy education. In *Virtual Reality Conference*, Costa Mesa, CA. doi: http://doi.ieeecomputersociety.org/10.1109/VR.2012.6180909 doi:10.1109/VR.2012.6180909

Bork, F., Barmaki, R., Eck, U., Yu, K., Sandor, C., & Navab, N. (2017). Empirical Study of Non-Reversing Magic Mirrors for Augmented Reality Anatomy Learning. *Paper presented at the 2017 IEEE International Symposium on Mixed and Augmented Reality (ISMAR)*. 10.1109/ISMAR.2017.33

Botella, C., Bretón-López, J., Quero, S., Baños, R., & García-Palacios, A. (2010). Treating cockroach phobia with augmented reality. *Behavior Therapy*, *41*(3), 401–413. doi:10.1016/j.beth.2009.07.002 PMID:20569788

Botella, C. M., Juan, M. C., Banos, R. M., Alcaniz, M., Guillen, V., & Rey, B. (2005). Mixing realities? An application of augmented reality for the treatment of cockroach phobia. *Cyberpsychology & Behavior*, *8*(2), 162–171. doi:10.1089/cpb.2005.8.162 PMID:15938656

Boyer, S. A. (2009). *SCADA: supervisory control and data acquisition*. International Society of Automation.

Carrino, F., Rizzotti, D., Gheorghe, C., Kabasu Bakajika, P., Francescotti-Paquier, F., & Mugellini, E. (2014). Augmented Reality Treatment for Phantom Limb Pain. In R. Shumaker & S. Lackey (Eds.), *Virtual, Augmented and Mixed Reality. Applications of Virtual and Augmented Reality* (pp. 248–257). Springer International Publishing. doi:10.1007/978-3-319-07464-1_23

Casas, S., Coma, I., Portalés, C., & Fernández, M. (2016). Towards a simulation-based tuning of motion cueing algorithms. *Simulation Modelling Practice and Theory*, *67*, 137–154. doi:10.1016/j.simpat.2016.06.002

Casas, X., Herrera, G., Coma, I., & Fernández, M. (2012). A Kinect-based augmented reality system for individuals with autism spectrum disorders. *Paper presented at the Computer Graphics Theory and Applications*, Rome, Italy.

Casas Yrurzum, S. (2014). *Mejoras en la generación de claves gravito-inerciales en simuladores de vehículos no aéreos [PhD thesis]*. Universitat de València.

Chan, B. L., Witt, R., Charrow, A. P., Magee, A., Howard, R., Pasquina, P. F., ... Tsao, J. W. (2007). Mirror Therapy for Phantom Limb Pain. *The New England Journal of Medicine*, *357*(21), 2206–2207. doi:10.1056/NEJMc071927 PMID:18032777

Chen, C.-H., Lee, I.-J., & Lin, L.-Y. (2015). Augmented reality-based self-facial modeling to promote the emotional expression and social skills of adolescents with autism spectrum disorders. *Research in Developmental Disabilities*, *36*, 396–403. doi:10.1016/j.ridd.2014.10.015 PMID:25462499

Chicchi Giglioli, I. A., Pallavicini, F., Pedroli, E., Serino, S., & Riva, G. (2015). Augmented reality: A brand new challenge for the assessment and treatment of psychological disorders. *Computational and Mathematical Methods in Medicine*. PMID:26339283

Chimes, G. P., Bernstein, C. D., Cortazzo, M. H., & Huber, L. M. (2009). Poster presentation. *PM & R*, *1*(9 Suppl.), S220. doi:10.1016/j.pmrj.2009.08.290

Chirico, A., Lucidi, F., De Laurentiis, M., Milanese, C., Napoli, A., & Giordano, A. (2016). Virtual Reality in Health System: Beyond Entertainment. A Mini-Review on the Efficacy of VR During Cancer Treatment. *Journal of Cellular Physiology*, *231*(2), 275–287. doi:10.1002/jcp.25117 PMID:26238976

Colomer, C., Noe, E., & Rodríguez, R. L. (2016). Mirror therapy in chronic stroke survivors with severely impaired upper limb function: a randomized controlled trial. *Paper presented at the European journal of physical and rehabilitation medicine*.

Connelly, L., Jia, Y., Toro, M. L., Stoykov, M. E., Kenyon, R. V., & Kamper, D. G. (2010). A pneumatic glove and immersive virtual reality environment for hand rehabilitative training after stroke. *IEEE Transactions on Neural Systems and Rehabilitation Engineering*, *18*(5), 551–559. doi:10.1109/TNSRE.2010.2047588 PMID:20378482

Connors, M. H., & Coltheart, M. (2011). On the behaviour of senile dementia patients vis-à-vis the mirror: Ajuriaguerra, Strejilevitch and Tissot (1963). *Neuropsychologia*, *49*(7), 1679–1692. doi:10.1016/j.neuropsychologia.2011.02.041 PMID:21356221

Correa, A. G. D., Ficheman, I. K., do Nascimento, M., & De Deus Lopes, R. (2009, 15-17 July 2009). Computer assisted music therapy: a case study of an augmented reality musical system for children with cerebral palsy rehabilitation. *Paper presented at the Ninth IEEE International Conference on Advanced Learning Technologies ICALT 2009*.

Cox, D. J., Davis, M., Singh, H., Barbour, B., Nidiffer, F. D., Trudel, T., ... Moncrief, R. (2010). Driving rehabilitation for military personnel recovering from traumatic brain injury using virtual reality driving simulation: A feasibility study. *Military Medicine*, *175*(6), 411–416. doi:10.7205/MILMED-D-09-00081 PMID:20572473

Cruz-Neira, C., Leigh, J., Papka, M., Barnes, C., Cohen, S. M., Das, S., . . . Siegel, L. (1993). Scientists in wonderland: A report on visualization applications in the CAVE virtual reality environment. *Paper presented at the IEEE 1993 Symposium on Research Frontiers in Virtual Reality*. 10.1109/VRAIS.1993.378262

Deconinck, F. J., Smorenburg, A. R., Benham, A., Ledebt, A., Feltham, M. G., & Savelsbergh, G. J. (2015). Reflections on mirror therapy: A systematic review of the effect of mirror visual feedback on the brain. *Neurorehabilitation and Neural Repair*, *29*(4), 349–361. doi:10.1177/1545968314546134 PMID:25160567

Desmond, D. M., O'neill, K., De Paor, A., McDarby, G., & MacLachlan, M. (2006). Augmenting the reality of phantom limbs: Three case studies using an augmented mirror box procedure. *JPO: Journal of Prosthetics and Orthotics*, *18*(3), 74–79.

Desmond, D. M., O'Neill, K., Paor, A. D., McDarby, G., & MacLachlan, M. (2006). Augmenting the Reality of Phantom Limbs: Three Case Studies Using an Augmented Mirror Box Procedure. *Journal of Prosthetics and Orthotics*, *18*(3), 74–79. doi:10.1097/00008526-200607000-00005

Díaz, D., Boj, C., & Portalés, C. (2016). HybridPLAY: A New Technology to Foster Outdoors Physical Activity, Verbal Communication and Teamwork. *Sensors (Basel)*, *16*(4), 586. doi:10.339016040586 PMID:27120601

Dohle, C., Pullen, J., Nakaten, A., Kust, J., Rietz, C., & Karbe, H. (2009). Mirror therapy promotes recovery from severe hemiparesis: A randomized controlled trial. *Neurorehabilitation and Neural Repair*, *23*(3), 209–217. doi:10.1177/1545968308324786 PMID:19074686

Doi, K. (2007). Computer-Aided Diagnosis in Medical Imaging: Historical Review, Current Status and Future Potential. *Computerized Medical Imaging and Graphics*, *31*(4-5), 198–211. doi:10.1016/j.compmedimag.2007.02.002

Dunleavy, M., & Dede, C. (2014). *Augmented reality teaching and learning. In Handbook of research on educational communications and technology* (pp. 735–745). Springer. doi:10.1007/978-1-4614-3185-5_59

Escribano, L. R., Herrera, G., Jordan, R., & Gimeno, J. (2010). Pictogram-Room: uso de la realidad aumentada para el aprendizaje visual de personas con Autismo. *Paper presented at the Investigaciones sobre autismo en español: problemas y perspectivas.*

Feintuch, U., Tuchner, M., Lorber-Haddad, A., Meiner, Z., & Shiri, S. (2009, June 29-July 2). VirHab - A virtual reality system for treatment of chronic pain and disability. *Paper presented at the Virtual Rehabilitation International Conference.*

Feltham, M. G., Ledebt, A., Deconinck, F. J. A., & Savelsbergh, G. J. P. (2010). Mirror visual feedback induces lower neuromuscular activity in children with spastic hemiparetic cerebral palsy. *Research in Developmental Disabilities*, *31*(6), 1525–1535. doi:10.1016/j.ridd.2010.06.004 PMID:20591615

Ferrari, M., & Matthews, W. S. (1983). Self-recognition deficits in autism: Syndrome-specific or general developmental delay? *Journal of Autism and Developmental Disorders*, *13*(3), 317–324. doi:10.1007/BF01531569 PMID:6196346

Fotopoulou, A., Jenkinson, P. M., Tsakiris, M., Haggard, P., Rudd, A., & Kopelman, M. D. (2011). Mirror-view reverses somatoparaphrenia: Dissociation between first- and third-person perspectives on body ownership. *Neuropsychologia, 49*(14), 3946–3955. doi:10.1016/j.neuropsychologia.2011.10.011 PMID:22023911

Fuchs, H., Livingston, M., Raskar, R., Colucci, D. n., Keller, K., State, A., . . . Meyer, A. (1998). Augmented reality visualization for laparoscopic surgery. In W. Wells, A. Colchester & S. Delp (Eds.), Medical Image Computing and Computer-Assisted Interventation — MICCAI'98 (pp. 934-943). Springer. doi:10.1007/BFb0056282

Gaitatzes, A., Christopoulos, D., & Roussou, M. (2001). Reviving the past: cultural heritage meets virtual reality. *Paper presented at the 2001 conference on Virtual reality, archeology, and cultural heritage.* 10.1145/584993.585011

Galatis, P., Gavalas, D., Kasapakis, V., Pantziou, G., & Zaroliagis, C. (2016). Mobile augmented reality guides in cultural heritage. *Paper presented at the 8th EAI International Conference on Mobile Computing, Applications and Services.* 10.4108/eai.30-11-2016.2266954

Gavish, N., Gutiérrez, T., Webel, S., Rodríguez, J., Peveri, M., Bockholt, U., & Tecchia, F. (2015). Evaluating virtual reality and augmented reality training for industrial maintenance and assembly tasks. *Interactive Learning Environments, 23*(6), 778–798. doi:10.1080/10494820.2013.815221

Gimeno, J., Fernández, M., Morillo, P., Coma, I., & Pérez, M. (2007). A reconfigurable immersive workbench and wall-system for designing and training in 3D environments. *Virtual Reality*, 458–467.

Gimeno, J., Morillo, P., Casas, S., & Fernández, M. (2011). An augmented reality (AR) CAD system at construction sites. In *Augmented Reality-Some Emerging Application Areas*. InTech.

Gimeno, J., Portalés, C., Coma, I., Fernández, M., & Martínez, B. (2017). Combining Traditional and Indirect Augmented Reality for Indoor Crowded Environments. A Case Study on the Casa Batlló Museum. *Computers & Graphics, 69*, 92–103. doi:10.1016/j.cag.2017.09.001

Giner Martínez, F., & Portalés Ricart, C. (2005, October 3-7). The Augmented User: A Wearable Augmented Reality Interface. *Paper presented at the International Conference on Virtual Systems and Multimedia (VSMM'05)*, Ghent, Belgium.

Gonzalez-Franco, M., Perez-Marcos, D., Spanlang, B., & Slater, M. (2010). The contribution of real-time mirror reflections of motor actions on virtual body ownership in an immersive virtual environment. *Paper presented at the 2010 IEEE Virtual Reality Conference (VR).* 10.1109/VR.2010.5444805

Gromala, D., Tong, X., Choo, A., Karamnejad, M., & Shaw, C. D. (2015). The Virtual Meditative Walk: Virtual Reality Therapy for Chronic Pain Management. *Paper presented at the 33rd Annual ACM Conference on Human Factors in Computing Systems*, Seoul, Republic of Korea. 10.1145/2702123.2702344

Groom, V., Bailenson, J. N., & Nass, C. (2009). The influence of racial embodiment on racial bias in immersive virtual environments. *Social Influence, 4*(3), 231–248. doi:10.1080/15534510802643750

Harmsen, W. J., Bussmann, J. B., Selles, R. W., Hurkmans, H. L., & Ribbers, G. M. (2015). A mirror therapy–based action observation protocol to improve motor learning after stroke. *Neurorehabilitation and Neural Repair*, *29*(6), 509–516. doi:10.1177/1545968314558598 PMID:25416737

Henriksen, B., Nielsen, R., Szabo, L., Evers, N., Kraus, M., & Geng, B. (2016). An affordable virtual reality system for treatment of phantom limb pain. *Paper presented at the 2016 Virtual Reality International Conference*. 10.1145/2927929.2927932

Herrador Colmenero, L., Perez Marmol, J. M., Martí-García, C., Querol Zaldivar, M. Á., Tapia Haro, R. M., Castro Sánchez, A. M., & Aguilar-Ferrándiz, M. E. (2017). Effectiveness of mirror therapy, motor imagery, and virtual feedback on phantom limb pain following amputation: A systematic review. *Prosthetics and Orthotics International*. PMID:29153043

Herrera, G., Jordan, R., & Gimeno, J. (2006). Exploring the advantages of augmented reality for intervention in autism spectrum disorders. *Paper presented at the Second World Autism Congress*, Cape Town, South Africa.

Hilbert, A., Tuschen-Caffier, B., & Vögele, C. (2002). Effects of prolonged and repeated body image exposure in binge-eating disorder. *Journal of Psychosomatic Research*, *52*(3), 137–144. doi:10.1016/S0022-3999(01)00314-2 PMID:11897232

Hildebrandt, T., Loeb, K., Troupe, S., & Delinsky, S. (2012). Adjunctive mirror exposure for eating disorders: A randomized controlled pilot study. *Behaviour Research and Therapy*, *50*(12), 797–804. doi:10.1016/j.brat.2012.09.004 PMID:23089085

Hoffman, H. G., Chambers, G. T., Meyer, I. I. I. W. J., Arceneaux, L. L., Russell, W. J., Seibel, E. J., ... Patterson, D. R. (2011). Virtual reality as an adjunctive non-pharmacologic analgesic for acute burn pain during medical procedures. *Annals of Behavioral Medicine*, *41*(2), 183–191. doi:10.100712160-010-9248-7 PMID:21264690

Ilusio. (2016). Augmented Reality Could Revolutionize Plastic Surgery. Retrieved from http://www.illusioimaging.com/

Ishii, H., Kobayashi, M., & Arita, K. (1994). Iterative design of seamless collaboration media. *Communications of the ACM*, *37*(8), 83–97. doi:10.1145/179606.179687

Jansen, A., Bollen, D., Tuschen-Caffier, B., Roefs, A., Tanghe, A., & Braet, C. (2008). Mirror exposure reduces body dissatisfaction and anxiety in obese adolescents: A pilot study. *Appetite*, *51*(1), 214–217. doi:10.1016/j.appet.2008.01.011 PMID:18342397

Jansen, A., Voorwinde, V., Hoebink, Y., Rekkers, M., Martijn, C., & Mulkens, S. (2016). Mirror exposure to increase body satisfaction: Should we guide the focus of attention towards positively or negatively evaluated body parts? *Journal of Behavior Therapy and Experimental Psychiatry*, *50*, 90–96. doi:10.1016/j.jbtep.2015.06.002 PMID:26117584

Javornik, A., Rogers, Y., Gander, D., & Moutinho, A. (2017). MagicFace: Stepping into character through an augmented reality mirror. *Paper presented at the 2017 CHI Conference on Human Factors in Computing Systems*. 10.1145/3025453.3025722

Johnsen, K., Dickerson, R., Raij, A., Lok, B., Jackson, J., Min, S., . . . Lind, D. S. (2005, March 12-16). Experiences in using immersive virtual characters to educate medical communication skills. *Paper presented at the IEEE Proceedings Virtual Reality*.

Juan, M. C., Alcaniz, M., Monserrat, C., Botella, C., Banos, R. M., & Guerrero, B. (2005). Using Augmented Reality to Treat Phobias. *IEEE Computer Graphics and Applications*, *25*(6), 31–37. doi:10.1109/MCG.2005.143 PMID:16315475

Key, A., George, C. L., Beattie, D., Stammers, K., Lacey, H., & Waller, G. (2002). Body image treatment within an inpatient program for anorexia nervosa: The role of mirror exposure in the desensitization process. *International Journal of Eating Disorders*, *31*(2), 185–190. doi:10.1002/eat.10027 PMID:11920979

Kilgus, T., Heim, E., Haase, S., Prüfer, S., Müller, M., Seitel, A., ... Schlemmer, H.-P. (2015). Mobile markerless augmented reality and its application in forensic medicine. *International Journal of Computer Assisted Radiology and Surgery*, *10*(5), 573–586. doi:10.100711548-014-1106-9 PMID:25149272

Kim, I.-J., Lee, H. J., & Kim, H.-G. (2004). Magic mirror: a new VR platform design and its applications. *Paper presented at the 2004 ACM SIGCHI International Conference on Advances in computer entertainment technology*, Singapore. 10.1145/1067343.1067394

Krijn, M., Emmelkamp, P. M. G., Olafsson, R. P., & Biemond, R. (2004). Virtual reality exposure therapy of anxiety disorders: A review. *Clinical Psychology Review*, *24*(3), 259–281. doi:10.1016/j.cpr.2004.04.001 PMID:15245832

Kugelmann, D., Stratmann, L., Nühlen, N., Bork, F., Hoffmann, S., Samarbarksh, G., ... Fallavollita, P. (2018). An Augmented Reality magic mirror as additive teaching device for gross anatomy. *Annals of Anatomy-Anatomischer Anzeiger*, *215*, 71–77. doi:10.1016/j.aanat.2017.09.011 PMID:29017852

Liao, Y.-Y., Yang, Y.-R., Cheng, S.-J., Wu, Y.-R., Fuh, J.-L., & Wang, R.-Y. (2015). Virtual reality–based training to improve obstacle-crossing performance and dynamic balance in patients with Parkinson's disease. *Neurorehabilitation and Neural Repair*, *29*(7), 658–667. doi:10.1177/1545968314562111 PMID:25539782

Lozano, J. A., Montesa, J., Juan, M. C., Alcañiz, M., Rey, B., Gil, J., . . . Morganti, F. (2005). VR-mirror: a virtual reality system for mental practice in post-stroke rehabilitation. *Paper presented at the International Symposium on Smart Graphics*. 10.1007/11536482_23

Lozano-Quilis, J.-A., Gil-Gomez, H., Gil-Gómez, J.-A., Albiol-Perez, S., Palacios, G., Fardoum, H. M., & Mashat, A. S. (2013). Virtual reality system for multiple sclerosis rehabilitation using KINECT. *Paper presented at the 2013 7th International Conference on Pervasive Computing Technologies for Healthcare (PervasiveHealth)*. 10.4108/icst.pervasivehealth.2013.252208

Lozano-Quilis, J.-A., Gil-Gómez, H., Gil-Gómez, J.-A., Albiol-Pérez, S., Palacios-Navarro, G., Fardoun, H. M., & Mashat, A. S. (2014). Virtual rehabilitation for multiple sclerosis using a kinect-based system: randomized controlled trial. *JMIR serious games, 2*(2).

Luethcke, C. A., McDaniel, L., & Becker, C. B. (2011). A comparison of mindfulness, nonjudgmental, and cognitive dissonance-based approaches to mirror exposure. *Body Image*, *8*(3), 251–258. doi:10.1016/j.bodyim.2011.03.006 PMID:21561817

Malloy, K. M., & Milling, L. S. (2010). The effectiveness of virtual reality distraction for pain reduction: A systematic review. *Clinical Psychology Review*, *30*(8), 1011–1018. doi:10.1016/j.cpr.2010.07.001 PMID:20691523

Marescaux, J., Rubino, F., Arenas, M., Mutter, D., & Soler, L. (2004, November 10). Augmented-reality-assisted laparoscopic adrenalectomy. *Journal of the American Medical Association*, *292*(18), 2214–2215. PMID:15536106

Mathur, A. S. (2015). Low cost virtual reality for medical training. *Paper presented at the 2015 IEEE Virtual Reality (VR)*. 10.1109/VR.2015.7223437

Mölbert, S., Thaler, A., Mohler, B., Streuber, S., Romero, J., Black, M., ... Giel, K. (2018). Assessing body image in anorexia nervosa using biometric self-avatars in virtual reality: Attitudinal components rather than visual body size estimation are distorted. *Psychological Medicine*, *48*(4), 642–653. doi:10.1017/S0033291717002008 PMID:28745268

Moro, C., Stromberga, Z., & Stirling, A. (2017). Virtualisation devices for student learning: Comparison between desktop-based (Oculus Rift) and mobile-based (Gear VR) virtual reality in medical and health science education. *Australasian Journal of Educational Technology*, *33*(6). doi:10.14742/ajet.3840

Mouraux, D., Brassinne, E., Sobczak, S., Nonclercq, A., Warzée, N., Sizer, P. S., ... Penelle, B. (2017). 3D augmented reality mirror visual feedback therapy applied to the treatment of persistent, unilateral upper extremity neuropathic pain: A preliminary study. *The Journal of Manual & Manipulative Therapy*, *25*(3), 137–143. doi:10.1080/10669817.2016.1176726 PMID:28694676

Müller, H., Michoux, N., Bandon, D., & Geissbuhler, A. (2004). A review of content-based image retrieval systems in medical applications—clinical benefits and future directions. *International Journal of Medical Informatics*, *73*(1), 1–23. doi:10.1016/j.ijmedinf.2003.11.024 PMID:15036075

Murray, C. D., Pettifer, S., Howard, T., Patchick, E., Caillette, F., & Murray, J. (2009). *Virtual solutions to phantom problems: Using immersive virtual reality to treat phantom limb pain. In Amputation, Prosthesis Use, and Phantom Limb Pain* (pp. 175–196). Springer.

Murray, C. D., Pettifer, S., Howard, T., Patchick, E. L., Caillette, F., Kulkarni, J., & Bamford, C. (2007). The treatment of phantom limb pain using immersive virtual reality: Three case studies. *Disability and Rehabilitation*, *29*(18), 1465–1469. doi:10.1080/09638280601107385 PMID:17729094

Orange España. (2012). Pictogram Room: juegos educativos para autism [YouTube video]. Retrieved from https://www.youtube.com/watch?v=5B4mKPdBbtE

Ortiz-Catalan, M., Sander, N., Kristoffersen, M. B., Håkansson, B., & Brånemark, R. (2014). Treatment of phantom limb pain (PLP) based on augmented reality and gaming controlled by myoelectric pattern recognition: A case study of a chronic PLP patient. *Frontiers in Neuroscience*, *8*, 24. doi:10.3389/fnins.2014.00024 PMID:24616655

Osumi, M., Ichinose, A., Sumitani, M., Wake, N., Sano, Y., Yozu, A., ... Morioka, S. (2017). Restoring movement representation and alleviating phantom limb pain through short-term neurorehabilitation with a virtual reality system. *European Journal of Pain (London, England), 21*(1), 140–147. doi:10.1002/ejp.910 PMID:27378656

Pan, Z., Cheok, A. D., Yang, H., Zhu, J., & Shi, J. (2006). Virtual reality and mixed reality for virtual learning environments. *Computers & Graphics, 30*(1), 20–28. doi:10.1016/j.cag.2005.10.004

Park, J.-Y., Chang, M., Kim, K.-M., & Kim, H.-J. (2015). The effect of mirror therapy on upper-extremity function and activities of daily living in stroke patients. *Journal of Physical Therapy Science, 27*(6), 1681–1683. doi:10.1589/jpts.27.1681 PMID:26180297

Paysant, J., Beis, J. M., Le Chapelain, L., & André, J. M. (2004). Mirror asomatognosia in right lesions stroke victims. *Neuropsychologia, 42*(7), 920–925. doi:10.1016/j.neuropsychologia.2003.12.001 PMID:14998706

Perpiñá, C., Botella, C., & Baños, R. (2003). Virtual reality in eating disorders. *European Eating Disorders Review, 11*(3), 261–278. doi:10.1002/erv.520

Portalés, C., Alonso-Monasterio, P., & Viñals, M. J. (2017). 3D virtual reconstruction and visualisation of the archaeological site Castellet de Bernabé (Llíria, Spain). *Virtual Archaeology Review, 8*(16). doi:10.4995/var.2017.5890

Portalés, C., Gimeno, J., Casas, S., Olanda, R., & Martínez, F. G. (2016). Interacting with Augmented Reality Mirrors. In Handbook of Research on Human-Computer Interfaces, Developments, and Applications (pp. 216–244). Hershey, PA: IGI Global.

Portalés Ricart, C. (2009). *Entornos multimedia de realidad aumentada en el campo del arte* [Doctoral Thesis]. Universidad Politécnica de Valencia, Valencia.

Probst, M. (2015). Body image therapy for patients with eating disorders: scientific and clinical perspectives.

Regenbrecht, H. T., Franz, E. A., McGregor, G., Dixon, B. G., & Hoermann, S. (2011). Beyond the Looking Glass: Fooling the Brain with the Augmented Mirror Box. *Presence, 20*(6), 559–576. doi:10.1162/PRES_a_00082

Richard, E., Billaudeau, V., Richard, P., & Gaudin, G. (2007, September 27-29). Augmented Reality for Rehabilitation of Cognitive Disabled Children: A Preliminary Study. *Paper presented at the Virtual Rehabilitation, 2007.*

Richards-Rissetto, H., Robertsson, J., von Schwerin, J., Agugiaro, G., Remondino, F., & Girardi, G. (2014). Geospatial virtual heritage: a gesture-based 3D GIS to engage the public with ancient maya archaeology. In Archaeology in the Digital Era (pp. 118-130).

Riva, G., Bacchetta, M., Baruffi, M., & Molinari, E. (2001). Virtual reality based treatment of body image disturbances in anorexia and bulimia nervosa: two pilot studies. *European Psychotherapy., 2*(3), 17.

Rizzo, A., Hartholt, A., Grimani, M., Leeds, A., & Liewer, M. (2014). Virtual reality exposure therapy for combat-related posttraumatic stress disorder. *Computer, 47*(7), 31–37. doi:10.1109/MC.2014.199

Rochat, P., & Zahavi, D. (2011). The uncanny mirror: A re-framing of mirror self-experience. *Consciousness and Cognition*, *20*(2), 204–213. doi:10.1016/j.concog.2010.06.007 PMID:20889353

Rodriguez, M. C., Aruanno, B., Bordegoni, M., Rossini, M., & Molteni, F. (2017). Immersive Virtual Reality System for Treatment of Phantom Limb Pain (PLP). *Paper presented at the ASME 2017 International Design Engineering Technical Conferences and Computers and Information in Engineering Conference*.

Roosink, M., Robitaille, N., McFadyen, B. J., Hébert, L. J., Jackson, P. L., Bouyer, L. J., & Mercier, C. (2015). Real-time modulation of visual feedback on human full-body movements in a virtual mirror: Development and proof-of-concept. *Journal of Neuroengineering and Rehabilitation*, *12*(1), 2. doi:10.1186/1743-0003-12-2 PMID:25558785

Rose, F. D., Brooks, B. M., & Rizzo, A. A. (2005). Virtual reality in brain damage rehabilitation [review]. *Cyberpsychology & Behavior*, *8*(3), 241–262. doi:10.1089/cpb.2005.8.241 PMID:15971974

Rossiter, H. E., Borrelli, M. R., Borchert, R. J., Bradbury, D., & Ward, N. S. (2015). Cortical mechanisms of mirror therapy after stroke. *Neurorehabilitation and Neural Repair*, *29*(5), 444–452. doi:10.1177/1545968314554622 PMID:25326511

Sato, H., Kitahara, I., & Ohta, Y. (2009). MR-mirror: a complex of real and virtual mirrors. *Paper presented at the International Conference on Virtual and Mixed Reality*. 10.1007/978-3-642-02771-0_54

Shuhaiber, J. H. (2004). Augmented reality in surgery. *Archives of Surgery (Chicago, Ill.)*, *139*(2), 170–174. doi:10.1001/archsurg.139.2.170 PMID:14769575

Sielhorst, T., Feuerstein, M., & Navab, N. (2008). Advanced Medical Displays: A Literature Review of Augmented Reality. *Display Technology. Journalism*, *4*(4), 451–467. doi:10.1109/jdt.2008.2001575

Stevens, J. A., & Stoykov, M. E. P. (2003). Using Motor Imagery in the Rehabilitation of Hemiparesis 1. *Archives of Physical Medicine and Rehabilitation*, *84*(7), 1090–1092. doi:10.1016/S0003-9993(03)00042-X PMID:12881842

Sucar, L. E., Orihuela-Espina, F., Velazquez, R. L., Reinkensmeyer, D. J., Leder, R., & Hernández-Franco, J. (2014). Gesture therapy: An upper limb virtual reality-based motor rehabilitation platform. *IEEE Transactions on Neural Systems and Rehabilitation Engineering*, *22*(3), 634–643. doi:10.1109/TNSRE.2013.2293673 PMID:24760913

Tang, S.-L., Kwoh, C.-K., Teo, M.-Y., Sing, N. W., & Ling, K.-V. (1998). Augmented reality systems for medical applications. *IEEE Engineering in Medicine and Biology Magazine*, *17*(3), 49–58. doi:10.1109/51.677169 PMID:9604701

Taylor, R. H., & Stoianovici, D. (2003). Medical robotics in computer-integrated surgery. *IEEE Transactions on* Robotics and Automation, *19*(5), 765–781. doi:10.1109/tra.2003.817058

Thieme, H., Mehrholz, J., Pohl, M., Behrens, J., & Dohle, C. (2012). Mirror therapy for improving motor function after stroke. *Cochrane Database of Systematic Reviews*, *14*(3). PMID:22419334

Thieme, H., Mehrholz, J., Pohl, M., Behrens, J., & Dohle, C. (2013). Mirror therapy for improving motor function after stroke. *Stroke*, *44*(1), e1–e2. doi:10.1161/STROKEAHA.112.673087 PMID:23390640

Thomas, D. J. (2016). Augmented reality in surgery: The computer-aided medicine revolution. *International Journal of Surgery*, *36*, 25. doi:10.1016/j.ijsu.2016.10.003 PMID:27741424

Trojan, J., Diers, M., Fuchs, X., Bach, F., Bekrater-Bodmann, R., Foell, J., ... Flor, H. (2014). An augmented reality home-training system based on the mirror training and imagery approach. *Behavior Research Methods*, *46*(3), 634–640. doi:10.375813428-013-0412-4 PMID:24338625

Tudor, S., Carey, S., & Dubey, R. (2015). Development and evaluation of a dynamic virtual reality driving simulator. *Paper presented at the 8th ACM International Conference on Pervasive Technologies Related to Assistive Environments*. 10.1145/2769493.2769593

Vargas González, A. N., Kapalo, K., Koh, S., & LaViola, J. (2017). Exploring the virtuality continuum for complex rule-set education in the context of soccer rule comprehension. *Multimodal Technologies and Interaction*, *1*(4), 30. doi:10.3390/mti1040030

Vural, S. P., Yuzer, G. F. N., Ozcan, D. S., Ozbudak, S. D., & Ozgirgin, N. (2016). Effects of mirror therapy in stroke patients with complex regional pain syndrome type 1: A randomized controlled study. *Archives of Physical Medicine and Rehabilitation*, *97*(4), 575–581. doi:10.1016/j.apmr.2015.12.008 PMID:26723854

Waltemate, T., Gall, D., Roth, D., Botsch, M., & Latoschik, M. E. (2018). The impact of avatar personalization and immersion on virtual body ownership, presence, and emotional response. *IEEE Transactions on Visualization and Computer Graphics*, *24*(4), 1643–1652. doi:10.1109/TVCG.2018.2794629 PMID:29543180

Windheim, K., Veale, D., & Anson, M. (2011). Mirror gazing in body dysmorphic disorder and healthy controls: Effects of duration of gazing. *Behaviour Research and Therapy*, *49*(9), 555–564. doi:10.1016/j.brat.2011.05.003 PMID:21726855

Won, A. S., Bailey, J., Bailenson, J., Tataru, C., Yoon, I. A., & Golianu, B. (2017). Immersive virtual reality for pediatric pain. *Children*, *4*(7), 52. doi:10.3390/children4070052 PMID:28644422

Wu, H.-K., Lee, S. W.-Y., Chang, H.-Y., & Liang, J.-C. (2013). Current status, opportunities and challenges of augmented reality in education. *Computers & Education*, *62*, 41–49. doi:10.1016/j.compedu.2012.10.024

Yantaç, A. E., Çorlu, D., Fjeld, M., & Kunz, A. (2015). Exploring diminished reality (DR) spaces to augment the attention of individuals with autism. *Paper presented at the 2015 IEEE International Symposium on Mixed and Augmented Reality Workshops (ISMARW)*.

Zanfir, A.-M., Georgescu, D. I., Turturica, S. C., Eczedi, M., & Mironiuc, A. (2017). Immersive VR in phantom limb pain therapy of amputee patients due to critical limb ischemia. *Acta Medica Marisiensis*, *63*(3), 115–120. doi:10.1515/amma-2017-0031

## KEY TERMS AND DEFINITIONS

**Augmented Reality Mirror:** An Augmented Reality application that follows the mirror metaphor, allowing users to see an image of themselves enhanced with virtual information.

**Face-To-Face Interaction:** Regarding to ARMs, to have direct visual contact with the own depicted face on the mirror-like surface.

**Image Blending:** Mixing two images. The output image is a combination of the corresponding pixel values of the input images.

**Regular Mirror:** A surface that reflects light. Regular mirrors have been traditionally used in medical therapy.

**Seamless Interaction:** Interaction free of functional, temporal, spatial or cognitive elements that force users to change the way in which they interact with the interface.

**Uncanny:** something that is so remarkable that it is beyond what is natural.

**Virtual Reality Mirror:** A Virtual Reality application that follows the mirror metaphor, allowing users to see an avatar of themselves.

# Chapter 8
# The State of Virtual and Augmented Reality Therapy for Autism Spectrum Disorder (ASD)

**Sinan Turnacioglu**
*Floreo, Inc., USA*

**Joseph P McCleery**
*Saint Joseph's University, USA & Children's Hospital of Philadelphia, USA*

**Julia Parish-Morris**
*University of Pennsylvania, USA & Children's Hospital of Philadelphia, USA*

**Vibha Sazawal**
*University of Maryland, USA*

**Rita Solorzano**
*Floreo, Inc., USA*

## ABSTRACT

*Autism spectrum disorder (ASD) is a heterogeneous neurodevelopmental condition affecting a growing number of individuals across the lifespan. It is characterized by observable impairments in social communication, as well as repetitive behaviors and restricted patterns of interests. Early, intensive behavioral interventions improve long-term outcomes in ASD, but are often expensive and hard to administer consistently. This chapter describes a new approach to autism intervention, using highly motivating virtual reality (VR) and augmented reality (AR) technologies that could soon support traditional autism therapies across ages and ability levels. The chapter begins by reviewing the ASD phenotype, followed by a review of the current landscape of research on VR and AR in ASD. A discussion of ASD-specific benefits and risks is followed by a presentation of new, harnessed immersive VR technology from Floreo, Inc. Finally, we propose a series of future research directions.*

DOI: 10.4018/978-1-5225-7168-1.ch008

## INTRODUCTION

Autism spectrum disorder (ASD) is a heterogeneous neurodevelopmental condition characterized by variable degrees of impairment in social communication and restricted and repetitive patterns of behavior (American Psychiatric Association, 2013). ASD prevalence is growing, and recent estimates range from 14.6 per 1000 children aged eight years (Christensen et al., 2016) to 2.24% in children aged 3 to 17 years (Zablotsky et al., 2015). It is a lifelong disorder, and the majority of adults with ASD continue to experience significant difficulties with socialization, independent living, employment, and mental health. A recent survey of young adults with ASD found that 24% reported social isolation, as well as high rates of anxiety, depression, and attention deficit hyperactivity disorder. In addition, 4 in 10 young adults with ASD were described as disconnected from work and continued education through their late teens and early twenties. Less than 20% of young adults with ASD lived independently (Roux et al., 2015).

Despite extensive research focused on behavioral and pharmacological treatments for the core symptoms of ASD, there remains a clear need for treatments to support social and emotional development and functional life skills in individuals with ASD which are both effective and cost-efficient. Reviews and meta-analyses have suggested that interventions for ASD as a whole show limited effectiveness, with few exceptions such as early intensive behavioral intervention and related types of applied behavior analysis-based programs. For example, a 2010 review evaluated the existing research base on comprehensive treatment models for ASD and found that such treatment models were weak in evidence of efficacy as a whole (Odom et al., 2010). A Technical Expert Panel developed guidelines for evidence-based interventions for ASD, with a primary finding that greater intensity and greater duration of treatment led to better outcomes (Maglione et al., 2012). Comprehensive intervention programs, such as applied behavior analysis-based interventions, are among the most effective for treating the core symptoms of ASD; however, these interventions as currently designed require significant clinical/educational oversight and tend to be both labor-intensive and costly, placing significant pressure on both human and financial resources related to serving this population. Other intervention programs have showed a lower strength of evidence. Furthermore, a 2015 review of evidence based practices for ASD found that the majority of intervention studies had focused on preschool-age and elementary school-age children. The authors recommended that research on interventions should expand to include an increased focus on adolescents and young adults with ASD (Wong et al., 2015).

The most recent National Standards Project from the National Autism Center, based in the United States, describes "Technology-based Intervention" as an Emerging intervention, warranting additional research (National Autism Center, 2015). Advances in immersive virtual reality (VR) and wearable augmented reality (AR) technology have provided new opportunities to design interventions targeting the core deficits associated with ASD and supporting optimal functional outcomes. The main objectives of this chapter are to: (1) Describe the autism phenotype, with a particular focus on domains amenable to intervention using VR and AR technologies; (2) Review what is known about using VR/AR in ASD; (3) Outline risks and benefits of AR/VR in ASD; (4) Present a new immersive VR platform developed by Floreo, Inc.; and (5) Describe future research directions in AR/VR intervention for ASD.

## BACKGROUND

### Autism Spectrum Disorder (ASD) and Technology

#### Autism and Technology-Based Interventions

Computer-based technology has long been recognized as a potentially very promising avenue for delivery of therapy to individuals with ASD. In some sense, it is inevitable that technology-based intervention and supports will become part of clinical and educational practices for this population, as technologies are becoming increasingly integrated into the lives of all individuals (McCleery, 2015). Computer-based systems provide a variety of benefits for intervention, including controlled environments for skill training. Developers and therapists can also adjust the intensity of stimuli in computerized environments to suit individual sensitivities, which can be critical for teaching and supporting populations with individual differences as varying as those with ASD and related conditions. External distractions can be minimized, or in some cases, introduced systematically as appropriate for a user's therapeutic needs. Similarly, computer-based lessons can be dynamically altered in systematic ways which promote generalization of skills across stimuli, environments, interactive partners, and situations. Technology can also be used to deliver therapies which include both rote repetition and controllable novelty of tasks and stimuli in ways that would not be feasible in real world environments.

##### *Preference for Technology*

Individuals with ASD have been noted to have particular preferences for computer-based and visually-based technologies, including VR. In an experimental study, 42 students with ASD were assigned to different visual presentation formats, and participants assigned to VR formats rated high levels of engagement with the material (Mineo et al., 2009). A review of computer technology for social communication teaching in ASD by Wainer and Ingersoll concluded that existing VR research supported the feasibility of this technology for individuals with ASD. Use of computer-based programs, including VR, was described as being rewarding for many research participants across studies. VR was also noted to have potential for direct targeting of expressive skills. The authors recognized that most of the publications in the intervention literature for social communication for ASD to date had been descriptive and exploratory as opposed to experimental (Wainer & Ingersoll, 2011). Experimental research, including randomized controlled clinical trials, on this topic is both active and needed.

Grynszpan in 2014 described some of the reasons why individuals with ASD may find technology-based programs particularly appealing (Grynszpan et al., 2014). These factors include consistency of a clearly defined task; a specific focus of attention that reduces distractions from unnecessary sensory stimuli; freedom from social demands during engagement with technology; provision of immediate, predictable, and repeatable responses; and visually cued instructions. These appealing elements need to be balanced with the potential for dependence on computer-based activities and possible isolation of individuals with ASD. Additionally, this meta-analysis of technology-based interventions for ASD supported the efficacy of this category of interventions while noting limitations of the existing literature, such as the relatively weak designs of some of the studies and lack of a strong body of randomized controlled trial (RCT) studies. Specifically, in regard to VR, the authors note that over ten years of research existed, but with little direct experimental evidence supporting efficacy, and they called for more studies in this specific area of technology research.

### *Computer-Assisted Learning in ASD*

Individuals with ASD appear to enjoy technology-based interventions and applications, but are they effective tools for learning? Odom and colleagues proposed a framework for evaluating research on technology-based programs for adolescents with ASD (Odom et al., 2015). This conceptual framework incorporated user characteristics, activities to be supported with a given technology, the context in which such technology support would be provided, and the specific type of technology to be used for instruction. Authors recommended that the overlap of these factors should be considered in evaluating issues such as effectiveness, ecological validity, and generalization of any interventions for adolescents with ASD developed using a technology platform.

In 2013, Ploog described the areas in which computer-assisted technologies have been studied in children with ASD, including support of language and reading skills, enhancement of face processing and emotion recognition, support of social skills such as communication, play and daily living skills. The authors addressed VR research specifically in the context of teaching social skills, and noted the limitations imposed historically on such research by the sophisticated nature of VR technology. However, they highlighted the promise of emerging computer-assisted technologies such as VR in supporting training of a diverse set of skills in individuals with ASD, along with the need for future research designs to include larger sample sizes as well as comparison control groups receiving intervention in traditional intervention programs (Ploog et al., 2013).

## Autism and Augmented/Virtual Reality

Augmented reality (AR) and virtual reality (VR) are both forms of technology that alter what the user sees. AR combines computer-generated content with the user's view of the real world in a three dimensional framework that is believable and encourages real time interactivity (Azuma, 1997). When the user should only interact with computer-generated content, and the real world is mostly occluded, we have VR (Norman, 2017). We first review the literature on AR in ASD, followed by an in-depth discussion of VR research in ASD.

## What Is Known About Augmented Reality in ASD?

Unique approaches have been studied to leverage AR to support individuals with ASD. Casas et al., (2012) used Microsoft Kinect to develop an augmented mirror for users to see themselves in a digital environment augmented with virtual objects. Another research group developed the Mobile Object Identification System (Mobis) that superimposes digital content on real objects (Escobedo et al., 2014).

The increasing availability of mobile phones, mobile tablets, and wearable technologies has created opportunities to develop novel approaches to therapy delivery using AR.

The availability of wearable AR technology in the form of Google Glass has spurred research into applications of AR in supporting social and emotional skills in individuals with ASD. Several groups have developed interventions using Google Glass to support social skills and emotion recognition in individuals with ASD. For example, several articles have been published exploring the potential of the Brain Power Autism System (BPAS) in supporting social communication skills in children and adults with ASD. BPAS uses Google Glass Explorer Edition and Glass Enterprise Edition to provide users with a smartglasses-based AR system. The system's social communication module provides gamified coaching on skills such as recognition of facial emotional expressions and attending to other people's faces. A feasibility study evaluated the ability of two male children with ASD to use BPAS in a single coaching session. Researchers found that participants tolerated use of the system with no noted adverse effects, and caregivers reported high levels of engagement (Liu et al., 2017).

Another study examining BPAS focused on acceptability of using a smartglasses product in school. In this study, eight children with ASD initially tried out BPAS in a controlled environment in order to explore different aspects of use of the system, and then the children and their parents participated in an interview session. Questions included the caregiver's opinion of their child's experience using BPAS and their child's enjoyment of the system and the child's interest in wearing such a device for one hour each day at their school. All study participants and caregivers provided positive responses to questions of acceptability of use in school and enjoyment of using BPAS (Sahin et al., 2017).

Safety and negative effects of BPAS were assessed in a study of 18 children and adults with ASD who experienced the system for a 1 to 1-½ hour session. Few negative effects were reported by participants, and those that were reported were minor in nature. No participants discontinued use of BPAS as a result of side effects, and there were no behavioral effects reported during use or when study participants were asked to stop using the smartglasses (Sahin et al., 2017). In a larger sample of BPAS in 21 children and adults with ASD, researchers assessed study participants' initial tolerability threshold, the user's ability to wear the smartglasses for one minute; the whole session tolerability threshold, the user's ability to wear the smartglasses for the full 1 to 1-½ hour session; and caregiver ratings of user tolerability. Study results indicated that most participants tolerated wearing the smartglasses for the full study session (Keshav et al., 2017).

Washington and colleagues reported on findings from a study of another Google Glass-based application, SuperpowerGlass (Washington et al., 2017). This platform focused on teaching facial expression recognition using real-time social cues to children with ASD. Several activities were used in the wearable therapy sessions, and families could review video from wearable therapy sessions in order to highlight key moments and longitudinal changes in behavior. Fourteen families participated in this pilot. Authors found that parents reported improved social behaviors in participating children when not wearing the device after the intervention, and made additional design conclusions such as accommodating for the functional level of users and augmenting video content from wearable therapy sessions with context about the reviewed content.

Researchers conducted a study on the usability and feasibility of the Google Glass-based application Holli (Kinsella et al., 2017). This application uses recorded user and interaction partner speech to generate suggested responses during a conversational exchange. Study participants included 15 children with ASD who engaged with a research assistant in a restaurant-themed practice conversation consisting of ten exchanges. Usability was assessed through measures of the system's effectiveness to accurately detect user and participant spoken utterances and efficiency of response time in providing suggested responses to the user, as well as responses to a user satisfaction questionnaire. Study results supported the usability of the Holli system with children with ASD and authors concluded that the system demonstrated value as an intervention modality for this population. Published research on the use of Google Glass-based AR technologies suggests that these systems may be safe for and well-tolerated by individuals with ASD, but additional research is needed to further assess their effectiveness for training of social, conversational, and facial expression recognition skills.

## What Is Known About Virtual Reality in ASD?

Researchers have addressed the unique features and potential of VR to support skill development in individuals with ASD. In 1997, Strickland described the elements of VR that could be helpful for teaching skills to this population (Strickland, 1997). These included: controllable input stimuli that can meet a user's individual sensory needs; modification of the virtual environment (VE) to support generalization; a safe learning situation to repetitively practice daily living skills; a primary visual and auditory world that fits the typical learning preferences of individuals with ASD; individualized treatment that can accommodate the spectrum of skills and needs of the population; preferred computer interactions that minimize the stress of complex social interactions; and body and head trackers that can monitor the physical activities of users.

Parsons and Mitchell extended existing behavioral and theory of mind interventions to examine the potential of VR in social skills training for teaching individuals with ASD (Parsons & Mitchell, 2002). Taking into account the beneficial aspects of such existing treatment approaches and their limitations, the authors proposed a set of elements to include in social skills interventions, allowing for repetition of target skills; rote learning of social skills; fading of prompts; verbal instructions of social skills; strategies to understand the impact of one's behavior on others; opportunity to practice skills across contexts and in realistic settings; role-playing of target skills; and accessibility and affordability. They acknowledged that there was the potential that certain aspects of VR might have an undesirable appeal to individuals with ASD, such as the obsessive potential of engaging with the technology due to predictability and the sense of control users may feel in a VE in contrast to the real world, but that these concerns could be minimized by the incorporation of flexible and unpredictable events in VEs. They recommended that VEs for social skills training should be used in collaboration with other people in order to minimize the isolation and lack of social engagement with solitary technology use which would be contradictory to the purpose of its use in social skill training. This article directed the focus of research to desktop platforms rather than immersive systems, due to contemporary concerns about cybersickness and expense.

In a qualitative review of research on the use of VR in rehabilitation of specific pediatric disabilities, authors concluded that VR was promising for treatment of deficits experienced by children with ASD. Research suggested that individuals with ASD are interested in and motivated to engage with VR experiences. Difficulties noted with use of VR with this clinical population included the ability of users to tolerate long sessions, cooperation with wearing a VR head-mounted display (HMD), and understanding and remaining engaged to tasks presented in the VR environment (Parsons et al., 2009).

In a follow up 2011 article on the state-of-the-art of VR technologies for children with ASD, Parsons and Cobb reviewed progress made up to that time on developing an evidence base for applications of VR in this population (Parsons & Cobb, 2011). The authors addressed key features of VR that make development of VR systems attractive to professionals working with populations with ASD. These include programming control of an individual's environment such as the level of stimuli and the nature of interactions in ways that are not possible in the real world. In addition, VR offers opportunities for repeated individual practice in a safe environment and use of gamification techniques to motivate users. Parsons and Cobb noted studies done on use and understanding of VEs, responses to "immersion" and feelings of "presence" in VR, and generalization of learning from the virtual to the real world. Research done up to that point indicated that children with ASD seem to like using VR, could use VR to learn new information, and responded in ways that suggested that they appreciated the representational aspects of VEs. Studies suggested that children with ASD did not find VR particularly aversive. Authors of the review noted that research was limited in demonstrating educational applications of VR technology for students with ASD, and they concluded that more work needed to be done to understand how best to use the unique features of VR to support the needs of children with ASD. They address two features of VR in particular that needed further investigation: whether the assumption that the more realistic a VE is, the greater the chance that users will generalize learning to the real world, and what are the specific and unique characteristics of VR technology that support learning in such environments for individuals with ASD.

In a recent review article, Parsons and colleagues complete a broader review of applications of VR in pediatric psychology (Parsons et al., 2017). In this review, they describe research conducted on different uses of VR in pediatric populations, including both typically developing children and children with developmental disabilities. The article covers key features of VR systems including immersion, presence, acceptance, and limited negative effects. The authors point out that while VR technology has become more affordable and available to larger numbers of people, there remains a need for ongoing research on effectiveness of VR-based interventions. In particular, they note a need for large scale randomized controlled trials, and for examinations of the ecological validity of VR implementation in appropriate pediatric settings. They also advised continued monitoring of safety issues related to children's use of VR.

## Non-Immersive VR

There are several approaches to delivering VR therapy, which can be separated into immersive and non-immersive systems. Immersive VR fully occludes the user's view of the real world with virtual content; whereas, non-immersive VR does not fully occlude the user's field of view. One of the earliest published studies on the use of VR with children with ASD employed an immersive VR system (Strickland, 1996). However, early-generation immersive displays raised concerns, such as the high cost of such systems, their weight in relation to sensory sensitivities common in individuals with ASD, and cybersickness concerns. Studies relying on non-immersive VR platforms have involved the use of traditional personal computers and game controllers which are used to interact with a three-dimensional world depicted on a conventional two-dimensional display, such as a television or laptop screen. Some systems use multiple televisions or computer monitors around the user to give the semblance of surrounding the user in content. Microsoft Kinect has also been used as a system for VR therapy delivery.

Researchers have used non-immersive VR approaches to study fire safety, job interview skills, street crossing, driving, and social competence and cognition in individuals with ASD. For example, Strickland and colleagues described a PC-based VR system to teach fire safety skills to children with ASD (Strickland et al., 2007). The VR intervention was provided to children either at home or at school. Fire safety skills were presented in a sequential manner. A virtual avatar demonstrated appropriate fire safety skills and then provided feedback after a child repeated the actions correctly or incorrectly. Fourteen children with ASD from 3 to 6 years of age participated in the study. Most participants were able to successfully demonstrate knowledge and generalization of skills to the real world following their experience with the VR-based fire safety skills program.

The potential of VR technology to support job interview skills has been studied in individuals with ASD, with a goal of improving opportunities for adult employment. Strickland and colleagues studied the effectiveness of an online job interviewing training program that incorporated a VR-based practice interview on interview-related behaviors in adolescents with high-functioning ASD (HFASD) (Strickland et al., 2013). The virtual platform used was an online, non-immersive environment consisting of a virtual office space with an "interviewer" who provided feedback to the study participant on both content- and delivery-specific interview-related behaviors. Twenty-two adolescents with HFASD or Asperger's disorder participated in this study, with half of the participants receiving the job interviewing training intervention and the other half serving as a contrast group with no active intervention. In this study, evaluators rated participants who received the job interviewing intervention higher on verbal content skills than those participants who did not receive virtual job interviewing support.

Another research group evaluated the VR job interview training for adults with ASD (Smith et al., 2014). The Virtual Reality Job Interview Training (VR-JIT) program is a computer and internet-based training simulation, which uses non-branching logic to present users with a unique interview experience based on responses to questions. VR-JIT was developed to improve job interview performance by allowing users to practice skills related to job-relevant interview content and interviewee performance. There were a variety of employment positions for which users could "apply" in the simulation, and users then experienced a simulated interview with a human resources representative avatar. Sixteen adults with ASD were randomized to VR-JIT and ten to treatment as usual. VR-JIT participants completed 20 training trials over five visits, and then were assessed through a questionnaires and role-play sessions. Results were promising for both feasibility of VR-JIT as well as effectiveness for improving job interview skills in adults with ASD.

In order to explore the potential of VR to support pedestrian safety skills in children with ASD, Josman and colleagues developed a desktop street-crossing VE (Josman et al., 2008). Six children with ASD between 8 and 16 years of age participated, with a control group of grade and gender-matched typically developing children. Researchers scored skills demonstrated while crossing the street in the VE as well as in a protected real street crossing scenario. Following the VR intervention, participants with ASD showed improvements in street-crossing skills both in the virtual street environment as well as in the real street scenario. More recently, another group explored the feasibility of a non-immersive VR system to support street crossing skills in seven adults with ASD (Saiano et al., 2015). The research platform included a VR environment projected on a screen, and study participants used a Microsoft Kinect system to interact with the VE. Caregivers reported an improvement in participants' street crossing skills following use of the VR platform.

Another area of work has involved examining driving simulators for use with individuals with ASD. Researchers developed a gaze-contingent VR driving simulator, VR Adaptive Driving Intervention Architecture (VADIA), and published results of a pilot study of system use (Wade et al., 2016). This simulator was a desktop-based platform designed to provide an individualized approach to teaching driving skills in individuals with ASD. The system was developed for performance-based and gaze-contingent modes of operation, as well as to collect physiological and EEG data. There was an observer assessment component for evaluation of driving skill progress in VADIA users. Twenty adolescents with

ASD participated in the pilot study, and results suggested that the simulator may be helpful in training driving skills in adolescents with ASD.

With regard to social skills, Parsons and colleagues studied the experience of adolescents with ASD using a desktop VE (Parsons et al., 2004). The authors noted that a desktop VE system was used due to concerns about the appropriateness of existing fully immersive VR systems for individuals with ASD. Study participants included 12 adolescents with ASD who were matched to comparison participants on verbal IQ and performance IQ. The procedure included a training session on the desktop VE followed by instructions to complete several tasks in a virtual cafe. Results indicated that users with ASD had similar use experiences as participants in the performance IQ-matched comparison group, and the adolescents with ASD seemed to understand that the VE was a representation of the real world. The authors concluded that such desktop VEs could serve as a useful approach for teaching social skills in adolescents with ASD. In a follow-up study, Mitchell, Parsons, and Leonard (2007) used a laptop VR application with a joystick and mouse for navigation within and interaction with the environment. Over a 6-week period, six study participants with ASD watched three sets of videos of real cafes and buses and provided information to researchers on social decision-making in these settings. At different points in between sets of videos, subjects engaged in the cafe VE over two sessions. The program provided feedback on behaviors that were rated as socially inappropriate. Following their experiences in the cafe VE, participants generally showed improvements in the information they provided researchers on social decision-making in the video cafe and bus settings, leading authors to conclude that VR has potential to support social skill development in individuals with ASD.

A Second Life-based desktop VR program was used for social interaction skill training in children with ASD (Ke & Im, 2013). Second Life was a popular virtual world with rich avatars that carry out various virtual life activities. This study involved four children with HFASD working with seven adult volunteers serving as facilitators and communication partners for the participating children. In this exploratory study, participants showed improved performance on measures of responding and interaction during VR sessions. The authors discussed the need to further study the potential to transfer skills learned in VR to real world situations.

One group has studied the feasibility of using a non-immersive computer platform, also using Second Life, to train social cognition skills (VR Social Cognition Training (VR-SCT); Didehbani et al., 2016). Researchers studied 30 participants, between 7 and 16 years of age, who engaged in one hour sessions, twice per week for five weeks. Participants demonstrated improved performance on emotion recognition tasks, suggesting that VR social cognition training is a feasible intervention for children with ASD.

Following up on this research, another group studied the use of functional MRI to predict treatment response to the VR-SCT system in young adults with ASD (Yang et al., 2017). In this study, subjects participated in two 1-hour sessions each week for five weeks. In the first three sessions, participants learned core social strategies, and in the other seven sessions, they practiced integrating these strategies. VR situations included dealing with confrontation, job interviewing, and blind dates. Seventeen young adults participated in the study. Participants were found to have improved emotion recognition scores following the VR-SCT intervention. Findings from this study also indicated that functional neuroimaging can be used to identify activated neural networks related to improved social emotional processing skills as trained through a VR intervention.

Lahiri and colleagues have published research on a VR-based social communication system that uses gaze patterns and eye physiology to provide feedback on user levels of engagement with a goal of supporting conversational skills. The VR platform is a desktop application with twenty-four social tasks involving an avatar narrating a personal story to users. Two different systems have been developed: one focused on performance of the social tasks, and a second system that is sensitive to engagement based on gaze patterns and eye physiological measures (fixation duration, blink rate, and pupil diameter). A 2015 paper described results of a usability study that compared the experiences of eight adolescent participants with ASD to the experiences of a pilot group of age-matched typically developing children (Lahiri et al., 2015). Participants with ASD showed improved performance on social communication tasks in the engagement-sensitive system, demonstrating both proof-of-concept of the technology and suggesting that this system has the potential to be an effective aid for individuals with ASD.

## Immersive VR

Immersive VR fully occludes the user's field of view, so that the user only sees virtual content. In practice, there are several types of technologies for immersive VR, including head-mounted displays (HMDs) which the user wears over the eyes, and whole-room systems called CAVEs. Many uses of immersive VR with regard to ASD intervention studies refer to CAVE environments. One of the advantages of these environments is that children do not need to put anything on their head. However, these rooms are usually expensive, custom-built, and exclusively used for VR. CAVE environments have been used to study feasibility and safety of use, as well as acquisition of emotional recognition, learning, and pedestrian crossing skills in individuals with ASD. With recent advances in VR technology, research efforts have shifted back to exploring applications of newer HMDs and VR platforms to support the needs of individuals with ASD. Today's HMDs are considerably lighter, much less expensive, and show higher-density visual content than those of the 1990s. Modern HMDs have been studied more broadly for their potential for commercial therapeutic application, including for the treatment of strabismus, anxiety, pain management, and pediatric road safety. In regard to use specifically with individuals with ASD, modern HMDs have been primarily assessed in studies using small numbers of children or adults.

As noted above, one of the earliest studies evaluating the feasibility of using VR technology with children with ASD employed an immersive VR system with an HMD. Strickland and colleagues conducted a study using an immersive VR HMD, published in 1996, to assess feasibility of using VR to teach pedestrian skills to children with ASD (Strickland et al., 1996). The intervention design was based on the Treatment and Education of Autistic and Related Communication-Handicapped Children (TEACCH) methodology of structured teaching and including parents as collaborators and cotherapists. Two subjects, a 7-½-year-old girl and a 9-year-old boy, used the VR system in multiple sessions over a five-week period, with sessions limited to five minutes at a time. Researchers found that the children accepted the HMD and repeatedly immersed themselves in the VE. They were able to track moving objects in the scene, and locate a stop sign in the VE. There was a suggestion of generalization, as the children were able to respond similarly in three different street scenes. Authors reported that this study was an opportunity to begin evaluating the experiences of individuals with ASD in VR and the potential of this technology to support the needs of this population.

Wallace and colleagues used an immersive "Blue Room" CAVE to study the responses of children with ASD to experiencing immersive VR (Wallace et al., 2010). Ten children with ASD, between 12 and 16 years of age, were compared to age-matched typically developing controls. The VEs presented in the Blue Room included residential street, school playground, and school corridor scenes. There were no significant differences between participants with ASD and typically developing controls in reporting of negative effects from experiencing VR. Additionally, children with ASD reported similar levels of a sense of presence in the VE to typically developing participants.

Some of the studies using modern HMDs have focused on the tolerance and feasibility of devices such as Oculus Rift in children and adults with ASD. While some individuals in these studies refused to wear the HMD or were unable to tolerate continued use of the HMD or the VR experience, most children and adults accepted the VR HMDs and reported enjoyment and interest in continued use of the systems. In one pilot study, 29 adults with ASD used an Oculus Rift HMD, first for 10 minutes, and then possibly for a longer session at a later date (Newbutt et al., 2016). While the content was not therapeutic, it was entertaining and offered similar physical effects to proposed theoretic content. Four of the 29 discontinued use of the VR HMD due to unwanted side effects, which included dizziness and tiredness.

Ehrlich and Munger conducted an experimental trial, also using the Oculus Rift, with a group of eight children with ASD and eleven neurotypical peers, recruited from a local school (Ehrlich & Munger, 2014). Children were asked to move to virtual objects using a typical gaming joystick. Researchers found that some of the lower functioning subjects with ASD refused to wear the HMD. Of note, the higher functioning subjects with ASD were very enthusiastic about using the VR technology. The authors concluded that the study was useful as a feasibility pilot, but advised that HMDs were "not appropriate for some children low on the spectrum".

A CAVE platform was used by Tzanavari and colleagues to assess the ability of children with ASD to learn pedestrian crossing skills (Tzanavari et al., 2015). In this study, six children with ASD used a CAVE over four days to practice street crossing skills. Following the intervention, authors noted that study participants demonstrated appropriate pedestrian crossing skills in a real street environment, with caregiver supervision.

In another study, researchers designed a semi-CAVE incorporating one wall and one floor display, to train emotional skills in students with ASD (Lorenzo et al., 2016). Two virtual scenes were presented to study participants. Forty children with ASD participated in this study, which lasted over three years with students using the system once per week. A robot-held camera was used to detect participant facial expressions. Participants demonstrated improvements in ratings of emotional responsiveness than what was seen in previous research using a desktop VR system.

Driving skills in individuals with ASD were also assessed through use of a semi-immersive VR driving simulation training (VRDST) program (Cox et al., 2017). The platform was a realistic driver's cockpit with the view projected onto a curved screen in front of the study participant. The simulator assessed driving-specific executive function skills and general tactical skills. In this study, 51 adolescents with ASD received either routine training or one form of VRDST for three months. Pre- and post-training evaluations showed significantly improved executive function and driving skills from baseline in study participants receiving the VRDST intervention as compared to routine training, leading authors to conclude that use of VRDST was feasible and potentially effective for training driving skills in individuals with ASD.

Two adolescents with ASD used Oculus Rift to experience three custom scenarios designed to support social interaction skills (Beach & Wendt, 2014). These were implemented in Second Life, and the authors played the role of the other characters as the adolescents used the simulation. Both participants reported enjoyment of the simulation and showed improved performance on real-world role-playing and other tasks.

One research group used the I-Glasses PC 3D Pro HMD to support social understanding and skills in children with ASD (Cheng et al., 2015). Three boys between 10 and 13 years of age participated in an experiment in which they engaged in virtual bus stop and classroom environments for five sessions. All subjects completed all sessions, and therapists reported that the treatment modality was motivating. Researchers concluded that this 3D-SU intervention system was effective in improving target social communication behaviors.

Researchers at Politecnico Milano have done a pilot study using supervised low-cost VR via Google Cardboard on a small sample of five children with intellectual disabilities (Garzotto et al., 2016; Gelsomini et al., 2016). The platform was a mobile application running on smartphones, and therapists supervised activities while using the application. The therapeutic content was a storytelling application that required the user to maintain eye contact with a virtual character for the story to continue. There was a personalization component that allowed the storytelling experience to address specific needs for each child. Study participants used the "Wildcard" storytelling system in eight individual therapeutic sessions lasting up to 180 seconds in duration each. Results were promising, as children in the study accepted the Google Cardboard HMD, and therapists found the platform easy to use and beneficial to the children. Researchers concluded that the device was acceptable to users and noted improvements in attention skills and visual contact.

## Risks and Benefits of VR/AR Interventions for ASD

The benefits of innovative technological innovations for treating the core impairments of ASD are beginning to emerge. However, when developing programs designed for use by individuals with ASD, it is critical to consider health and safety concerns specific to the use of VR and AR in this population. Core features of ASD may adversely impact users' experiences with AR and immersive VR technology. For example, sensory hypersensitivities are part of the current diagnostic criteria for ASD (American Psychiatric Association, 2013). These sensory issues may increase the likelihood that somebody with ASD may experience symptoms of cybersickness while using VR or AR. The potential for cybersickness, a form of motion or simulator sickness related to sensory mismatch or conflict, is one of the more common concerns related to the use of AR and immersive VR technologies in the general population (Kiryu & So, 2007). Symptoms include dizziness, nausea, eye strain and fatigue, and these effects may cause somebody experiencing them to discontinue use of VR or AR applications prematurely or to avoid such experiences altogether.

Another key factor when considering the experiences of individuals with ASD using AR and VR technologies is that the social communication deficits that are a fundamental aspect of the condition may impact an individual's ability to relay side effects or other health information to caregivers or educators and other professionals working with the user. For example, many individuals with ASD have limited expressive language skills, and may be unable to effectively relay feelings related to cybersickness or other side effects, such as migraines or visual discomfort, experienced during or after use of an AR or VR system (Ely et al., 2016).

Migraine headaches can be triggered by bright lights, loud sounds, or sensory mismatch (Charles, 2013). Many migraine sufferers are also prone to motion sickness (Cuomo-Granston & Drummond, 2010), and migraines in children have been reported to be triggered by video games and concentration with visual fixation (Neut et al., 2012). Migraine sufferers may be more sensitive to VR environments than individuals who are not predisposed to migraines. While there is no literature supporting an increased risk of migraine in individuals with ASD, there remains concern that AR or VR users with ASD may not effectively communicate premonitory symptoms of a migraine or the pain associated with a migraine headache caused by use of a VR or AR system.

The exacerbation of visual problems is another concern related to use of VR and AR systems by individuals with ASD. Strabismus, a condition in which the eyes are not properly aligned, is a condition which may be impacted by premature or excessive use of VR and AR in children. In younger children, there is a critical period of visual development, during which the brain is particularly sensitive to the visual input it receives. After this critical period, the brain is considerably less plastic. The outcome of ocular conditions such as strabismus is affected by the timing of the initial misalignment between the two eyes, and untreated strabismus after this critical period may result in loss of vision in the misaligned eye (Daw, 1997). Children with ASD have a higher rate of strabismus than the general population (Anketell et al., 2013; Ikeda et al., 2013). There is also evidence that children with ASD experience higher rates of convergence insufficiency, which may also contribute to visual strain while using VR and AR systems (Milne et al., 2009).

Visual discomfort could be related to use of medications with anticholinergic effects, such as antihistamines, tricyclic antidepressants, and antipsychotics, which are all used by individuals with ASD (Green et al., 2006; Oswald & Sonenklar, 2007). This is a particular challenge in younger children or individuals with limited expressive language, who may have difficulty reporting eye strain or blurry or double vision that may be related to medication side effects exacerbated by VR or AR use.

Also of concern, is for individuals with ASD using VR or AR systems, is the risk of seizures occurring in people with photosensitivity, abnormal sensitivity to light stimuli (Rubboli et al., 2004). Exposure to such photic activity can cause dizziness, headaches, and seizures in susceptible individuals. Photosensitivity is associated with a variety of epileptic syndromes in children and adults (Covanis, 2005; Lu et al., 2008). Photic seizures have been reported in association with television viewing (Shoja et al., 2007), as well as with video game players (Ferrie et al., 1994; Inoue et al., 1999). In many cases, the cause is likely some sort of photic stimulus as with television, but in other cases seizures were reported in individuals with epilepsy without visual sensitivity (Millett et al., 1999).

There is thus a theoretical risk that VEs may trigger seizure activity in users with photosensitive epilepsy. Several studies have reported that individuals with ASD have a higher prevalence of epilepsy than seen in the general population (Buckley & Holmes, 2016; McCue et al., 2016; Thomas et al., 2017). This increased baseline rate of seizure disorder raises a concern that VR or AR use may exacerbate an underlying seizure disorder.

There are several recommendations for safe use of VR and AR in this population. First, children and adults with ASD and a known history of seizure activity should generally not use VR or AR applications, and individuals with a history of photosensitivity response on electroencephalogram (EEG) testing should also avoid VR and AR. People with a family history of seizures or photosensitivity should use VR and AR with caution.

Another recommendation is to consider vision screening or a full evaluation by an optometrist or ophthalmologist to identify any existing vision problems prior to first use. Users should also ensure a proper fit of the VR HMD or wearable AR system, considering in particular ensuring that the HMD's display matches the user's inter-pupillary distance or IPD. Failure to calibrate the HMD properly can lead to eye strain.

There should also be a limit on the length of VR and AR sessions, since short sessions reduce the amount of time that the eye is under strain. Because of ongoing development of visual systems in younger children, concerns remain regarding use of VR and AR technology over long periods of time, such as lengthy sessions or recurrent use over months to years, in this population, and the impact of long-term use on visual development needs to be closely monitored in order to minimize the potential for visual impairment related to VR or AR use.

## A Real-Time Tethered Approach to VR Interventions in ASD

The Floreo VR platform uses modern lightweight HDMs, the availability of mobile VR, and Wi-Fi connectivity to create a unique approach to supporting the needs of individuals with ASD. Floreo is an innovative downloadable application that provides a supervised VR experience. The application is run by a user on a smartphone with a dedicated HMD providing the VE, while a monitor uses a tablet or phone to observe the user's field of vision in the VE and thus supervise the training experience. Figure 1 displays the use of the Floreo VR platform by a user and supervising monitor. The platform allows for smoother and more direct integration of existing evidence-based ASD intervention strategies with an immersive VR experience. Specifically, the linked iPad-based monitoring and supervision by a therapist allows for direct feedback and support to be provided to the learner in vivo, ultimately allowing for existing applied behavior analytic and cognitive-behavioral intervention methods and procedures to be directly implemented in the context of dynamic immersive VR experiences. Advantages to this approach include teaching and learning environments and experiences which integrate a variety of computer-automated and therapist-mediated procedures, dynamic environments which can be altered to change and respond based upon therapist-driven clinical/educational decision-making, and computer-generated environments which can increase learner motivation and engagement to maximize learning.

*Figure 1. Floreo VR with smartphone and head-mounted display paired with tablet*

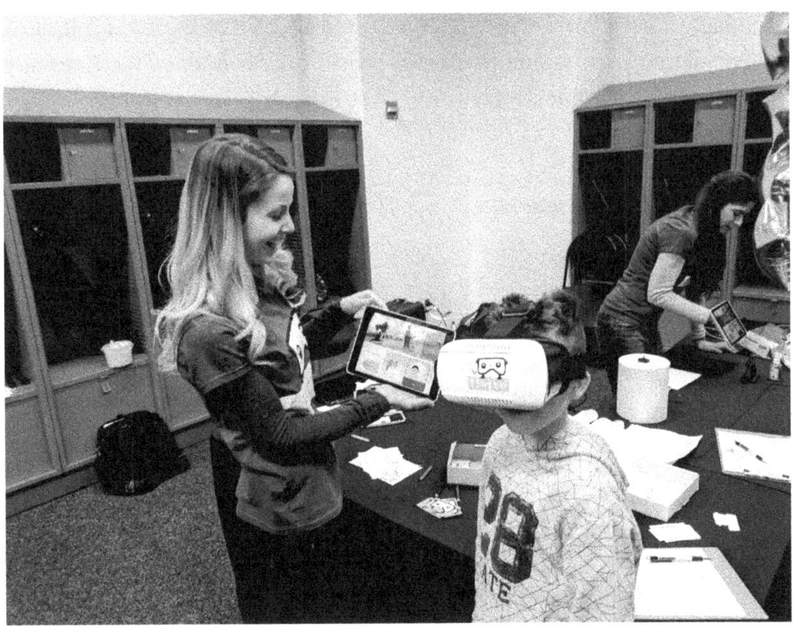

The National Institute of Mental Health has provided funding to Floreo and the Children's Hospital of Philadelphia for a Small Business Technology Transfer Research (STTR) project to establish feasibility and safety of a mobile Floreo VR module for training police safety skills in adolescents and adults with ASD. Figure 2 shows a screenshot of the VE designed for Floreo's Police Safety Module. In addition, a pilot study assessing feasibility and tolerability of Floreo's Joint Attention Module (JAM) was conducted with students with ASD at a private special education school. Twelve participants, between 9 and 16 years of age, underwent up to 14 VR sessions over a five-week period. Most of the participants were able to complete all of the VR sessions, and monitors provided high ratings of tolerability, enjoyment, and value of using Floreo's JAM application with the participating students. Mild side effects were reported in a small number of instances, and side effects did not lead to any participants withdrawing from the pilot. Results suggested that use of the JAM was feasible and well-tolerated by special education students with ASD (Ravindran et al., 2017). The study team plans to conduct further research on feasibility and tolerability as well as the effectiveness of the JAM using larger sample sizes and a randomized controlled trial study design.

## FUTURE RESEARCH DIRECTIONS

In addition to continuing and expanding current efforts to experimentally examine the effectiveness of VR and AR-based interventions for individuals with ASD, future research should consider and examine the following. First, what are the relationships between VR and AR and existing evidence-based interventions? For example, how, and to what degree, can AR or immersive VR be integrated with existing applied behavior analytic, developmental-behavioral, and cognitive-behavioral intervention methods and approaches? Second, what methods can be developed, and which methods are necessary, for generalization of skills trained in VR or AR to meaningful improvements in real-world functioning in individuals with ASD? For example, will AR or immersive VR training consistently result in transfer of skills immediately to real-world environments in this population? If not, can AR or immersive VR based lessons be conducted in parallel with separate sessions of live therapist implemented training, to produce robust and consistent improvements in real-world functioning? Third, researchers will want to determine the proper dosing schedules for various AR or immersive VR intervention protocols, both

*Figure 2. Screenshot of virtual environment for Floreo VR's Police Safety Module*

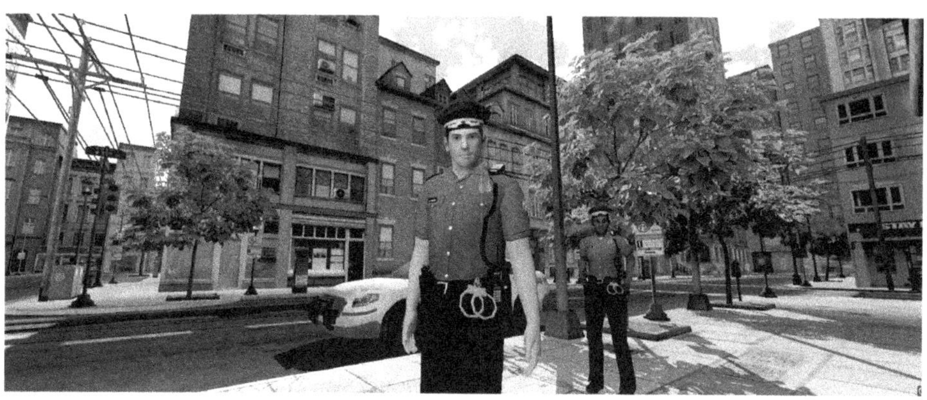

in terms of rapidity of skill acquisition and in terms of maintenance of trained skills over time. Finally, regarding immersive VR specifically, a major advantage of this approach is the capacity to incorporate early training of generalization across environments, people, and stimuli, through relatively easy incorporation of multiple environments (VR playground, VR classroom, VR store, etc.), multiple virtual human interactants, and multiple examplars of environmentally and contextually representative stimuli. Thus, while generalization of taught skills to real-world activities may be challenging in some cases, generalization across these other factors may be relatively easier for immersive VR based training.

## CONCLUSION

There is a growing body of research on the use of innovative VR and AR technologies with children and adults with ASD. Although many of the studies to date have been conducted using small numbers of participants or as descriptive and feasibility pilot studies, preliminary results from recent and ongoing experimental studies also provide support that VR can be used to effectively implement and support teaching and learning in individuals with ASD. Recent progress in the development of immersive HMD-based VR systems and wearable AR systems has provided opportunities to explore the impact of such technology on the lives and well-being of individuals with ASD. It is critical that future research efforts define the health and safety profile of long-term use of VR and AR for educational purposes and training of social communication and daily living skills in this population. Furthermore, future research must utilize high quality experimental clinical research designs, including randomized controlled trials, to determine the effectiveness of interventions delivered using such platforms. Further research needs to be conducted specifically on the safe use of VR and AR for long-term therapy for children with ASD. Considering the current status of technology-based development and integration into all of our daily lives, along with the increasing flexibility, lowering costs, and increasing technological capacities associated with VR and related technologies, we are highly optimistic that we are on the threshold of making dramatic breakthroughs regarding the development and testing of VR-based interventions which are both highly effective and cost-efficient for individuals with ASD.

## ACKNOWLEDGMENT

This research was supported by the National Institutes of Mental Health [1R42MH115539-01]; we gratefully acknowledge the individuals and families that participated in our research.

## REFERENCES

American Psychiatric Association. (2013). *Diagnostic and Statistical Manual of Mental Disorders* (5th ed.). Washington, DC.

Anketell, P., Saunders, K., Gallagher, S., Bailey, C., & Little, J. A. (2013). Visual findings in children with Autistic Spectrum Disorder. *Investigative Ophthalmology & Visual Science*, *54*(15), 569–569.

Azuma, R. T. (1997). A survey of augmented reality. *Presence*, *6*(4), 355–385. doi:10.1162/pres.1997.6.4.355

Beach, J., & Wendt, J. (2014). *Social Interaction Development through Immersive Virtual Environments*. International Association for Development of the Information Society.

Buckley, A. W., & Holmes, G. L. (2016). Epilepsy and autism. *Cold Spring Harbor Perspectives in Medicine*, *6*(4), a022749. doi:10.1101/cshperspect.a022749 PMID:26989064

Casas, X., Herrera, G., Coma, I., & Fernández, M. (2012). *A Kinect-based Augmented Reality System for Individuals with Autism Spectrum Disorders* (pp. 440–446). GRAPP/IVAPP.

Charles, A. (2013). The evolution of a migraine attack–a review of recent evidence. *Headache*, *53*(2), 413–419. doi:10.1111/head.12026 PMID:23278169

Cheng, Y., Huang, C. L., & Yang, C. S. (2015). Using a 3D immersive virtual environment system to enhance social understanding and social skills for children with autism spectrum disorders. *Focus on Autism and Other Developmental Disabilities*, *30*(4), 222–236. doi:10.1177/1088357615583473

Christensen, D. L., Baio, J., Braun, K. V. N., Bilder, D., Charles, J., Constantino, J. N., ... Yeargin-Allsopp, M. (2016). Prevalence and characteristics of autism spectrum disorder among children aged 8 years — autism and developmental disabilities monitoring network, 11 sites, United States, 2012. *MMWR. Surveillance Summaries*, *65*(3), 1–23. doi:10.15585/mmwr.ss6503a1 PMID:27031587

Covanis, A. (2005). Photosensitivity in idiopathic generalized epilepsies. *Epilepsia*, *46*(s9), 67–72. doi:10.1111/j.1528-1167.2005.00315.x PMID:16302877

Cox, D. J., Brown, T., Ross, V., Moncrief, M., Schmitt, R., Gaffney, G., & Reeve, R. (2017). Can youth with autism spectrum disorder use virtual reality driving simulation training to evaluate and improve driving performance? An exploratory study. *Journal of Autism and Developmental Disorders*, *47*(8), 2544–2555. doi:10.100710803-017-3164-7 PMID:28540452

Cuomo-Granston, A., & Drummond, P. D. (2010). Migraine and motion sickness: What is the link? *Progress in Neurobiology*, *91*(4), 300–312. doi:10.1016/j.pneurobio.2010.04.001 PMID:20416353

Daw, N. W. (1997). Critical periods and strabismus: What questions remain? *Optometry and Vision Science*, *74*(9), 690–694. doi:10.1097/00006324-199709000-00002 PMID:9380366

Didehbani, N., Allen, T., Kandalaft, M., Krawczyk, D., & Chapman, S. (2016). Virtual Reality Social Cognition Training for children with high functioning autism. *Computers in Human Behavior*, *62*, 703–711. doi:10.1016/j.chb.2016.04.033

Ehrlich, J., & Munger, J. (2012). Utilizing head mounted displays as a learning tool for children with autism. In Proceedings of 4th European Immersive Education Summit, Vienna, Austria.

Ely, E., Chen-Lim, M. L., Carpenter, K. M. II, Wallhauser, E., & Friedlaender, E. (2016). Pain assessment of children with autism spectrum disorders. *Journal of Developmental and Behavioral Pediatrics*, *37*(1), 53–61. doi:10.1097/DBP.0000000000000240 PMID:26703326

Escobedo, L., Tentori, M., Quintana, E., Favela, J., & Garcia-Rosas, D. (2014). Using augmented reality to help children with autism stay focused. *IEEE Pervasive Computing*, *13*(1), 38–46. doi:10.1109/MPRV.2014.19

Zablotsky, B., Black, L. I., Maenner, M. J., Schieve, L. A., & Blumberg, S. J. (2015). Estimated prevalence of autism and other developmental disabilities following questionnaire changes in the 2014 National Health Interview Survey (National health statistics reports; no 87). Hyattsville, MD: National Center for Health Statistics.

Ferrie, C. D., De Marco, P., Grünewald, R. A., Giannakodimos, S., & Panayiotopoulos, C. P. (1994). Video game induced seizures. *Journal of Neurology, Neurosurgery, and Psychiatry*, *57*(8), 925–931. doi:10.1136/jnnp.57.8.925 PMID:8057115

Garzotto, F., Gelsomini, M., Clasadonte, F., Montesano, D., & Occhiuto, D. (2016). Wearable Immersive Storytelling for Disabled Children. In *Proceedings of the International Working Conference on Advanced Visual Interfaces - AVI '16* (pp. 196–203). New York, NY: ACM Press.

Gelsomini, M., Garzotto, F., Montesano, D., & Occhiuto, D. (2016, August). Wildcard: A wearable virtual reality storytelling tool for children with intellectual developmental disability. In *2016 IEEE 38th Annual International Conference of the Engineering in Medicine and Biology Society (EMBC)* (pp. 5188-5191). IEEE. 10.1109/EMBC.2016.7591896

Green, V. A., Pituch, K. A., Itchon, J., Choi, A., O'Reilly, M., & Sigafoos, J. (2006). Internet survey of treatments used by parents of children with autism. *Research in Developmental Disabilities*, *27*(1), 70–84. doi:10.1016/j.ridd.2004.12.002 PMID:15919178

Grynszpan, O., Weiss, P. L., Perez-Diaz, F., & Gal, E. (2014). Innovative technology-based interventions for autism spectrum disorders: A meta-analysis. *Autism*, *18*(4), 346–361. doi:10.1177/1362361313476767 PMID:24092843

Ikeda, J., Davitt, B. V., Ultmann, M., Maxim, R., & Cruz, O. A. (2013). Brief report: Incidence of ophthalmologic disorders in children with autism. *Journal of Autism and Developmental Disorders*, *43*(6), 1447–1451. doi:10.100710803-012-1475-2 PMID:22350452

Inoue, Y., Fukao, K., Araki, T., Yamamoto, S., Kubota, H., & Watanabe, Y. (1999). Photosensitive and Nonphotosensitive Electronic Screen Game-Induced Seizures. *Epilepsia*, *40*(s4), 8–16. doi:10.1111/j.1528-1157.1999.tb00900.x PMID:10487167

Jarrold, W., Mundy, P., Gwaltney, M., Bailenson, J., Hatt, N., McIntyre, N., ... Swain, L. (2013). Social attention in a virtual public speaking task in higher functioning children with autism. *Autism Research*, *6*(5), 393–410. doi:10.1002/aur.1302 PMID:23696132

Josman, N., Ben-Chaim, H. M., Friedrich, S., & Weiss, P. L. (2008). Effectiveness of virtual reality for teaching street-crossing skills to children and adolescents with autism. *International Journal on Disability and Human Development*, *7*(1), 49–56. doi:10.1515/IJDHD.2008.7.1.49

Ke, F., & Im, T. (2013). Virtual-reality-based social interaction training for children with high-functioning autism. *The Journal of Educational Research*, *106*(6), 441–461. doi:10.1080/00220671.2013.832999

Keshav, N. U., Salisbury, J. P., Vahabzadeh, A., & Sahin, N. T. (2017). Social communication coaching smartglasses: Well tolerated in a diverse sample of children and adults with autism. *JMIR mHealth and uHealth*, *5*(9), e140. doi:10.2196/mhealth.8534 PMID:28935618

Kinsella, B. G., Chow, S., & Kushki, A. (2017). Evaluating the usability of a wearable social skills training technology for children with autism spectrum disorder. *Frontiers in Robotics and AI*, *4*, 31. doi:10.3389/frobt.2017.00031

Kiryu, T., & So, R. H. (2007). Sensation of presence and cybersickness in applications of virtual reality for advanced rehabilitation. *Journal of Neuroengineering and Rehabilitation*, *4*(1), 34. doi:10.1186/1743-0003-4-34 PMID:17894857

Lahiri, U., Bekele, E., Dohrmann, E., Warren, Z., & Sarkar, N. (2015). A physiologically informed virtual reality based social communication system for individuals with autism. *Journal of Autism and Developmental Disorders*, *45*(4), 919–931. doi:10.100710803-014-2240-5 PMID:25261247

Liu, R., Salisbury, J. P., Vahabzadeh, A., & Sahin, N. T. (2017). Feasibility of an autism-focused augmented reality smartglasses system for social communication and behavioral coaching. *Frontiers in Pediatrics*, *5*, 145. doi:10.3389/fped.2017.00145 PMID:28695116

Lorenzo, G., Lledó, A., Pomares, J., & Roig, R. (2016). Design and application of an immersive virtual reality system to enhance emotional skills for children with autism spectrum disorders. *Computers & Education*, *98*, 192–205. doi:10.1016/j.compedu.2016.03.018

Lu, Y., Waltz, S., Stenzel, K., Muhle, H., & Stephani, U. (2008). Photosensitivity in epileptic syndromes of childhood and adolescence. *Epileptic Disorders*, *10*(2), 136–143. PMID:18539564

Maglione, M. A., Gans, D., Das, L., Timbie, J., & Kasari, C. (2012). Nonmedical interventions for children with ASD: Recommended guidelines and further research needs. *Pediatrics*, *130*(Suppl. 2), S169–S178. doi:10.1542/peds.2012-0900O PMID:23118248

McCleery, J. P. (2015). Comment on technology-based intervention research for individuals on the autism spectrum. *Journal of Autism and Developmental Disorders*, *45*(12), 3832–3835. doi:10.100710803-015-2627-y PMID:26537909

McCue, L. M., Flick, L. H., Twyman, K. A., Xian, H., & Conturo, T. E. (2016). Prevalence of non-febrile seizures in children with idiopathic autism spectrum disorder and their unaffected siblings: A retrospective cohort study. *BMC Neurology*, *16*(1), 245. doi:10.118612883-016-0764-3 PMID:27894273

Millett, C. J., Fish, D. R., Thompson, P. J., & Johnson, A. (1999). Seizures During Video-Game Play and Other Common Leisure Pursuits in Known Epilepsy Patients Without Visual Sensitivity. *Epilepsia*, *40*(s4), 59–64. doi:10.1111/j.1528-1157.1999.tb00908.x PMID:10487175

Milne, E., Griffiths, H., Buckley, D., & Scope, A. (2009). Vision in children and adolescents with autistic spectrum disorder: Evidence for reduced convergence. *Journal of Autism and Developmental Disorders*, *39*(7), 965–975. doi:10.100710803-009-0705-8 PMID:19224351

Mineo, B. A., Ziegler, W., Gill, S., & Salkin, D. (2009). Engagement with electronic screen media among students with autism spectrum disorders. *Journal of Autism and Developmental Disorders*, *39*(1), 172–187. doi:10.100710803-008-0616-0 PMID:18626761

Mitchell, P., Parsons, S., & Leonard, A. (2007). Using virtual environments for teaching social understanding to 6 adolescents with autistic spectrum disorders. *Journal of Autism and Developmental Disorders, 37*(3), 589–600. doi:10.100710803-006-0189-8 PMID:16900403

National Autism Center. (2015). *Findings and conclusions: National standards project, phase 2*. Randolph, MA: Author.

Neut, D., Fily, A., Cuvellier, J. C., & Vallée, L. (2012). The prevalence of triggers in paediatric migraine: A questionnaire study in 102 children and adolescents. *The Journal of Headache and Pain, 13*(1), 61–65. doi:10.100710194-011-0397-2 PMID:22042255

Newbutt, N., Sung, C., Kuo, H. J., Leahy, M. J., Lin, C. C., & Tong, B. (2016). Brief report: A pilot study of the use of a virtual reality headset in autism populations. *Journal of Autism and Developmental Disorders, 46*(9), 3166–3176. doi:10.100710803-016-2830-5 PMID:27272115

Norman, K. L. (2017). *Cyberpsychology: An introduction to human-computer interaction*. Cambridge University Press. doi:10.1017/9781316212554

Odom, S. L., Boyd, B. A., Hall, L. J., & Hume, K. (2010). Evaluation of comprehensive treatment models for individuals with autism spectrum disorders. *Journal of Autism and Developmental Disorders, 40*(4), 425–436. doi:10.100710803-009-0825-1 PMID:19633939

Odom, S. L., Thompson, J. L., Hedges, S., Boyd, B. A., Dykstra, J. R., Duda, M. A., ... Bord, A. (2015). Technology-aided interventions and instruction for adolescents with autism spectrum disorder. *Journal of Autism and Developmental Disorders, 45*(12), 3805–3819. doi:10.100710803-014-2320-6 PMID:25468409

Oswald, D. P., & Sonenklar, N. A. (2007). Medication use among children with autism spectrum disorders. *Journal of Child and Adolescent Psychopharmacology, 17*(3), 348–355. doi:10.1089/cap.2006.17303 PMID:17630868

Parsons, S., & Cobb, S. (2011). State-of-the-art of virtual reality technologies for children on the autism spectrum. *European Journal of Special Needs Education, 26*(3), 355–366. doi:10.1080/08856257.2011.593831

Parsons, S., Mitchell, P., & Leonard, A. (2004). The use and understanding of virtual environments by adolescents with autistic spectrum disorders. *Journal of Autism and Developmental Disorders, 34*(4), 449–466. doi:10.1023/B:JADD.0000037421.98517.8d PMID:15449520

Parsons, T. D., Riva, G., Parsons, S., Mantovani, F., Newbutt, N., Lin, L., ... Hall, T. (2017). Virtual reality in pediatric psychology. *Pediatrics, 140*(Suppl. 2), S86–S91. doi:10.1542/peds.2016-1758I PMID:29093039

Parsons, T. D., Rizzo, A. A., Rogers, S., & York, P. (2009). Virtual reality in paediatric rehabilitation: A review. *Developmental Neurorehabilitation, 12*(4), 224–238. doi:10.1080/17518420902991719 PMID:19842822

Ploog, B. O., Scharf, A., Nelson, D., & Brooks, P. J. (2013). Use of computer-assisted technologies (CAT) to enhance social, communicative, and language development in children with autism spectrum disorders. *Journal of Autism and Developmental Disorders, 43*(2), 301–322. doi:10.100710803-012-1571-3 PMID:22706582

Ravindran, V., Sazawal, V., Solorzano, R., & Turnacioglu, S. (2017). Experiences with virtual reality-based training for joint attention: a usability and initial feasibility pilot of FloreoVR's Joint Attention Module in a special education school setting.

Roux, A. M., Shattuck, P. T., Rast, J. E., Rava, J. A., & Anderson, K. A. (2015). National Autism Indicators Report: Transition into Young Adulthood. Philadelphia, PA: Life Course Outcomes Research Program, A.J. Drexel Autism Institute, Drexel University.

Rubboli, G., Parra, J., Seri, S., Takahashi, T., & Thomas, P. (2004). EEG diagnostic procedures and special investigations in the assessment of photosensitivity. *Epilepsia*, *45*(s1), 35–39. doi:10.1111/j.0013-9580.2004.451002.x PMID:14706044

Sahin, N. T., Keshav, N. U., Salisbury, J. P., & Vahabzadeh, A. (2017). Cool enough for school: Second version of Google Glass rated by children facing challenges to social integration as desirable to wear at school.

Sahin, N. T., Keshav, N. U., Salisbury, J. P., & Vahabzadeh, A. (2017). An augmented reality social communication aid for children and adults with autism: User and caregiver report of safety and lack of negative effects.

Saiano, M., Pellegrino, L., Casadio, M., Summa, S., Garbarino, E., Rossi, V., ... Sanguineti, V. (2015). Natural interfaces and virtual environments for the acquisition of street crossing and path following skills in adults with Autism Spectrum Disorders: A feasibility study. *Journal of Neuroengineering and Rehabilitation*, *12*(1), 17. doi:10.118612984-015-0010-z PMID:25885279

Shoja, M. M., Tubbs, R. S., Malekian, A., Jafari Rouhi, A. H., Barzgar, M., & Oakes, W. J. (2007). Video game epilepsy in the twentieth century: A review. *Child's Nervous System*, *23*(3), 265–267. doi:10.100700381-006-0285-2 PMID:17211654

Smith, M. J., Ginger, E. J., Wright, K., Wright, M. A., Taylor, J. L., Humm, L. B., ... Fleming, M. F. (2014). Virtual reality job interview training in adults with autism spectrum disorder. *Journal of Autism and Developmental Disorders*, *44*(10), 2450–2463. doi:10.100710803-014-2113-y PMID:24803366

Strickland, D. (1997). Virtual reality for the treatment of autism. *Studies in Health Technology and Informatics*, 81–86. PMID:10184809

Strickland, D., Marcus, L. M., Mesibov, G. B., & Hogan, K. (1996). Brief report: Two case studies using virtual reality as a learning tool for autistic children. *Journal of Autism and Developmental Disorders*, *26*(6), 651–659. doi:10.1007/BF02172354 PMID:8986851

Strickland, D. C., Coles, C. D., & Southern, L. B. (2013). JobTIPS: A transition to employment program for individuals with autism spectrum disorders. *Journal of Autism and Developmental Disorders*, *43*(10), 2472–2483. doi:10.100710803-013-1800-4 PMID:23494559

Strickland, D. C., McAllister, D., Coles, C. D., & Osborne, S. (2007). An evolution of virtual reality training designs for children with autism and fetal alcohol spectrum disorders. *Topics in Language Disorders*, *27*(3), 226–241. doi:10.1097/01.TLD.0000285357.95426.72 PMID:20072702

Thomas, S., Hovinga, M. E., Rai, D., & Lee, B. K. (2017). Brief report: prevalence of co-occurring epilepsy and autism spectrum disorder: the US National Survey of Children's Health 2011–2012. *Journal of Autism and Developmental Disorders*, *47*(1), 224–229. doi:10.100710803-016-2938-7 PMID:27752862

Tzanavari, A., Charalambous-Darden, N., Herakleous, K., & Poullis, C. (2015). Effectiveness of an immersive virtual environment (CAVE) for teaching pedestrian crossing to children with PDD-NOS. In *2015 IEEE 15th International Conference on Advanced Learning Technologies (ICALT)* (pp. 423-427). IEEE.

Wade, J., Zhang, L., Bian, D., Fan, J., Swanson, A., Weitlauf, A., ... Sarkar, N. (2016). A gaze-contingent adaptive virtual reality driving environment for intervention in individuals with autism spectrum disorders. *ACM Transactions on Interactive Intelligent Systems*, *6*(1), 3. doi:10.1145/2892636

Wainer, A. L., & Ingersoll, B. R. (2011). The use of innovative computer technology for teaching social communication to individuals with autism spectrum disorders. *Research in Autism Spectrum Disorders*, *5*(1), 96–107. doi:10.1016/j.rasd.2010.08.002

Wallace, S., Parsons, S., Westbury, A., White, K., White, K., & Bailey, A. (2010). Sense of presence and atypical social judgments in immersive virtual environments: Responses of adolescents with Autism Spectrum Disorders. *Autism*, *14*(3), 199–213. doi:10.1177/1362361310363283 PMID:20484000

Washington, P., Voss, C., Kline, A., Haber, N., Daniels, J., Fazel, A., ... Wall, D. (2017). SuperpowerGlass: A wearable aid for the at-home therapy of children with autism. *Proceedings of the ACM on Interactive, Mobile, Wearable and Ubiquitous Technologies, 1*(3), 112. 10.1145/3130977

Wong, C., Odom, S. L., Hume, K. A., Cox, A. W., Fettig, A., Kucharczyk, S., ... Schultz, T. R. (2015). Evidence-based practices for children, youth, and young adults with autism spectrum disorder: A comprehensive review. *Journal of Autism and Developmental Disorders*, *45*(7), 1951–1966. doi:10.100710803-014-2351-z PMID:25578338

Yang, Y. D., Allen, T., Abdullahi, S. M., Pelphrey, K. A., Volkmar, F. R., & Chapman, S. B. (2017). Brain responses to biological motion predict treatment outcome in young adults with autism receiving Virtual Reality Social Cognition Training: Preliminary findings. *Behaviour Research and Therapy*, *93*, 55–66. doi:10.1016/j.brat.2017.03.014 PMID:28384509

## KEY TERMS AND DEFINITIONS

**Augmented Reality:** technology that adds computer-generated content to the user's view of the real world.

**Autism Spectrum Disorder:** a neurodevelopmental condition with core symptoms of social communication impairment and restricted and repetitive patterns of behavior.

**Avatar:** a computer-generated representation of an individual in a virtual environment.

**Cybersickness:** a form of motion or simulator sickness related to sensory mismatch or conflict; symptoms include dizziness, nausea, eye strain and fatigue.

**Head-Mounted Display:** a device worn over a user's head, providing a visual display in front of one or both of the user's eyes.

**Immersive Virtual Reality:** VR platforms designed to create a sense in the user that he or she is actually in the VE; the platform fully occludes the user's view of the real world with virtual content.

**Non-Immersive Virtual Reality:** VR experiences that typically use desktop or laptop screens to present the VE to a user, so the user does not experience the sense of actually being in the VE; the platform does not fully occlude the user's field of view.

**Virtual Reality:** technology that provides computer-generated content, in which a user can engage directly with the VE or with avatars within the VE.

**Wearable Technology:** electronic devices that are worn on the body and often include tracking information related to fitness or health.

# Chapter 9
# Virtual Reality (VR) for School Children With Autism Spectrum Disorder (ASD):
## A Way of Rethinking Teaching and Learning

**Giuliana Guazzaroni**
*Università Politecnica delle Marche, Italy*

**Anitha S. Pillai**
*Hindustan Institute of Technology and Science, India*

## ABSTRACT

*Various medical and technological organizations are working on the development of unconventional solutions such as therapy and assistance for people with autism spectrum disorder (ASD). Different organizations, researchers and educators have been involved in the study and realization of virtual reality (VR) solutions to be used as therapy, training, and support for these individuals. Previous researches and experiments showed that it is possible to ameliorate the level of concentration, coordination, socialization, communication, self-awareness, and memory in school children treated with these tools. VR environments may offer a total physical involvement of the ASDs that may see the world through virtual immersion and active practice. This chapter presents a way of rethinking teaching and learning.*

## INTRODUCTION

Autism spectrum disorders (ASD) present impairments in three important domains: social skills, communication and behaviour. It is important to help ASD individuals with proper strategies (American Psychiatric Association, 2013; Bellani et al., 2011; Parsons & Mitchell, 2002). Virtual reality (VR) for these users has been studied and developed for over two decades (Newbutt et al., 2016). VR is a simulation of everyday real world based on computer 3D immersive graphics and 360-degree videos. VR

DOI: 10.4018/978-1-5225-7168-1.ch009

immersive environments may be helpful for educators and therapists to offer the opportunity to access a protected, tailor made and repeatable learning environment (Bellani et al., 2011; Kandalaft et al., 2013; Newbutt et al., 2016). An immersive learning environment is a virtual environment where students can connect, interact, find 360-degree learning objects and complete educational tasks wearing a special head-mounted display. These learning spaces can reproduce real existence, can invent totally new virtual worlds, can offer tailor made experiences useful to understand and perform specific tasks (Bellani et al., 2011). The literature is progressively accepting the benefits of VR facilities in teaching ASD individuals, especially related to social skills (Parsons & Mitchell, 2002; Bellani et al., 2011; Kandalaft et al., 2013; Didehbani et al., 2016; Newbutt et al., 2016). In fact, children with autism experience fundamental difficulties in the social domain. This impairment interferes with the process of creating relationships, participating and integrating with peers (Parsons & Mitchell, 2002; Kandalaft et al., 2013). Core difficulties in communication is one of the critical limitations of ASD children. According to Halabi et al. (2017), these children 'commonly demonstrate difficulties in initiating as well as responding to social interactions'. In a social situation ASDs experience limitations in processing context, dialogue and non-verbal communication. Many studies have investigated the use of VR technology in the education process of autistic children. The nature of VR learning environments is positive as it induces controlled verbal and non-verbal stimuli, allow to monitor children's behavior and permit the repetition of the proposed task (Halabi et al., 2017; Newbutt et al., 2016; Bellani et al., 2011; Parsons & Mitchell, 2002). Moreover, children in the autism spectrum usually present impairments and delay in understanding symbolism and symbolic play. VR facilities may offer a further opportunity for these children to understand and manipulate symbols, for teaching pretend play and for understanding imagination (Herrera et al., 2008) with the purpose, for example, to teach numbers and alphabets. ASD children present a developmental delay in the acquisition of self-recognition. Autistic individuals are impaired in accessing autobiographical memories and events happened in the past (Uddin, 2011). The autobiographical memory in children with autism is marked by errors of omission, and it seems poor especially for early-life events (Crane et al., 2009; Uddin, 2011; Lyons & Fitzgerald, 2013). Another relevant characteristics of autism is the lack of empathy and emotional engagement with peers. ASD pupils cannot interpret emotions in the right way, they cannot process their own emotions and have difficulties with the emotional engagement with other people as they are generally focused on their own concerns (Lyons & Fitzgerald, 2013). For ASD schoolboys and girls an immersive virtual scenario can be an attractive learning environment because it releases their pressure. There is less physical inflection involved in VR animation or in a 360-degree movies than within real human interactions, and for ASDs this simplification can help reduce their confusion and anxiety. In this context, VR learning tools offer the potential to create a training and treatment environment, immersive and dynamic, allowing interaction, behavioral tracking, and performance recording (Rizzo & Kim, 2005). In this chapter, the authors outline how a proper use of VR educational facilities ia a new a way of rethinking teaching and learning, and it is useful to improve concentration, coordination, socialisation, numbers and words learning, self-awareness and memory in ASD pupils.

## A WAY OF RETHINKING TEACHING AND LEARNING FOR ASD CHILDREN

### Teaching and Training ASD Children Using VR Facilities

VR is used in teaching and training ASD pupils. Different studies (Parsons & Cobb, 2011; Bellani et al., 2011; Rizzo & Kim, 2005) pointed out that this technology is advantageous for people with cognitive and perceptual impairments, including autism, because VR can support in planning, problem-solving and management of behaviour. Moreover, VR offers an effective communication help for children with limited language (Parsons & Cobb). Rizzo and Kim (2005), affirmed that VR is a powerful learning resource. According to them, VR presents the strengths of stimulus control and consistency, self-guided exploration and independent practice, interface modification on user's impairments, safe testing in a special training environment and gaming factors to enhance motivation to learn etc. (Rizzo & Kim, 2005). The use of VR for skill development requires interaction with virtual representation of a person/animal (avatar). For a really successful design of VR learning, avatars and their specific role in a virtual space should be interpreted by an ASD child. Basic emotions embodied by avatars should be appropriately understood and facial expressions should be informative for autistic children (Parsons & Cobb, 2011). A research (Ramachandiran et al., 2015) designed a VR learning environment for autistic pupils by developing a virtual space devoted to picture exchange communication system (PECS) methodology for data collection. PECS is a communication method that does not require speech as it is based on exchanging real object photos with the aim to deliver a message efficaciously. Exchanging the proper pictures, ASD children start an important act of communication. A total of 41 parents and 41 ASD children participated in the experiment. The role of the parents using the PECS methodology was to facilitate their children to communicate and choose the objects (e.g. Objects/specimens related to a toilet virtual environment). Autistic children need an effective learning tool not only to improve their knowledge, but also their behaviours. In fact, they may develop unusual fears which limit their daily life activities. In this experiment, the height of the sitting toilet was a real concern for parents as a number of autistic children suffer from acrophobia, the fear of height. The authors concluded that there are different VR based learning tools available today, but only a small selections of these tools are useful for ASDs. In fact, VR environments for teaching autism spectrum children should be designed to minimise their level of fear (Ramachandiran et al., 2015). Unusual fears have long been recognized as common in autism. In a sample of 1033 children with autism, unusual fears were reported by 421 (41%) of the children (Mayers et al., 2013). The most common unusual fear was the fear of toilets, the fear of vacuum cleaners, the elevators, the mechanical toys, the swings and the wind. Children with autism perceive, experience and react to the world differently than those without. Common experiences for most children (e.g. A change in their daily routine) is terrifying and distressing for a child with autism (Mayers et al., 2013). A VR head-mounted display (VR-HMD) is an important tool to plunge in a real VR immersive environment. Nevertheless, VR-HMD may represent a fearful device for an autistic pupil. A study (Newbutt et al., 2016) revealed that all ASD participants were willing to wear a VR-HMD. Each user's verbal and non verbal behavioral reactions to the HMD were recorded and observed. All the participants were disposed to plunge in at least two of the three preselected VR environments proposed. They generally accepted the HMD and were willing to complete the tasks associated with the VR scenarios. In addition, the involved users with ASD reported higher spatial presence, engagement and ecological validity within the VR environment, and lower level of negative effects (Newbutt et al., 2016). VR facilities are encouraging tools for teaching and training ASDs, a 360 degrees real world, or a safe recreated one, can be repeated to provide experiences that can help students understand specific concept and learn to perform required tasks (Bellani et al., 2011).

## VR for Reading Numbers and Words

Literature review shows that children with autism are relatively better at visual processing. It is observed that children with autism usually find difficulties in reading textual information (numbers and words), but excel in instruction that is accompanied by visual component. Saadatzi et al. (2018) developed a tutoring system using VR and Robots that featured a virtual teacher instructing words and another robot emulating a peer. Results indicated that participants acquired, maintained and generalized 100% of the words explicitly instructed to them, made fewer errors while learning the words common between them and the robot peer, and vicariously learned 94% of the words solely instructed by the robot (Saadatzi et al., 2018). According to the authors percent of correct reading responses for words in explicit learning (EL) and explicit-plus-vicarious learning (EVL) groups across baseline, instructional sessions, and post-instruction probes showed improvement Prior to the intervention, none of the participants read EL or EVL words correctly (Saadatzi et al., 2018).

## Improving Concentration in ASD Children Using VR

Concentration is very important in learning. By concentration we mean paying attention or focussing on one thing and ignoring or putting other things out of our minds. Children should concentrate in class to learn/understand what a teacher is teaching, One of the main problem faced by children with ASD is lack of ability to concentrate and listen for a long period of time. In addition to the social, communicative and behavioral symptoms that define the disorder, individuals with ASD have difficulty re-orienting attention quickly and accurately (Chukoskie et al., 2017). Literature review points out that a child with autism may have an unflinching ability to concentrate on activities that are interesting to them and concentration seems to be fleeting when they are involved in activities that are not interesting to them. Atypical gaze and attention are among the earliest symptoms observed in ASD and disruption of these foundation skills critically affects the development of higher level cognitive and social behaviour (Chukoskie et al., 2017).

## VR for Strengthening Coordination

Coordination plays an important role in carrying out our day to day activities. A specific study (Muneer et al., 2015) explored the use of VR games not just for enjoyment but also to improve skills in children with developmental disabilities. The main aim of this study was targeted at the enhancement of motor skills. The children's communication, cognitive and social/emotional skills were also monitored as part of this study. Therapists guided 5 children (4 boys with ASD and 1 girl with Learning Disability) while they played carefully chosen games on the Xbox-Kinect, in individual sessions (Muneer et al., 2015).

Each child was made to undergo between 4 and 6 sessions over a period of one month. A 4-point rating scale was used to evaluate motor, communication, cognitive and social skills at the beginning of the session, and after completing it. From these scores authors found that there was good progress not only in motor skills but also in cognitive and social skills. Initial findings indicate that VR games provide a useful platform for building interventions for children with developmental disabilities (Muneer et al., 2015). The different ways in which children with varied developmental profiles might benefit from virtual reality-based interventions were also put forth by the authors. Six unique VR training scenarios with corresponding training protocols are designed, implemented and being delivered to over 100 school-aged children with normal-ranged IQ (IQ > 70) via a 4-side fully immersive CAVE™ VR installation in 28 sessions (14 weeks) (Ip et al., 2016). Ip et al. (2016) pointed out that the results of their study showed significant improvements in three major designated aspects, including emotion recognition, affective expression and social reciprocity.

## Better Socialising With the Help of VR

ASD is a neurodevelopmental disorder characterized by deficits in social interaction and communication and is accompanied by restricted patterns of interest and behavior (Psychiatry Online: DSM Library, n.d.). Children with ASD find it difficult to socialise even with kids of their age. They find it difficult to initiate as well as respond in social interactions. As a result of this, they do not interact and stay away from others. These difficulties include processing the situation and dialogue surrounding them, inability understanding nonverbal aspects of communication, lack of human engagement, and inability generalizing between environments (Lahiri et al, 2011; Kuriakose et al., 2013). Virtual environments offer a new and exciting perspective on social skills training for people with ASD (Parsons & Mitchell, 2002). Deficits in social communication and difficulty inhibiting thoughts and regulating emotions can lead to social isolation and low self-esteem (Didehbani et al., 2016). Researchers from the Center for Brainhealth at the University of Texas at Dallas identified thirty young people ages 7 to 16 with high-functioning autism and divided them into two groups. The teams were given 10, one-hour sessions of virtual reality training over a 5-week period to learn strategies and practice social situations such as meeting a peer for the first time, confronting a bully, and inviting someone to a party. Children were made to interact with two clinicians through virtual avatars. One clinician served as a coach, providing instructions and guidance, while the other was the conversational partner who played a classmate, bully, teacher or others, depending on the scenario in the video-game-like world (Didehbani et al., 2016). Researchers observed relationships in life grow from virtual world conversations and saw a lot of growth in their ability to initiate and maintain a conversation, interpret emotions and judge the quality of a friendship. Their study also saw improvements in diverse domains including emotion recognition, making social attribution, and executive functions and they concluded that core social skills can be enhanced using VR. Authors (Ke & Im, 2013) examined the implementation and potential effect of a virtual-reality-based social interaction program on the interaction and communication performance of children with high functioning autism. Collection of data for the study was collected from behaviour observation and analysis, questionnaires and interviewing. According to Ke and Im (2013), children who participated in the study showed improvements in performance of responding, initiation, greeting and positive conversation-ending during the intervention, and the social competence measures after the intervention also showed progress. The study highlighted the importance of a virtual-reality-based learning environment for learners with special needs. The application of Collaborative Virtual Environment (CVE) technology in ASD intervention brings advantages in providing a safe, flexible, and collaborative environment (Zhao et al., 2016). VR technology may be an ideal tool for allowing participants to practise behaviours in role-play situations, whilst also providing a safe environment for rule learning and repetition of tasks (Parsons & Mitchell, 2002). According to the authors role-play within virtual environments stimulate the mental simulation of social events and also encourages a more flexible approach to social problem solving. VR providing a simulated environment that could be used for training people with special needs by exposing them which to a simulated version of the workplace they will be working at. This will help them overcome social awkwardness as they would become more comfortable with the workplace environment (Rahaman et al., 2017). Children with ASD often suffer from deficits in communication and social interaction, which lead to various social challenges in interacting with peers in collaborative tasks (Zhao et al., 2016). Research geared at utilizing technology to mend social and communication impairments in children with autism is actively underway. Immersive VR is a relatively recent technology that has the potential of being an effective therapeutic tool for developing various skills in autistic children (Halabi et al., 2017). A research presents a scenario-based interactive VR system to improve the communications skills of autistic children using speech recognition, natural interaction and role-play. In the experiments conducted, participants showed a better performance with a computer augmented virtual environment (CAVE) than with a head-mounted display (HMD) or a normal desktop. The results indicate that immersive VR could be more satisfactory and motivational than desktop for children with ASD (Halabi et al., 2017).

## Self-Awareness in ASD Children

Research revealed evidence for altered self-representation, or intrapersonal cognition, in ASD individuals. (Uddin, 2011). Self-related cognition may also be altered in ASD children. Typically developing children at the age of two can recognize themselves in a mirror. In contrast, infants with autism present a delay in the acquisition of this ability (Uddin, 2011; Lind & Bowler, 2009). The ability of self-face recognition in the mirror is considered a test for self-awareness. Research data on recognition of one's own face disclosed that ASDs children have deficits of self-awareness. As measured by a specific test, they have little interest in their own mirror images (Lyons & Fitzgerald, 2013). The prefrontal cortex, particularly the Right Hemisphere (RH), has a crucial role in self-face identification. Face recognition studies in ASDs point out a lack of body awareness. Autistic individuals are impaired in differentiating between self and others (Lyons & Fitzgerald, 2013). Language difficulties are common in autism spectrum disorder. Stereotypical verbal behaviours are commonly observed including repetitive language, idiosyncratic phrases, difficulties with pronouns and echolalia (American Psychiatric Association, 2013; Lyons & Fitzgerald, 2013; Gernsbacher et al., 2016; Brignell et al., 2018). Gernsbacher et al. (2016) reported that autistic children's difficulties with pronouns were interpreted by some studies as unawareness of personal identity. Duff and Flattery (2014) recently interpreted autistic children's problem with pronouns as a deficit in the understanding the self and other relationship. According to Lyons and Fitzgerald (2013), language difficulties have a negative effects on mental process and reduce specific aspects of ASD children self-awareness. Inner speech is consequently impaired in pupils with autism, they are 'visual thinkers' and 'rely heavily on visualization to process information' (Lyons & Fitzgerald, 2013). A teaching methodology in students diagnosed with ASD should be specifically designed to develop positive self-awareness and joint attention (JA) strategies (Duff & Flattery, 2014).

## Memory and Narrative Self in ASD Children

Individuals create their own identity by 'constructing autobiographical narratives or life stories' (Lyons & Fitzgerald, 2013). Huang et al. (2017) affirmed that there are impairments in the psychological self in individuals with ASD and they generally have limited awareness in the self and others. The development of self is associated with the autobiographical memory. The components that form an autobiographical memory system are impaired in ASD individuals (Lyons & Fitzgerald, 2013; Uddin, 2011). A study demonstrated as individuals with autism generated fewer memories than those without as they present difficulty in using past experiences to improve the self (Crane et al., 2009; Uddin, 201). ASD children's autobiographical memory is 'marked by error of omission, and memory is particularly poor for early-life events' (Uddin, 2011). According to Lyons and Fitzgerald (2013), ASDs remember their real-life experiences less well than other individuals and they generally present episodic and poor memory. ASD children have great difficulties in creating their 'self-narrative' as 'the narrative of individuals with ASD, and the self that is represented in this narrative, is quite vague and not representing the true self' (Lyons & Fitzgerald, 2013). Researches regarding the characteristics of the self in ASD are important to develop crucial interventions to help this population better handle challenges in life (Andersen, 2016; Huang et al., 2017). Effective intervention programs are needed to ameliorate social communication impairments in ASD students to improve self-competence and the quality of their life (Huang et al., 2017). ASDs should have more opportunities to develop their skills and be offered proper feedback on their behaviors, since children usually acquire self-awareness and knowledge by interacting with their environments and peers (Duff & Flattery, 2014; Huang et al., 2017). In this context, VR may represent a valid tool to teach ASD students crucial skills as emphasized by many authors; the evidence of results suggest that VR is a useful facility with unique potential for ASD learners (Parsons & Mitchell, 2002; Herrera et al., 2008; Aiello et al., 2012; Bellani et al., 2011; Parsons & Cobb, 2011; Didehbani et al., 2016; Halabi et al., 2017).

## FUTURE PROSPECTS

### Cybersickness and VR Side Effects

According to Parsons and Mitchell (2002), there are some ethical concerns using 'fully immersive' VR technology as it requires head-mounted displays (HMD). Thanks to the advance in technology, VR head-mounted display (VR-HMD) are now cheaper than the expensive displays considered by Parsons and Mitchell in 2002. For example, the Google Cardboard is a cheap and useful VR-HMD, easy to use with ASD children. This platform is a low-cost system to encourage interest and development in VR applications. Users can build their own viewer using specifications published by Google, or purchase a pre-manufactured one. The other ethical concern pointed out by some authors is 'cybersickness', described as nausea, headaches and dizziness (Cobb et al. 1999; Parsons & Mitchell, 2002). Researches (Tiiro, 2018) regarding cybersickness in VR indicate that higher visual realism causes more cybersickness than lower visual realism. A greater level of detail in high visual realism graphics causes more visual flow and stronger sensory mismatches that causes cybersickness. Studies are devoted to minimize cybersickness effects as it is widely accepted that VR side effects cannot be eliminated (Tiiro, 2018). VR-HMD industry and software developers have worked hard to avoid it because cybersickness may

*Figure 1. A VR learning session with a student*

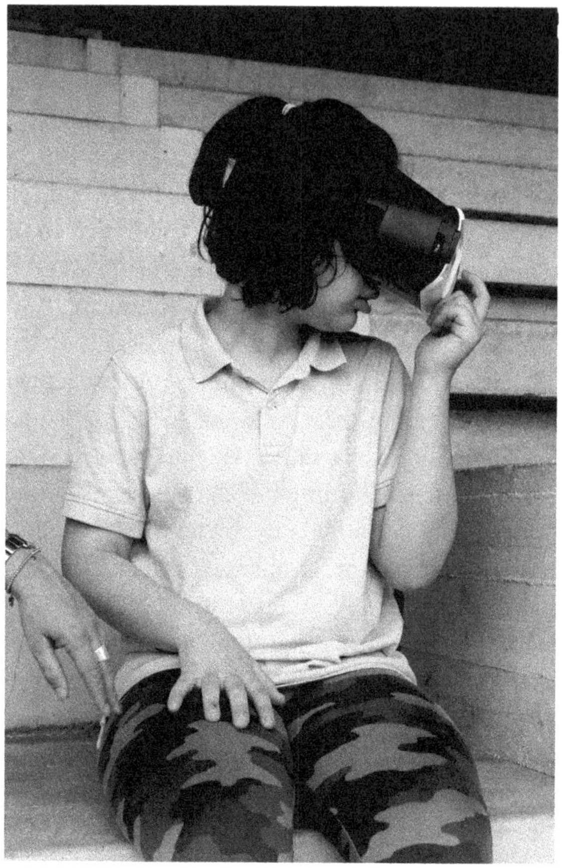

represent a deterrent to mass adoption of VR (Mason, 2017). Cybersickness can be limited by knowing its causes, specific measures should be taken to fix VR side effects. Studies indicated methods to prevent cybersickness, including a correct calibration of VR technology and customization to students' needs to offer ASDs a natural user interface (UI). Techniques to reduce cybersickness while navigating in virtual environments were proposed by Kemeny et al. (2017). An example is to reduce the field of view (FOV) and the immersion level. Most VR headset manufacturers say HMD are not suitable for children under age 12 or 13 (Mukamal, 2017). Although there are no long-term studies and ophthalmologists agree there is no reason to be concerned that VR headsets will damage eye development. In fact, age limitations for VR technology might make sense for the content a child may access online without adult supervision. Moreover, staring at a VR-HMD screen, or any digital device, for a protracted period may cause eye fatigue (Mukamal, 2017). Appropriate, research-based and ethical regulations should be planned to enhance the benefits and minimize the potential harm of VR technology. Parents, educators and teachers should handle media and digital literacy best practices. This includes being involved and informed of their children's use of media, encouraging critical thinking regarding their VR educational experiences. In truth, most stimulating and creative uses of VR should come from an open dialogue between educators, teachers and their students (Darvasi, 2016).

## VR Active Learning for ASD Children

Future work considering VR active learning for young students with an ASD should use flexible and accessible tools and approaches based on well-researched evidence-based practice to be implemented at home, in school and/or other suitable places (Parsons & Cobb, 2011). A VR learning environment should be active, easy to use, and helpful for educators and parents ‘to enhance the daily life social behaviours of individuals with autism’ (Bellani et al., 2011). Future research in VR technology for training ASDs should take advance of facial tracking and movement of the avatar, allow naturalistic and real-time facial expressions (Kandalaft, 2013) and emotions. As in the real world, VR environments should offer ‘total body involvement’, which allows people to see the world through ‘sensorimotor learning’ as ‘experiential component is one of the stages of a process that leads to the world’s symbolic representation’ (Aiello et al., 2012). The result should be an active learning environment that enables ‘active experimentation’ where learning ‘comes from acting, experiencing, observing’ (Aiello et al., 2012). VR facilities should be designed in such a way that users would find it difficult to tell the difference from what is a real experience and what is not (Guazzaroni, 2017). Learning from experiences is impossible in most cases at school, but VR technologies can allow direct interaction with VR environments and objects. It was reported that experiential learning in a VR learning environment is identical to an experience in the real world (Maraj et al., 2017). Moreover, it was determined that the enhanced vividness and interactivity in a VR environment allows students to recognize the experience as being closer to a direct experience (Kwon et al., in press). Implementing a VR learning experience should involve the exploration of unusual pedagogical and technological boundaries. VR technology is immersive and users need viewers to block out the external world and plunge themselves in a digital realm (Guazzaroni, 2017). The spatial immersion in a virtual world is a perception of being physically present in a non-physical world that provides a very absorbing environment (Freina & Ott, 2015). Consequently, VR should allow first-person experience in virtual worlds as the possibility to visit special places and views. For instance, dangerous zones where a student cannot go. VR viewers, like Google Cardboard, represent a cheap HMD to start using fully immersive VR with ASD children. VR-HMD has the potential to enhance the classroom, or the single student, by providing concrete knowledge, based on real experience, authentic and engaging learning (Oigara, 2018). The use of proper VR technology in education can be an opening to the informal learning environments. Furthermore, these technologies should help the transition from the ‘Learning work’ to the ‘Learning adventure’. In other words, a positive class atmosphere where students’ activities are aimed to satisfy a personal desire of acquiring knowledge (Leo et al., 2010). VR facilities should be used as a proper and valid aid to teach ASD students crucial skills as reported by many researches. The evidence of results suggest that VR offer unique potential for ASD learners (Parsons & Mitchell, 2002; Herrera et al., 2008; Aiello et al., 2012; Bellani et al., 2011; Parsons & Cobb, 2011; Ramachandiran et al., 2015; Didehbani et al., 2016; Halabi et al., 2017). Future work should also consider to use virtual worlds and immersive VR to help the integration of the ASD students with their peers, to improve empathy and friendship between students in the class. A stimulating and creative use of VR facilities should be encouraged and come from an open dialogue between parents, teachers and their students (Darvasi, 2016).

## CONCLUSION

The use of immersive technology is taking an increasingly prominent role in research and teaching practice related to ASD. Technological advances can potentially lead to more effective strategies and enhance the quality of life for people with ASD and their families (Bölte et al., 2010). The potential of VR technology is to facilitate the learning processes and to avoid problems characterizing traditional teaching/learning methods. Researchers considered VR based learning effective for autistic children to facilitate their teaching/learning process (Ramachandiran et al., 2015). Studies revealed that VR is advantageous for ASD learners to teach safety skills, to hold their interest, to monitor eye gaze, to help learning of pretend play, to make sense of emotions of avatars (Kandalaft et al., 2013). Impairments in communication is one of the most important lack of autistic children as they commonly demonstrate difficulties in initiating and responding to social interactions (Halabi et al., 2017). VR technology has been proved to be effective and handful to improve social skills in children with autism. Consequently, VR facilities should be used in the future to provide an efficient, flexible and affordable support for autistic school children (Halabi et al., 2017; Catren, 2017; Kandalaft et al., 2013; Parsons & Mitchell, 2002).

## REFERENCES

Aiello, P., D'Elia, F., Di Tore, S., & Sibilio, M. (2012). A constructivist approach to virtual reality for experiential learning. *E-Learning and Digital Media*, *9*(3), 317–324. doi:10.2304/elea.2012.9.3.317

American Psychiatric Association. (2013). *Diagnostic and statistical manual of mental disorders: DSM-5*. Washington, DC: American Psychiatric Publishing.

Andersen, M. (2016). A conceptual framework for understanding characteristics of self-awareness associated with autism spectrum disorder. *Scandinavian Journal of Child and Adolescent Psychiatry and Psychology*, *4*(3), 109–114. doi:10.21307jcapp-2016-017

Bellani, M., Fornasari, L., Chittaro, L., & Brambilla, P. (2011). Virtual reality in autism: State of the art. *Epidemiology and Psychiatric Sciences*, *20*(3), 235–238. doi:10.1017/S2045796011000448 PMID:21922965

Bölte, S., Golan, O., Goodwin, M. S., & Zwaigenbaum, L. (2010). What can innovative technologies do for Autism Spectrum Disorders? *Autism*, *14*(3), 155–159. doi:10.1177/1362361310365028 PMID:20603897

Brignell, A., Morgan, A. T., Woolfenden, S., Klopper, F., May, T., Sarkozy, V., & Williams, K. (2018). A systematic review and meta-analysis of the prognosis of language outcomes for individuals with autism spectrum disorder. *Autism & Developmental Language Impairments*. Retrieved July 3, 2018 from http://journals.sagepub.com/doi/10.1177/2396941518767610

Catren, N. R. (2017). *Virtual reality may be a help to autistic children in the classroom*. Retrieved March 5, 2018 from http://www.independent.co.uk/news/science/virtual-reality-may-be-a-help-to-autistic-children-in-the-classroom-a7676391.html

Chukoskie, L., Westerfield, M., & Townsend, J. (2017). A novel approach to training attention and gaze in ASD: A feasibility and efficacy pilot study. *Developmental Neurobiology*, *78*(5), 546–554. doi:10.1002/dneu.22563 PMID:29218791

Cobb, S., Nichols, S. C., Ramsey, A., & Wilson, J. (1999). Virtual reality induced symptoms and effects (VRISE). *Presence (Cambridge, Mass.)*, *8*(2), 169–186. doi:10.1162/105474699566152

Crane, L., Goddard, L., & Pring, L. (2009). Specific and general autobiographical knowledge in adults with autism spectrum disorders: The role of personal goals. *Memory (Hove, England)*, *17*(5), 557–576. doi:10.1080/09658210902960211 PMID:19499459

Darvasi, P. (2016). *Five ethical considerations for using virtual reality with children and adolescents.* Retrieved July 3, 2018 from https://www.kqed.org/mindshift/46103/five-ethical-considerations-for-using-virtual-reality-with-children-and-adolescents

Didehbani, N., Allen, T., Kandalaft, M., Krawczyk, D., & Chapman, S. (2016). Virtual reality social cognition training for children with high functioning autism. *Computers in Human Behavior*, *62*, 703–711. doi:10.1016/j.chb.2016.04.033

Duff, C. K., & Flattery, J. J. (2014). Developing mirror self awareness in students with autism spectrum disorder. *Journal of Autism and Developmental Disorders*, *44*(5), 1027–1038. doi:10.100710803-013-1954-0 PMID:24077784

Freina, L., & Ott, M. (2015). A literature review on immersive virtual reality in education: state of the art and perspectives. In *The International Scientific Conference eLearning and Software for Education* (vol. 1, pp. 133-141). Bucharest: eLSE.

Gernsbacher, M. A., Morson, E. M., & Grace, E. J. (2016). Language and speech in autism. *Annual Review of Linguistics*, *2*(1), 413–425. doi:10.1146/annurev-linguistics-030514-124824 PMID:28127576

Guazzaroni, G. (2017). The impact of augmented reality and virtual reality study material in the future of learning: a teamwork experience. In G. Kurubacak & H. Altinpulluk (Eds.), *Mobile Technologies and Augmented Reality in Open Education* (pp. 77–94). Hershey, PA: IGI Global. doi:10.4018/978-1-5225-2110-5.ch004

Halabi, O., El-Seoud, S. A., Alja'am, J. M., Alpona, H., Al-Hemadi, M., & Al-Hassan, D. (2017). Immersive virtual reality in improving communication skills in children with autism. *International Journal of Interactive Mobile Technologies*, *2*(11). Retrieved from http://online-journals.org/index.php/i-jim/article/view/6555/4365

Herrera, G., Alcantud, F., Jordan, R., Blanquer, A., Labajo, G., & De Pablo, C. (2008). Development of symbolic play through the use of virtual reality tools in children with autistic spectrum disorders: Two case studies. *Autism*, *12*(2), 143–157. doi:10.1177/1362361307086657 PMID:18308764

Huang, A. X., Hughes, T. L., Sutton, L. R., Lawrence, M., Chen, X., Ji, Z., & Zeleke, W. (2017). Understanding the self in individuals with autism spectrum disorders (ASD): A review of literature. *Frontiers in Psychology*, *8*, 1422. doi:10.3389/fpsyg.2017.01422 PMID:28878717

Ip, H. H., Wong, S. W., Chan, D. F., Byrne, J., Li, C., Yuan, V. S., & Wong, J. Y. (2016). Virtual Reality Enabled Training for Social Adaptation in Inclusive Education Settings for School-Aged Children with Autism Spectrum Disorder (ASD). *Lecture Notes in Computer Science Blended Learning: Aligning Theory with Practices,* 94-102.

Kandalaft, M. R., Didehbani, N., Krawczyk, D. C., Allen, T. T., & Chapman, S. B. (2013). Virtual reality social cognition training for young adults with high-functioning autism. *Journal of Autism and Developmental Disorders*, *43*(1), 34–44. doi:10.100710803-012-1544-6 PMID:22570145

Ke, F., & Im, T. (2013). Virtual-reality-based social interaction training for children with high-functioning autism. *The Journal of Educational Research*, *106*(6), 441–461. doi:10.1080/00220671.2013.832999

Kemeny, A., George, P., & Mérienne, F. (2017). New VR Navigation Techniques to Reduce Cybersickness. *Electronic Imaging, The Engineering Reality of Virtual Reality*, *6*, 48-53. Retrieved April 29, 2018 from http://www.ingentaconnect.com/contentone/ist/ei/2017/00002017/00000003/art00009?crawler=true&mimetype=application/pdf

Kuriakose, S., Kunche, S., Narendranath, B., Jain, P., Sonker, S., & Lahiri, U. (2013). A step towards virtual reality based social communication for children with Autism. *2013 International Conference on Control, Automation, Robotics and Embedded Systems (CARE).* 10.1109/CARE.2013.6733744

Lahiri, U., Welch, K. C., Warren, Z., & Sarkar, N. (2011). Understanding psychophysiological response to a Virtual Reality-based social communication system for children with ASD. *2011 International Conference on Virtual Rehabilitation*. 10.1109/ICVR.2011.5971841

Leo, T., Manganello, F., & Chen, N. S. (2010). From the learning work to the learning adventure. *Proceedings of EDEN 2010.*

Lind, S. E., & Bowler, D. M. (2009). Delayed self-recognition in children with autism spectrum disorder. *Journal of Autism and Developmental Disorders*, *39*(4), 643–650. doi:10.100710803-008-0670-7 PMID:19051001

Lyons, V., & Fitzgerald, M. (2013). Atypical sense of self in autism spectrum disorders: a neuro-cognitive perspective. In M. Fitzgerald (Ed.), *Recent Advances in Autism Spectrum Disorders* (vol. 1). INTECH Open Access Publisher. Retrieved April 9, 2018 from https://mts.intechopen.com/books/recent-advances-in-autism-spectrum-disorders-volume-i/atypical-sense-of-self-in-autism-spectrum-disorders-a-neuro-cognitive-perspective

Maraj, C. S., Martinez, S. G., Badillo-Urquiola, K. A., Stevens, J. A., & Maxwell, D. B. (2016). Preliminary review of a virtual world usability questionnaire. In S. Lackey & R. Shumaker (Eds.), Lecture Notes in Computer Science: Vol. 9740. *Virtual, Augmented and Mixed Reality. VAMR 2016* (pp. 35–46). Cham: Springer. doi:10.1007/978-3-319-39907-2_4

Mason, B. (2017). *Virtual reality has a motion sickness problem.* Retrieved April 29, 2018 from https://www.sciencenews.org/article/virtual-reality-has-motion-sickness-problem

Mayes, S. D., Calhoun, S. L., Aggarwal, R., Baker, C., Mathapati, S., Molitoris, S., & Mayes, R. D. (2013). Unusual fears in children with autism. *Research in Autism Spectrum Disorders*, *7*(1), 151–158. doi:10.1016/j.rasd.2012.08.002

Mukamal, R. (2017). *Are virtual reality headsets safe for eyes?* Retrieved July 5, 2018 from https://www.aao.org/eye-health/tips-prevention/are-virtual-reality-headsets-safe-eyes

Muneer, R., Saxena, T., & Karanth, P. (2015.). *Virtual Reality Games as an Intervention for Children: A Pilot Study*. Retrieved July 5, 2018 from http://dcidj.org/article/view/456

Newbutt, N., Sung, C., Kuo, H. J., Leahy, M. J., Lin, C. C., & Tong, B. (2016). Brief report: A pilot study of the use of a virtual reality headset in autism populations. *Journal of Autism and Developmental Disorders*, 1–11. PMID:27272115

Oigara, J. N. (2018). Integrating virtual reality tools into classroom instruction. In J. Keengwe (Ed.), *Handbook of Research on Mobile Technology, Constructivism, and Meaningful Learning* (pp. 147–159). Hershey, PA: IGI Global. doi:10.4018/978-1-5225-3949-0.ch008

Parsons, S., & Cobb, S. (2011). State-of-the art of virtual reality technologies for children on the autism spectrum. *European Journal of Special Needs Education*, *26*(3), 355–366. doi:10.1080/08856257.2011.593831

Parsons, S., & Mitchell, P. (2002). The potential of virtual reality in social skills training for people with autistic spectrum disorders. *Journal of Intellectual Disability Research*, *46*(5), 430–443. doi:10.1046/j.1365-2788.2002.00425.x PMID:12031025

Psychiatry Online | DSM Library. (n.d.). Retrieved May 20, 2018 from https://dsm.psychiatryonline.org/doi/book/10.1176/appi.books.9780890425596

Rahaman, S., Ansari, Z., Biswas, P., & Memon, S. B. (n.d.). *Virtual Reality for combating social awkwardness in Special Needs*. Retrieved March 10, 2018 from https://www.scitechnol.com/peer-review/virtual-reality-for-combating-social-awkwardness-in-special-needs-twPN.php?article_id=6674

Ramachandiran, C. R., Jomhari, N., Thiyagaraja, S., & Maria, M. (2015). Virtual reality based behavioural learning for autistic children. *The Electronic Journal of e-Learning*, *13*(5), 357-365.

Rizzo, A., & Kim, G. J. (2005). A SWOT analysis of the field of virtual reality rehabilitation and therapy. *Presence (Cambridge, Mass.)*, *14*(2), 119–146. doi:10.1162/1054746053967094

Saadatzi, M. N., Pennington, R. C., Welch, K. C., & Graham, J. H. (2018). Small-Group Technology-Assisted Instruction: Virtual Teacher and Robot Peer for Individuals with Autism Spectrum Disorder. *Journal of Autism and Developmental Disorders*. doi:10.100710803-018-3654-2 PMID:29926295

Tiiro, A. (2018). *Effect of Visual Realism on Cybersickness in Virtual Reality* (Unpublished Master's thesis). University of Oulu, Finland. Retrieved July 16, 2018 from http://jultika.oulu.fi/files/nbnfioulu-201802091218.pdf

Uddin, L. Q. (2011). The self in autism: An emerging view from neuroimaging. *Neurocase*, *17*(3), 201–208. doi:10.1080/13554794.2010.509320 PMID:21207316

Zhao, H., Swanson, A., Weitlauf, A., Warren, Z., & Sarkar, N. (2016). A Novel Collaborative Virtual Reality Game for Children with ASD to Foster Social Interaction. Universal Access in Human-Computer Interaction. Users and Context Diversity Lecture Notes in Computer Science, 276-288.

## ADDITIONAL READING

Bashiri, A., Ghazisaeedi, M., & Shahmoradi, L. (2017). The opportunities of virtual reality in the rehabilitation of children with attention deficit hyperactivity disorder: A literature review. *Korean Journal of Pediatrics*, *60*(11), 337–343. doi:10.3345/kjp.2017.60.11.337 PMID:29234356

Bethel, D. M. (1973). *Makiguchi the Value Creator: Revolutionary Japanese Educator and Founder of Soka Gakkai*. New York, Tokyo: John Weatherhill.

Blake, E. H., & Winterbottom, C. (2008). Constructivism, virtual reality and tools to support design. In *Proceedings of the 7th ACM conference on Designing interactive systems*, (pp. 230-239), New York, NY: ACM.

Botella, C., Fernández-Álvarez, J., Guillén, V., García-Palacios, A., & Baños, R. (2017). Recent Progress in Virtual Reality Exposure Therapy for Phobias: A Systematic Review. *Current Psychiatry Reports*, *19*(7), 42. doi:10.100711920-017-0788-4 PMID:28540594

Bronack, S. C. (2011). The role of immersive media in online education. *Journal of Continuing Higher Education*, *59*(2), 113–117. doi:10.1080/07377363.2011.583186

Burke, S. L., Bresnahan, T., Li, T., Epnere, K., Rizzo, A., Partin, M., ... Trimmer, M. (2018). Using Virtual interactive Training Agents (ViTA) with adults with autism and other developmental disabilities. *Journal of Autism and Developmental Disorders*, *48*(3), 905–912. doi:10.100710803-017-3374-z PMID:29168090

Casas, X., Herrera, G., Coma, I., & Fernández, M. (2012). A kinect-based augmented reality system for individuals with autism spectrum disorders. In *Proceedings of the International Conference on Computer Graphics Theory and Applications and International Conference on Information Visualization Theory and Applications* (vol. 1. pp. 440-446). GRAPP, (VISIGRAPP 2012).

Damasio, A. R. (2010). *L'Autre moi-même – Les nouvelles cartes du cerveau, de la conscience et des emotions*. Paris, F: Odile Jacob.

De Bono, E. (1995). *Six thinking hats*. Boston, USA: Little Brown and Company.

Dewey, J. (1966, first published 1916). Democracy and education: an introduction to the philosophy of education. New York, USA: Free Press.

El Sayed, N. A. M., Zayed, H. H., & Sharawy, M. I. (2011). ARSC: Augmented reality student card. An augmented reality solution for the education field. *Computers & Education*, *56*(4), 1045–1061. doi:10.1016/j.compedu.2010.10.019

Forbes contributors, 2018. The Difference Between Virtual Reality, Augmented Reality And Mixed Reality. Retrieved July 10, 2018 from Freeman, D. & Freeman, J. 2017. Why virtual reality could be a mental health gamechanger. Retrieved July 10, 2018 from:Freeman, D., Reeve, S., Robinson, A., Ehlers, A., Clark, D., Spanlang, B., & Slater, M. (2017). Virtual reality in the assessment, understanding, and treatment of mental health disorders. *Psychological Medicine*, *47*(14), 2393–2400. doi:10.1017/S003329171700040X PMID:28325167

Freina, L., & Ott, M. (2015). A literature review on immersive virtual reality in education: state of the art and perspectives. In *The International Scientific Conference eLearning and Software for Education* (vol 1, pp. 133-141), Bucharest, RO: eLSE.

Gardner, H. (2006). *Five minds for the future*. Boston, USA: Harvard Business School Press.

Guazzaroni, G. (2012). Emotional mapping of museum augmented places (EMMAP). In M. Pieri (Ed.) Mobile Learning. Esperienze e Riflessioni "Made in Italy". Bari, IT: Progedit.

Guazzaroni, G. (2013, October). Street poetry in augmented reality. In S. Leone (Ed.), *Synergic Integration of Formal and Informal E-Learning Environments for Adult Lifelong Learners*. Hershey, PA: IGI Global.

Guazzaroni, G. (2013, October). The ritual and the rhythm: interacting with augmented reality, visual poetry and storytelling across the streets of scattered L'Aquila. In eLearning Papers on Design for Learning Spaces and Innovative Classrooms (34).

Guazzaroni, G. (2013). Emotional mapping of the archaeologist game. In M. Lytras, P. Ordoñez De Pablos and F.J. García-Peñalvo (Eds.), Advanced Human-Computer Interaction: Computers in Human Behavior, Elsevier, 29 (2) 335-344. doi:10.1016/j.chb.2012.06.008

Guazzaroni, G. (2015). Realtà aumentata un'opportunità di apprendimento. In L. Salvucci (Ed.), Strumenti per la Didattica della Matematica. Ricerche, esperienze, buone pratiche (pp. 145-152). Milano, IT: Franco Angeli.

Guazzaroni, G. (2018). Walking eight. Archaeology of the next future. In M. G. Ullate (Ed.), *Proceedings of Cultural Management and Governance for European Pilgrimage Routes and Religious Tourism and Thermal Tourism – Cultour plus – Cori. IT*.

Guazzaroni, G., & Leo, T. (2011). Emotional mapping of a place of interest using mobile devices for learning. In I. Arnedillo Sánchez, & P. Isaías (Eds.), *Proceedings of IADIS International Conference on Mobile Learning* (pp. 277-281). Avila, E. March 10-13 2011.

Happé, F., Booth, R., Charlton, R., & Hughes, C. (2006). Executive function deficits in autism spectrum disorders and attention-deficit/hyperactivity disorder: Examining profiles across domains and ages. *Brain and Cognition*, *61*(1), 25–39. doi:10.1016/j.bandc.2006.03.004 PMID:16682102

Howlin, P. (1997). *Autism: Preparing for adulthood*. London, United Kingdom: Routledge. doi:10.4324/9780203426913

Kulman, R. (2018). Virtual Reality (VR) assessment of ADHD. Retrieved March 5, 2018 from http://learningworksforkids.com/2018/01/virtual-reality-vr-assessment-adhd

Kwon, C. (in press). Verification of the possibility and effectiveness of experiential learning using HMD-based immersive VR technologies. *Virtual Reality (Waltham Cross)*.

Lave, J., & Wenger, E. (1991). *Situated Learning: Legitimate Peripheral Participation*. Cambridge, UK: Cambridge University Press. doi:10.1017/CBO9780511815355

Lee, J. M., Cho, B. H., Ku, J. H., Kim, J. S., Lee, J. H., Kim, I. Y., & Kim, S. I. (2001). A study on the system for treatment of ADHD using virtual reality. In *Engineering in Medicine and Biology Society. Proceedings of the 23rd Annual International Conference of the IEEE* (vol. 4, pp. 3754-3757) Istanbul, TR: IEEE. 10.1109/IEMBS.2001.1019654

Leone, S., & Guazzaroni, G. (2010). Pedagogical sustainability of interoperable formal and informal learning environments. In F. Lazarinis, S. Green, & E. Pearson (Eds.), *Developing and Utilizing E-Learning Applications*. Hershey, PA: IGI Global. doi:10.4018/978-1-61692-791-2.ch001

Mathew, P. S., & Pillai, A. S. (2015). Big data challenges and solutions in healthcare: A survey. *Advances in Intelligent Systems and Computing Innovations in Bio-Inspired Computing and Applications,* 543-553.

Mathew, P. S., Pillai, A. S., & Palade, V. (2017). Applications of IoT in healthcare. *Cognitive Computing for Big Data Systems Over IoT Lecture Notes on Data Engineering and Communications Technologies,* 263-288.

Mühlberger, A., Jekel, K., Probst, T., Schecklmann, M., Conzelmann, A., Andreatta, M., ... Romanos, M. (2016). The influence of methylphenidate on hyperactivity and attention deficits in children with ADHD: A virtual classroom test. *Journal of Attention Disorders*. doi:10.1177/1087054716647480 PMID:27178061

Murphy, K. (2015). Feeling woozy? It may be cyber sickness. Retrieved April 29, 2018 from https://well.blogs.nytimes.com/2015/11/14/feeling-woozy-it-may-be-cyber-sickness

Piaget, J. (1998). *The origin of intelligence in the child. Jean Piaget: Selected Works*. London, United Kingdom: Routledge.

Radu, I. (2014). Augmented reality in education: A meta-review and cross-media analysis. *Personal and Ubiquitous Computing*, *18*(6), 1533–1543. doi:10.100700779-013-0747-y

Schank, R. C. (1995). What we learn when we learn by doing. In *Technical Report No. 60*. Northwestern University, Institute for Learning Sciences.

Scheeren, A. M., Begeer, S., Banerjee, R., Terwogt, M. M., & Koot, H. M. (2010). Can you tell me something about yourself? Self-presentation in children and adolescents with high-functioning autism spectrum disorder in hypothetical and real life situations. *Autism*, *14*(5), 457–473. doi:10.1177/1362361310366568 PMID:20841344

Schmid Mast, M., Kleinlogel, E. P., Tur, B., & Bachmann, M. (2018). The future of interpersonal skills development: Immersive virtual reality training with virtual humans. *Human Resource Development Quarterly*, *29*(2), 125–141. doi:10.1002/hrdq.21307

Squire, K., & Klopfer, E. (2007). Augmented reality simulations on handheld computers. *Journal of the Learning Sciences*, *16*(3), 371–413. doi:10.1080/10508400701413435

Tambovtsev, D., Floksy, N., & Peshé, O. (2016). How to avoid the effect of motion sickness in VR. Retrieved March 9, 2018 from https://vrscout.com/news/avoid-motion-sickness-developing-for-vr

Temurnikar, A. (2018). New age classrooms are the future of education (Interview). Retrieved May 5, 2018 from http://bweducation.businessworld.in/article/New-Age-Classrooms-are-the-Future-of-Education-/10-04-2018-146020/

The Guardian. (2017). The Party: a virtual experience of autism – 360 video. Retrieved March 9, 2018 from https://www.theguardian.com/technology/2017/oct/07/the-party-a-virtual-experience-of-autism-360-video

The National Autistic Society. (2016). Too much information. Retrieved March, 9 2018 from http://www.autism.org.uk/vr

Virtual reality training improves social skills of individuals on the autism spectrum. (2016, September 20). Retrieved April 10, 2018 from https://www.sciencedaily.com/releases/2016/09/160920141800.htm

Whalon, K. (2018, March 20). Enhancing the Reading Development of Learners with Autism Spectrum Disorder. Retrieved from https://www.thieme-connect.com/products/ejournals/abstract/10.1055/s-0038-1628366

Winn, W. (1993). *A conceptual basis for educational applications of virtual reality. Human Interface Technology Laboratory*. USA: Washington Technology Center. University of Washington.

Wu, H. K., Lee, S. W.-L., Chang, H. Y., & Liang, J. C. (2013). Current status, opportunities and challenges of augmented reality in education. *Computers & Education*, *62*, 41–49. doi:10.1016/j.compedu.2012.10.024

Zahavi, D. (2010). Complexities of self. *Autism*, *14*(5), 547–551. doi:10.1177/1362361310370040 PMID:20841340

## KEY TERMS AND DEFINITIONS

**Augmented Reality (AR):** The possibility to overlay computer graphics or computer audio onto the real world and augment, in this way, human perceptions.

**Autism Spectrum Disorder (ASD):** A developmental disorder that affects communication and behavior.

**Avatar:** A computer-generated representation of an individual in a virtual reality environment.

**Cybersickness:** Typically occurs during or after immersion in a virtual environment. A form of motion or simulator sickness related to sensory mismatch or conflict. The symptoms include dizziness, nausea, and eye fatigue.

**Head-Mounted Display (HMD):** A device worn over a user's head, providing a visual display in front of one or both of the user's eyes.

**Immersive Learning Environment:** A virtual environment where students can connect, interact, find 360-degree learning objects and complete educational tasks wearing a special head-mounted display.

**Learning Adventure:** The adventure of learning is directed to satisfy a personal desire of acquiring knowledge, and it is aimed at providing expertise in some specific domain.

**Learning Environment:** A digital space where students can connect, interact, find learning content, and complete educational tasks.

**Virtual Reality (VR):** The possibility to immerse in a completely virtual world using special goggles to visualize computer graphics or computer sound.

# Chapter 10
# Virtual Reality (VR) for Children Diagnosed With Autism Spectrum Disorder (ASD):
## Interventions to Train Social and Everyday Living Skills

**Ali Adjorlu**
*Aalborg University – Copenhagen, Denmark*

**Stefania Serafin**
*Aalborg University – Copenhagen, Denmark*

## ABSTRACT

*Children and adolescents diagnosed with autism spectrum disorder (ASD) have significant difficulties with communication and social skills. Consequently, children diagnosed with ASD are often victims of social rejection and targets of bullying, which have an adverse impact on their emotional and mental wellbeing. Social anxiety, depression, and poor academic achievement are some of the consequences that can harm their whole lives. This chapter will begin with an elaboration of the challenges facing children and adolescents diagnosed with ASD. This will be followed by an introduction to virtual reality (VR) and its advantages for extending the capabilities of some of the traditional interventions developed to teach social and everyday living skills to children and adolescents diagnosed with ASD.*

## AUTISM SPECTRUM DISODER

Leo Kanner coined the term autism in 1943 (Kanner, 1943), describing an individual's inability to create regular emotional contact with others. This definition has throughout the years evolved into Autism Spectrum Disorder (ASD) with the term "spectrum" indicating the variety of communicative and social interaction challenges facing individuals diagnosed with this developmental disorder.

DOI: 10.4018/978-1-5225-7168-1.ch010

The fifth and latest edition of the Diagnostic and Statistical Manual of Mental Disorders (American Psychiatric Association, 2013) describes ASD as a range of pervasive and lifelong neurodevelopmental disorders, characterized by severe deficits in social and communicative skills of individuals diagnosed with it. These impairments exist in both the non-verbal and verbal communication skills, with the verbal limitation including difficulties with initiating or responding to social interaction and participating in a regular back and forth conversation and the non-verbal deficits resulting in a hard time understanding gestures and facial expressions or keeping eye contact with others.

Consequently, developing, maintaining and understanding relationships with others is a difficult task, resulting in a hard time having personal relations with friends or partners. Furthermore, these deficits lead to adversities in various adaptive skills such as using the public transportation, shopping in the supermarket or buying food in a workplace or school cantina (Matson, 2009).

DSM-5 divides the severity levels of ASD into three groups. The third level includes the low functioning individuals with severe deficits in communication skills, who are only able to use few words of intelligible speech and rarely initiate or responds to social interactions. The first level includes the high functioning individuals who are capable of communication using full sentences while still having noticeably impaired social skills.

These deficits result in a wide range of consequences throughout the lives of individuals diagnosed with ASD. Studies indicate that children diagnosed with ASD are at higher risk of being bullied (Bitsika & Sharpley, 2014; Schrooten et al., 2017). Being bullied during childhood can lead to depression and suicidal thoughts, with the primary coping strategy of children diagnosed with ASD against bullying being withdrawal from school altogether, which has significant consequences on their academic career and future independence. Studies indicate that school refusal is far more common among students with ASD than in general population. Approximately 40% to 50% of students with ASD show school refusal behavior compared to only 5% to 28% of children and adolescents without ASD (Havik et al., 2015; Munkhaugen et al., 2017; Kearney, 2001). In addition to bullying, social anxiety, lower social motivation and depression are some of the main reasons for the school refusal behavior observed in children and adolescents diagnosed with ASD (Munkhaugen et al., 2017).

Upon adulthood, according to some studies, 50% or more of participants diagnosed with ASD depend entirely or to a large extent on parents or caretakers for living arrangement and employment (Billstedt et al., 2005; Cederlund et al., 2008; Howlin et al., 2013). The socio-economic cost during the lifespan of an individual diagnosed with ASD is estimated to be around 1.4 million dollars in the United States of America and 0.9 million pounds in the United Kingdom (Buescher et al., 2014). These costs consisted mainly of adult care services and loss of productivity. According to a study conducted by Leigh and Du, the annual medical- and non-medical economical cost of ASD in the United States of America will rise from 268 billion dollars in 2015 to 461 billion dollars in 2025 (Leigh & Du, 2015).

Approximately 1 out of every 50 children is diagnosed with ASD (Xu et al., 2018), further underlining the importance and agency of interventions to teach social and everyday living skills to children and adolescents diagnosed with ASD, helping them towards independent adulthood.

Wang and Spillance conducted a literature review of evidence-based interventions to teach social skills to children diagnosed with ASD (Wang & Spillance, 2009). Five different categories of social skills training interventions emerged from their review of 38 studies: Social Stories, Peer-Mediated Interventions, Video Modelling, cognitive behavior therapy and Others.

Social stories, an intervention developed by Gray and Garand is a method in which short stories, often written by teachers, therapist or parents are designed with the purpose of teaching children diagnosed with ASD about how to behave in different social contexts that they find challenging (Gray & Garand, 1993). As previously mentioned, one of the primary deficits of individuals diagnosed with ASD is language skills. Thus, social stories often include a combination of text and pictures. Illustrations are used to describe the social context, where it takes place, who is involved and what is the appropriate behavior in that specific context.

The peer-mediated social skills intervention is a method that involves teaching social interaction strategies such as sharing, encouraging, guiding or praising to normally developed peers. These peers are then asked to interact with children diagnosed with ASD, trying to promote appropriate social behavior (Wang et al., 2011). According to Strain et al., (2008) peer-mediated interventions can limit the problem of generalization and transfer of knowledge experienced in adult-mediated social skills interventions since this method often take place in that specific location (playgrounds, classrooms etc.) in which the child diagnosed with ASD is supposed to apply these skills.

Video modelling is a method that involves filming an appropriate behavior performed by a peer, an adult or an individual diagnosed child him or herself. The child diagnosed with ASD is than supposed to watch the video and try to replicate the proper behavior displayed in the video (Wang & Spillance, 2009). According to the literature review conducted by Wang and Spillane (2009), video-modelling has demonstrated the highest effectiveness in teaching social skills to children diagnosed with ASD. Charlop-Christy and Daneshvar argue that the reason for the efficacy of video-modelling interventions is that children diagnosed with ASD attend more to characters in a video compare to real people due to the level of distress and anxiety they feel when trying to understand real people (Charlop-Christy & Daneshvar, 2003).

Cognitive Behavioral therapy (CBT) is a method where therapist challenges irrational thoughts that promote maladaptive behavior while motivating logical strategies that encourage appropriate behavior (Wood et al., 2009). These cognitive strategies promoted by the therapists are then hierarchically rehearsed in real life by the child as homework. CBT is often applied to treat social anxiety in children diagnosed with ASD (Wood et al. 2009). By challenging the negative feelings the child experiences about certain social situations that lead to fear and isolation, the therapist attempts to promote strategies to cope with the adverse cognition.

VR has the potential for supporting all the above approaches for teaching social and everyday living skills to children diagnosed with ASD. Social stories and video modelling are learning interventions that communicate knowledge via visual information due to the ASD populations language skills impairment. Peer-mediated interventions rely on rehearsing social skills with the peers of the child diagnosed with ASD in natural environments such as classrooms and playgrounds while CBT provides the child with appropriate coping strategies and encourage repetitive, hierarchal rehearsal. VR enables the creation of interactive and immersive virtual environments such as classrooms or playgrounds within which children diagnosed with ASD can rehearse a variety of social and everyday living skills.

## VIRTUAL REALITY FOR AUTISM

Virtual Reality refers to immersive virtual environments presented to its users via head-mounted displays, cave automatic virtual environments or desktop screens (Adjorlu, 2018). By substituting the users' real world sensory information with digitally generated once, VR can be applied to create controllable simulations tailored to treat a variety of mental disorders and disabilities.

Some of the first applications for VR to attend mental disabilities were interventions to treat simple phobias such as claustrophobia and Acrophobia (Williford et al., 1993; North & North, 1994). VR can by exposing individuals with anxiety disorders to virtual environments, seek to provoke anxiety and then remove that anxiety via repetitive hierarchal exposure to the controlled virtual environments.

In 1992, Williford et al. conducted case studies using virtual environments to expose patients to heights such as walking across footbridges, looking out from high balconies or ascending in elevators (Williford et al., 1993). Lamson and Meisner (1994) exposed 30 participants with acrophobia to a simulated height in VR. A post-study conducted thirty months later showed that 90% of those participants with acrophobia were able to ride in a glass elevator.

Another early VR intervention to treat anxiety disorder attempt to address the fear of flying (North & North, 1994). Traditional in-vivo exposure therapy to treat fear of flying is expensive and cumbersome while VR can be used to treat the patients in the safe environments of the therapist's office.

Strickland et al. conducted one of the first published studies on VR as a learning tool for children diagnosed with ASD (Strickland et al, 1996). Two case studies were designed to determine whether children diagnosed with ASD would tolerate VR equipment such as head-mounted displays and respond to the virtual environment in a meaningful way. A Division Inc. ProVision 100 head-mounted display was used to render a street setting with colored moving cars. No 3D pedestrian avatars were included in the VR intervention due to the technical limitation of the hardware and software of the time. Two children both diagnosed with ASD participated in the study, both trying the VR application for approximately half to one hour sessions over a period of seven days for one child and four days for the other child. During these sessions, the head-mounted displays were used for a maximum of 5 minutes at a time to avoid discomfort. The children were instructed to keep track of the cars in the scene and report back the color of the cars by saying it out loud. The results of the case studies indicate that both of the children diagnosed with ASD accepted the VR head-mounted display while being able to fulfil the tasks of tracking the virtual cars with their head, body and gestures while verbally labelling their colors. Results of these interventions were promising, creating an early hype for VR interventions to treat mental disabilities and disorders. Some of the initial studies described above were low-fidelity virtual environments that could extremely costly to develop or purchase the required equipment for (Rizzo & Koenig, 2017). Consequently, the enthusiasm for head-mounted display based VR flagged due to hardware performance limitation in addition to their high prices. Therefore, most of the studies investigating the effectiveness of Virtual Environments to teach social and everyday living skills to children diagnosed with ASD used desktop and laptop computers.

Mitchel et al. (2007) investigated if a virtual environment consisting of a virtual café could be used to teach social skills to children diagnosed with ASD. Six children diagnosed with ASD participated in the study. The main task in the Virtual Café was to find an appropriate place to seat. The participants could navigate around the café using a joystick and a mouse. A hierarchal approach was taken by dividing the Virtual Café experience into four levels of difficulty. Higher levels would increase the number of people in the virtual café as well as the ambient noise while decreasing the number of empty tables. The participants started by the till with food and drink on a tray and were told to "find a place to sit" on one of the six tables available. Once the participant moved to a table and pressed the mouse button, a set of options would appear. If the table was already occupied by virtual avatars, the participant would have the options of either sit-down at the table anyways or ask the avatar a question from a list of three questions presented to him in a graphical user interface. One of these questions was "Is this seat available?" while the two other questions were irrelevant and included questions such as "What is your name?". If the participants choose one of the irrelevant questions, they would be told by the program that the question was not appropriate for this specific task.

The sessions were run by a teacher who adapted to the participant's individual needs, replicating the way that the teacher and their pupil usually use a computer or more interestingly, the way a teacher facilitates a traditional social story. The teacher could discuss the social context with the child, give advice or even repeat a session if he felt that the child has not learned sufficiently from the first attempt. Each session lasted approximately 40 minutes where the child completed all four levels. Each child went through two sessions of training with the virtual café in two successive days. Six children, three male and three females participated in the study. Four of the participants made the error of sitting at an occupied table without asking if the seat was taken in the first session. However, during the second virtual café session on the second day only one of participant made that similar error. Pre- and post-measurements of the participants obtained social skills was conducted using video footage. Two of these footages included cafés with a variety of available seats, and three of the videos were of buses to investigate whether the participants could generalize their training to a different environment. Each clip lasted approximately 30 seconds, and a facilitator asked the participant about where he would seat and why. Each of the six participants went through three video sessions. Three of the participants experienced the two virtual café sessions between video session one and two, and the other three of the participants experienced the virtual café sessions between video session two and three. Results indicated a clear improvement in the judgment of the participants in choosing a place to seat in the video session that followed right after a virtual café session. There was only a minor improvement in video sessions that followed another video session, indicating that the non-interactive video training and rehearsal was less effective than the interactive virtual café. Furthermore, the participants also illustrated some improvement in the video of the bus, showing that the training in a virtual café has the potential to be generalised to other contexts.

More studies have investigated the use of non-immersive VR via computer screens, keyboards and mouse to teach social skills to children diagnosed with ASD. Didehbani et al. (2016) examined the impact of social cognition training in virtual environments on thirty children in the age range between 7-16 all diagnosed with ASD. Didehbani et al. call the intervention used in their study the Virtual Reality Social Cognition Training (VR-SCT). The VR-SCT was developed via the openly available SecondLife software and was designed by licensed psychologists and pathologist at the centre for BrainHealth at Texas University. Two participants and two trained clinicians were involved in each VR-SCT session. The lead clinicians act as the "coach" while the confederate clinician played various roles in the virtual environment. The coach moderated each session and provided individual feedback to the participants. Once the participants logged into the system, the coach directed them to the specific location of one of the designed social-scenarios designed to emphasize a target social learning objective in different contexts. These were social scenarios such as meeting new people, being approached by a bully, bonding with a peer and handling a variety of social dilemmas. The confederate clinician played the various roles such as the bully or the new friends, controlling the avatars on a computer located in a different room. The confederate therapist approached the participants via loosely-scripted conversations and morphed her voice to match the gender, age and race of the avatar she was controlling in each social scenario. As an example, in one of the scenes, the confederate clinician played the role of a child in a park who had just lost her puppy. Using her avatar, she would approach the participants' avatar and tell them that she has lost her puppy and that she was very sad and waited for a response. If the participants were unable to respond, the confederate therapist would initiate open-ended comments for the participants to follow and initiate a response. The "lost puppy" scenario would last for about ten minutes, followed by five minutes feedback from the coach therapist. The therapist would ask structured questions about the participants' awareness of the social context such as: "Why was she sad?" and "How could you have cheered her up?". The coach would then provide individuals educational feedback about how to behave in similar social situations. Each participant completed ten VR-SCT sessions, two per week, at the Center for BrainHealth at the University of Texas. Pre- and post-measurements of the participants' social skills were conducted using NEPSY second edition-facial affect recognition (Korkman et al., 2007), Social attribution Task (Abell et al., 2000) and The Developmental Neuropsychological Assessment Second Edition (NEPSY-II)-Auditory Attention and Response Set (Korkman et al., 2007).

The results illustrated an improvement in the participants' measure of affect recognition, the theory of mind and analogical reasoning.

Significant improvements in the performance of microprocessors, as well as the availability of cheaper head-mounted display hardware, have revived the interest in head-mounted based virtual reality as a mean to treat mental disorders and disabilities. Today, head-mounted display hardware such as the Oculus Rift and the HTC Vive provide their users with much higher frame rate, resolution, field of view and intuitive controllers for significantly lower prices compare to head-mounted display hardware available in the 90s.

Adjorlu et al. developed a VR intervention for the HTC Vive hardware, designed to train shopping skills of children and adolescents diagnosed with ASD (Adjorlu et al., 2017). The participants would navigate through a virtual supermarket and pick up items listed on a virtual shopping list. In order to achieve a low-road towards the transfer of knowledge to the real-world, the virtual supermarket was designed to look similar to a real-world supermarket located close to the participants' school. The users could move around in a 1;1 version of the virtual supermarket by walking within the Vive base-station area or via VR teleportation. The Vive base-stations send out infrared light signals that are captured via the infrared sensors on the Vive head-mounted display and controllers. This data is then triangulated to determine the position of the user within the virtual environment. VR teleportation works by using the controller to point at a specific location and pressing a button which will then teleport the user to that particular location. Total of 32 products was modelled, textured and place on the shelves. One of the Vive controllers was attached to a real-world shopping basket so that the user would have a real shopping basket in one hand and a VIVE controller in the other hand which could be used to view the virtual shopping list, grabbing objects from the selves and VR teleportation. The user could walk towards a specific item and grab it using the VIVE controller and place it inside the virtual shopping basket which was moved around in the virtual environment by moving the real shopping basket. Nine participants diagnosed with ASD ranging in age between 12 to 15 year participated in the study. Five of the participants were part of the experiment group, going through seven VR supermarket training sessions in a two-week period while four of the participants were used in a control group, receiving shopping skills training via the regular shopping trips to the real supermarket. These VR training sessions were facilitated by a teacher at the Valhøj school in Copenhagen. Pre- and post-measurements of the participants shopping skills were conducted in a real-world supermarket by measuring the effectivity (Number of right product picked up in the real supermarket) and efficiency (the time they spent finishing their real-world shopping session). The experiment group scored lower in both efficiency and effectivity in the real supermarket compare to the control group during the pre-VR training measurements, while they performed better on both efficiency and effectivity on the post-VR measurements. The highlight of the study was one of the participants in the experiment group who refused to walk into the real supermarket on his own during the pre-VR training measurement. One of the teachers had to take his hand and follow him around the supermarket for him to finish his tasks. However, after the seven VR training sessions, during the post-VR training measurement at the real supermarket, he completed his real-world shopping task on his own. This study shows the potential of VR interventions to teach everyday living skills to children and adolescents diagnosed with ASD, helping them towards independent adulthood as well as showing some potentials in bridging the gap between training in VR environment and performing the trained skills in a real-world context.

Recent studies have also investigated the potential of head-mounted display based VR interventions to teach social skills to children diagnosed with ASD. Inspired by the social stories method described earlier, a Virtual Reality Social Story intervention was designed to teach children diagnosed with ASD skills about sharing (Adjorlu et al., 2018). A virtual classroom was designed based on a real classroom for children with mental disorders at Valhøj school in Copenhagen. The VR social story intervention included three scenarios each designed to teach sharing skills. The scenarios were facilitated by a teacher who could communicate with the participants using a microphone which reproduced his voice via a teacher avatar in the virtual classroom. The three scenarios in the VR environment were as followed:

- The participant is standing in the virtual classroom. A virtual child is playing a game on a computer in front of him. The teacher will then tell the participant to try to play on the virtual child's computer. The participant could then walk towards the virtual child and use his Vive controller grab the computer. This action would trigger the virtual child to look sad and say "I was not done playing". The teacher could then pause everything in VR simulation except his teacher avatar and discuss the social story with the participant.
- The participant is now playing on the virtual computer himself. A simple color game is designed for this purpose. Colors on the computer screen will change between green, blue and red. There are three buttons in front of the computer each with one of these colors. The child must press the button with the same color as the one appearing on the computer screen. Once the teacher feels that the participant is sufficiently engaged in the game, he can press a button, and a virtual child will take the computer away from the participant without asking for permission first. The teacher could again pause the VR simulation and discuss the situation with the participant.
- In the third scenario, the participant once again observed a virtual child playing on the virtual computer. This time he is asked by the teacher to verbally ask the virtual child if he can borrow his computer. The teacher could then press J button on the keyboard, triggering the avatar to say "Yes, you might borrow the computer" or the N button which would trigger the avatar to say "No, I am not done playing yet".

The simulation was tested by two teachers at Valhøj school in Copenhagen who used it to run VR social story sessions on five of their students diagnosed with ASD. After the sessions, the teachers filled out questionnaires reporting the level of effectiveness of the VR social story intervention as a tool to teach social skills to children diagnosed with ASD. This was followed by a semi-structured interview conducted by the authors. The results of this exploratory study indicate that the children were able to relate to the social story while being able to have a productive discussion with the teacher about the social scenario during and after the sessions. Both of the studies above were developed through user-centred design approach, involving the teachers that work with children diagnosed with ASD early in the design process. By including the stakeholders, the needs and preferences of people with ASD, their teachers and their families can be pinpointed by designers, developers and researchers, who can develop solutions to meet these needs.

Studies on VR as an intervention for children and adolescents show promising results even though its full potential has not yet been explored. Most of the studies are obscure and seldom live up to the standard of clinical research, thus making VR teach social and everyday living skills to children diagnosed with ASD ripe for future research. The promising results illustrated in the studies above show that VR has several strong advantages in teaching social and everyday living skills to children and adolescents diagnosed with ASD.

## ADVANTAGES OF VIRTUAL REALITY TRAINING FOR CHILDREN DIAGNOSED WITH AUTISM SPECTRUM DISORDER

Albert "Skip" Rizzo, the director of the Medical Virtual Reality Lab at the University of Southern California and Sebastian Thomas Koenig, the director of the Katana Simulations Pty. Ltd. argues that VR interventions for treatment and training of individuals diagnosed with mental disorders have the potential of being a revolutionary tool, by combining the controlled environment of laboratory setting with the ecological validity of real-world interventions (Rizzo & Koenig, 2017). Due to the development of cheap high fidelity VR products being developed so rapidly these days, Rizzo & Koenig predict that VR devices will become like "toasters". Not everyone will use them every day, but everyone will have a set at home. VR technology can become an indispensable tool in the toolbox of teachers, therapist and psychologists of future working with children and adolescents diagnosed with ASD. In this section, we will present seven main advantages of using VR as a tool to teach everyday and social living skills to children and adolescents diagnosed with ASD.

### Ecological Validity of the Training

Traditional intervention to train and teach individuals with mental disorders have been criticised for having limited ecological validity (Neisser, 1982; Parsons et al., 2017). Ecological validity defines the degree of similarity of an intervention to the real world and its effectivity in improving real-world behavior. This view challenges analogue methods such as CBT and social stories ability to teach children diagnosed with ASD skills on how to behave in complex social contexts without training and learning that take place in similar complex social contexts. By designing virtual environments to replicate real-world scenarios, earlier examples have enhanced the ecological validity of VR interventions to teach social and everyday living skills to children diagnosed with ASD. These examples include the virtual supermarket to teach shopping skills (Adjorlu et al., 2017), Virtual classroom to teach sharing skills (Adjorlu et al., 2018) or the virtual park to teach social skills to children and adolescents diagnosed with ASD (Didehbani et al., 2016). Importance of ecological validity is especially essential for children diagnosed with ASD due to their inability to generalise knowledge gained in one context to a different setting (Arnold-Saritepe et al., 2009). Behavioral analysts Stokes & Bear suggests to include as many as possible stimulus from the real-world environment of the desired skill to its training environment (Stokes & Baer, 1977). Therefore, it's not only the creation of graphical similarity to the real world that is important but also the actual activities that are going to take place in these virtual training environments. In the virtual supermarket described above, the authors attempted to provide stimuli from the real world in the training intervention by giving an actual shopping basket (with a sensor attached to it) to the users instead of an HTC Vive controller. In the virtual classroom designed to teach sharing skills, the users had to verbally ask the virtual child about whether they could borrow the computer from them instead of choosing what to say from a list of dialogues on a graphical user interface as done in the virtual café. (Mitchell et al., 2007).

High fidelity graphical realism is not necessary for increasing the ecological validity of therapeutic or training interventions in VR. In interactive virtual environments, humans tend to illustrate a high "Suspension of disbelief", believing that they are actually inside the digital environment (Dede, 2009). Merely resembling the real world, including real-world challenges and having an intuitive user interaction is more important than having realistic graphics for the ecological validity of VR interventions. VR exposure therapy interventions with low-fidelity graphics have still managed to activate significant emotional responses (Bordnick et al., 2013; Norrholm et al., 2016).

## Motivation Towards Training

As mentioned earlier, the primary deficit of individuals diagnosed with ASD is verbal and non-verbal communication with others. This weakness makes it difficult to motivate children diagnosed with ASD to participate in interventions that require human interaction. Therefore, as early as 1968, computers were used as a tool to teach communication skills to children diagnosed with ASD (Colby, 1968). The advantages of computer-based learning interventions over human-mediated interventions for the ASD population have been reported in several studies (Chen & Bernard-Optiz, 1993; Zarr, 1994). Grandin & Acariano state that the thought process of autistic individuals is mainly visual (Lewin, 1986) while it is argued that learning interventions that apply visual cues are more useful than verbally mediated instructions (National Research Council, 2001). Gamification of the VR interventions can further increase the motivation of children diagnosed with ASD and keeping them engaged. A study conducted by Strickland shows that children diagnosed with ASD were very motivated when using a VR training application she developed that incorporated gaming elements (Strickland, 2011). Children with Attention Deficit Hyperactivity Disorder (ADHD) often have a fascination for computer games (Greenhill, 1998), being able to keep focus during gaming sessions while having a hard time paying attention to a lecture given in a real classroom. Prensky argues that children today, being part of the "Digital native" who have grown up with technologies are more motivated towards using learning intervention that applies gaming element to keep them engaged compare to traditional classroom-based teaching interventions (Prensky, 2003).

## Individualized Training

ASD described a spectrum of disorders within which individuals diagnosed with it can have a varying set of strengths and weaknesses. Given the non-homogeneity of the ASD population, it is essential to design individualized and personalized interventions. Through a user-centered approach, by involving all of the stakeholder (the diagnosed individual, parents, teachers etc.) researchers can develop personalized VR training interventions. In the traditional social and everyday living skills training methods such as social stories or cognitive behavioral therapy, the therapists or teachers can provide personalized feedback to the diagnosed individual (Wang & Spillance, 2009). In Didehbani et al. (2016), social skills training intervention, the therapist could give feedback on the social scenarios after each training session. In the sharing skill intervention developed by Adjorlu et al. the teacher was able to pause the VR social story session and communicate with the users via his in-game avatar using a microphone. Everything in the scene would freeze except the teacher's avatar to have the child's full attention for the personalised feedback. Thereby, VR interventions can be developed by researchers as a tool to extend the abilities of therapist and teachers instead of replacing them. The ability to pause the intervention can enable the therapist to intervene strategically with the purpose of enhancing the clients learning, decision making, coping behaviors, language or cognitive structuring (Rizzo & Koenig, 2017). Feedback delivery is believed to be essential for learning in Virtual Environments (Levin et al., 2015; Sohlberg & Mateer, 2017).

Furthermore, VR interventions can be designed to include cueing stimulus that can be used to guide user performance and help in avoiding errors. In the VR supermarket described earlier a three-dimensional arrow would appear pointing at the location of the next product on the user's shopping list by the press of a button on the HTC Vive controller. This function was activated by the teacher who was running the VR training sessions if he felt that error-free learning was required for that specific child.

## Hierarchal Delivery of Training

VR enables the creation of simulations within which children diagnosed with ASD can train and rehearse a variety of social and everyday living skills. The tasks in these VR simulations can be delivered hierarchically across a range of difficulty levels, beginning at the most attainable and comfortable for the particular user.

By creating a balance between the abilities of the users and the challenges provided to them by the VR intervention, researchers can induce the users to the state called Flow (*Csikszentmihalyi*, 1997). Flow is described as the primary key to fun experiences and motivation towards learning. As an example, the virtual café scenario included four different levels of difficulty, where the user would start having to choose a place to seat in an almost empty café in level one while level four included a crowded virtual café with lots of background noise. Furthermore, a hierarchal delivery of VR training intervention will give the therapist or teachers the opportunity to provide feedback based on individuals' performance across each level.

## Safety

A virtual environment provides a safe context for developing skills associated with daily living such as the street crossing or fire safety training VR interventions developed by Strickland (2001; Strickland et al., 1996). Mistakes in such environments are less catastrophic, and the stimulus that represents the consequences of failure can be controlled or removed altogether. This asset served as the driving force for early studies applying VR as a treatment method for individuals with mental disorder and disabilities. Fear of height and fear of simulation interventions allowed the user to receive exposure therapy in a safe and controllable environment.

Rizzo and Koenig describe the potential that the rehearsal of dangerous activities in virtual environments might create a false sense of safety and omnipotence which can put the user at risk when acting in the real world (Rizzo & Koenig, 2017). Therefore, it is suggested to closely monitoring the user's behavior with the purpose of recognizing the risk-taking practice that can put him or her at risk in the real world.

## Independent Training Outside Schools and Clinics

In Cognitive Behavioral Therapy, One of the described methods to teach appropriate behavior to children diagnosed with ASD, the therapist often require "homework" from their clients (Wood et al., 2009). Thus, children diagnosed with ASD are encouraged to engage in activities recommended by the clinician at home and in their spare time. The availability of affordable and high-fidelity VR equipment provides the opportunity to implement homework as part of VR social and everyday living skills training interventions. However, as this availability of VR hardware is still in its early stage, very little research has been conducted on the effects of home-based independent VR training for children diagnosed with ASD. Future research should measure the effect of independent home-based training sessions in VR. Online tracking of user performance by clinicians/teachers during VR homework might also provide new opportunities to guide the users and should be explored by future research. The possibility to produce and distribute digital copies of identical virtual environments designed for training social and everyday living skills further supports the possibility of including "homework" in future interventions. While the initial costs of producing a VR application can be high, it can be distributed to a large number of users, bringing the costs down compare to relying on costly physical environments for in vivo therapy and training.

### Training Data

VR enables the therapist or teachers to capture and review a complete set of data from the users' performance and behavior during the training session. The VR supermarket automatically gathered quantitative data on the number of times the user grabbed different items from the shelves and time they spent navigating in the virtual supermarket. In the sharing skills training intervention, the teacher could view the training session live from the users' perspective. Live footage of the users' performance is possible from any desire camera angle in VR training interventions. Furthermore, today VR head-mounted displays can be equipped with eye trackers that can provide valuable data on what the users are gazing at in the virtual environment. One of the central deficits of individuals diagnosed with ASD is difficulties keeping eye contact with others, a skill that can be rehearsed in VR using eye tracking hardware. Systematic analysis of children diagnosed with ASD's performance in VR social and everyday living skills interventions can help improve our understanding

## CONCLUSION

Virtual Reality interventions have the potential of amplifying the effectivity of traditional evidence-based interventions to teach social and everyday living skills to children and adolescents diagnosed with ASD. By studying and getting inspired by evidence-based interventions such as social stories and video-modeling, researchers, designers, and developers can create VR training applications that can break down the communication barriers children with ASD experience while interacting with real people.

Furthermore, by adding gamification elements, VR interventions can even be motivated to use, especially for training applications that require repetition. Social stories, a method that attempts to present social situations via illustrations (Wang & Spillane, 2009) can be replicated in immersive and interactive three-dimensional VR environments. Similar to traditional social stories, teachers can facilitate VR social stories, providing individual feedback to the children during the training session. The teachers and therapists can even participate in the VR environment, controlling a virtual character, playing different roles depending on the specific social skill they are trying to teach.

One of the main advantages of peer-mediated interventions to teach social skills is the fact that the social interaction strategies are explained to the children diagnosed with ASD by their peers in their specific contexts such as playgrounds, classrooms, and cantinas (Wang et al., 2011). VR affords the possibility to not only place the children in these specific social contexts in which they have to learn the required social behavior but also to put virtual avatars of their peers in these virtual environments. Homework is often part of the Cognitive Behavioral Therapy interventions. Virtual Environments can also be designed by developers so that the child can independently rehearse right behavior in the safe and comfortable environment of their homes. Designers of future VR interventions for children diagnosed with ASD should, therefore, start by looking at what already works for this target group by studying these traditional interventions and trying to use VR as a means to amplify their effect.

The first known study on VR as an intervention for children diagnosed with ASD was published 21 years ago (Strickland et al., 1996) Moreover, the first known study on VR as a tool to design intervention for individuals with mental disorders was conducted only 26 years ago (Williford et al., 1993). VR hardware and software have just recently reached the maturity required to create high-fidelity interventions with intuitive user interfaces and high graphical capabilities. This can explain the lack of the systematic research on larger sample sizes. Rizzo and Koenig make a sharp point by arguing that considering that psychology as science for studying human behavior has existed for approximately 125 years, it does make sense that VR need a few more years to evolve to help people with behavioral problems (Rizzo & Koenig, 2017). The emergence of affordable VR hardware as well as the availability of developmental software such as game engines unity3D or Unreal Engine, is having a dominant effect on the growth of the VR development community. These tools have found their way to high school and university students who now have access to VR development software for free and can start creating applications as part of their school projects or as a hobby. This momentum can lead to a future with a wide range of VR training interventions for individuals with special needs such as children diagnosed with ASD.

Healthcare budget is the second largest cost in the USA government budget after the military (Rizzo & Koenig, 2017) and second most significant part of the Danish government's budget after social investments (Finansministeriet, 2017). This can further support the momentum for the development and research of VR interventions for individuals with mental disorder and disabilities.

However, designers and researchers of these interventions should carefully consider the side-effects VR might induce, such as cybersickness and aftereffects.

Cybersickness describes a form of motion sickness that occurs when there is a conflict between the sensory input received by our visual, auditory, proprioceptive, and vestibular modalities (Kennedy et al., 1994). In virtual environments, this conflict occurs when there is an incongruency between the visual and auditory information delivered by the VR system and what is felt by our body. Consequently, motion sickness induced by VR can result in vomiting, nausea, ataxia, eyestring and vertigo and disorientation. High fidelity VR hardware such as the Oculus Rift and the HTC Vive enables the developers to create VR interventions with natural interaction schemes that provide visual feedback to the users based on their physical movement in the real world. Furthermore, the high frame rate that hardware such as the Oculus Rift and HTC Vive provide can further reduce the risk of motion sickness. None of the participants in the supermarket or social story VR interventions that used the HTC Vive reported experiencing any motion sickness.

Aftereffect is described as a consequence of imperfect replica of the VR intervention to the real world that can result in disturbed locomotion, changes in postural control, perceptual-motor disturbances, drowsiness, fatigue and lower arousal (Rizzo & Rothbaum, 2002). This is another side effect that should be carefully considered by researchers, designers, and developers of future VR training applications for children and adolescents diagnosed with ASD. Finally, further research is needed to investigate the physiological consequences of HMD based VR usage for a prolonged period by children and adolescents.

Albert "Skip" Rizzo and Sebastian Thomas Koenig, two of the most influential researchers within the emerging field of VR for therapeutic interventions argue that VR can become an indispensable tool in the toolbox of psychological researchers (Rizzo & Koenig, 2017).

For this to happen, researchers should attempt to answer questions such as treatment dose requirements of VR, what modalities should they use to provide feedback, the complexity of VR tasks, what graphical style works best and most importantly what interactions schemes should be designed to achieve the best possible usability and user experience.

Most of the studies on using VR to teach social and everyday living skills to children and adolescents diagnosed with ASD have been designed for and evaluated on children on the high functioning side of the Autism Spectrum Disorder (Parsons, 2016). Therefore, future research should focus more on children across the whole spectrum of autism, attempting to find out what interventions and interaction schemes work for who, in which context and for what skills.

While current findings seem to show promising results on the potentials of VR to teach social and everyday living skills to children diagnosed with ASD, reviews on the topic recommend more controlled and systematic research with larger sample sizes. There seems to be no study that systematically investigates what aspects of VR work for who. Furthermore, future research should involve all of the stakeholders including parents and teachers of children diagnosed with ASD in making decisions about what is needed and in what way. User-centered design should be the central methodology in the design process of VR interventions, involving all of the end users in the process of mapping the requirement specifications for future VR interventions.

## REFERENCES

Abell, F., Happe, F., & Frith, U. (2000). Do triangles play tricks? Attribution of mental states to animated shapes in normal and abnormal development. *Cognitive Development*, *15*(1), 1–16. doi:10.1016/S0885-2014(00)00014-9

Adjorlu, A. (2018). Virtual Reality Therapy. In *Encyclopedia of Computer Graphics and Games (ecgg)*. Springer. doi:10.1007/978-3-319-08234-9_244-1

Adjorlu, A., Høeg, E. R., Mangano, L., & Serafin, S. (2017, October). Daily Living Skills Training in Virtual Reality to Help Children with Autism Spectrum Disorder in a Real Shopping Scenario. In *Mixed and Augmented Reality (ISMAR-Adjunct), 2017 IEEE International Symposium on* (pp. 294-302). IEEE. 10.1109/ISMAR-Adjunct.2017.93

Adjorlu, A., Hussain, A., Mødekjær, C., & Warming Austad, N. (2018). Head-Mounted Display-Based Virtual Reality Social Story as a Tool to Teach Social Skills to Children Diagnosed with Autism Spectrum Disorder. In *K-12 Embodied Learning through Virtual & Augmented Reality (KELVAR), 2018 IEEE Virtual Reality Workshop on* (pp. 1-4). IEEE.

American Psychiatric Association. (2013). *Diagnostic and statistical manual of mental disorders (DSM-5®)*. American Psychiatric Pub.

Arnold-Saritepe, A. M., Phillips, K. J., Mudford, O. C., De Rozario, K. A., & Taylor, S. A. (2009). Generalization and maintenance. In *Applied behavior analysis for children with autism spectrum disorders* (pp. 207–224). Springer. doi:10.1007/978-1-4419-0088-3_12

Billstedt, E., Gillberg, C., & Gillberg, C. (2005). Autism after adolescence: Population-based 13-to 22-year follow-up study of 120 individuals with autism diagnosed in childhood. *Journal of Autism and Developmental Disorders*, *35*(3), 351–360. doi:10.100710803-005-3302-5 PMID:16119476

Bitsika, V., & Sharpley, C. F. (2014). Understanding, experiences, and reactions to bullying experiences in boys with an autism spectrum disorder. *Journal of Developmental and Physical Disabilities*, *26*(6), 747–761. doi:10.100710882-014-9393-1

Bordnick, P. S., Yoon, J. H., Kaganoff, E., & Carter, B. (2013). Virtual reality cue reactivity assessment: A comparison of treatment-vs. nontreatment-seeking smokers. *Research on Social Work Practice*, *23*(4), 419–425. doi:10.1177/1049731513482377

Buescher, A. V., Cidav, Z., Knapp, M., & Mandell, D. S. (2014). Costs of autism spectrum disorders in the United Kingdom and the United States. *JAMA Pediatrics*, *168*(8), 721–728. doi:10.1001/jamapediatrics.2014.210 PMID:24911948

Cederlund, M., Hagberg, B., Billstedt, E., Gillberg, I. C., & Gillberg, C. (2008). Asperger syndrome and autism: A comparative longitudinal follow-up study more than 5 years after original diagnosis. *Journal of Autism and Developmental Disorders*, *38*(1), 72–85. doi:10.100710803-007-0364-6 PMID:17340200

Charlop-Christy, M. H., & Daneshvar, S. (2003). Using video modeling to teach perspective taking to children with autism. *Journal of Positive Behavior Interventions*, *5*(1), 12–21. doi:10.1177/10983007030050010101

Chen, S. S. A., & Bernard-Opitz, V. (1993). Comparison of personal and computer-assisted instruction for children with autism. *Mental Retardation*, *31*(6), 368. PMID:8152382

Colby, K. M. (1968). Computer-aided language development in nonspeaking children. *Archives of General Psychiatry*, *19*(6), 641–651. doi:10.1001/archpsyc.1968.01740120001001 PMID:4177129

Csikszentmihalyi, M. (1997). *Finding flow: The psychology of engagement with everyday life*. Basic Books.

Dede, C. (2009). Immersive interfaces for engagement and learning. *Science, 323*(5910), 66-69.

Didehbani, N., Allen, T., Kandalaft, M., Krawczyk, D., & Chapman, S. (2016). Virtual reality social cognition training for children with high functioning autism. *Computers in Human Behavior*, *62*, 703–711. doi:10.1016/j.chb.2016.04.033

Finansministeriet. (2017). *Udgiftslofter og statens finanser.* Center for udgiftspolitik og modernisering.

Gray, C. A., & Garand, J. D. (1993). Social stories: Improving responses of students with autism with accurate social information. *Focus on Autistic Behavior*, *8*(1), 1–10. doi:10.1177/108835769300800101

Greenhill, L. L. (1998). Diagnosing attention-deficit/hyperactivity disorder in children. *The Journal of Clinical Psychiatry*, *59*, 31–41. PMID:9680051

Havik, T., Bru, E., & Ertesvåg, S. K. (2015). Assessing reasons for school non-attendance. *Scandinavian Journal of Educational Research*, *59*(3), 316–336. doi:10.1080/00313831.2014.904424

Howlin, P., Moss, P., Savage, S., & Rutter, M. (2013). Social outcomes in mid-to later adulthood among individuals diagnosed with autism and average nonverbal IQ as children. *Journal of the American Academy of Child and Adolescent Psychiatry*, *52*(6), 572–581. doi:10.1016/j.jaac.2013.02.017 PMID:23702446

Kanner, L. (1943). Autistic disturbances of affective contact. *Nervous Child*, *2*(3), 217–250.

Kearney, C. A. (2001). *School refusal behavior in youth: A functional approach to assessment and treatment*. American Psychological Association. doi:10.1037/10426-000

Kennedy, R. S., Berbaum, K. S., & Drexler, J. (1994, June). Methodological and measurement issues for identification of engineering features contributing to virtual reality sickness. In *Image 7*. Tucson, AZ: Conference.

Korkman, M., Kirk, U., & Kemp, S. (2007). NEPSY–Second Edition (NEPSY-II). San Antonio, TX: The Psychological Corporation.

Lamson, R., & Meisner, M. (1994, June). *The effects of virtual reality immersion in the treatment of anxiety, panic and phobia of heights. In Virtual reality and persons with disabilities.* Paper presented at the 2nd Annual International Conference, San Francisco, CA.

Leigh, J. P., & Du, J. (2015). Brief report: Forecasting the economic burden of autism in 2015 and 2025 in the United States. *Journal of Autism and Developmental Disorders*, *45*(12), 4135–4139. doi:10.100710803-015-2521-7 PMID:26183723

Levin, M. F., Weiss, P. L., & Keshner, E. A. (2015). Emergence of virtual reality as a tool for upper limb rehabilitation: Incorporation of motor control and motor learning principles. *Physical Therapy*, *95*(3), 415–425. doi:10.2522/ptj.20130579 PMID:25212522

Lewin, J. E. (1986). Emergence: Labeled Autistic. *The American Journal of Occupational Therapy*, *40*(7), 503–503. doi:10.5014/ajot.40.7.503b

Matson, J. L., Rivet, T. T., Fodstad, J. C., Dempsey, T., & Boisjoli, J. A. (2009). Examination of adaptive behavior differences in adults with autism spectrum disorders and intellectual disability. *Research in Developmental Disabilities*, *30*(6), 1317–1325. doi:10.1016/j.ridd.2009.05.008 PMID:19540717

Mitchell, P., Parsons, S., & Leonard, A. (2007). Using virtual environments for teaching social understanding to 6 adolescents with autistic spectrum disorders. *Journal of Autism and Developmental Disorders*, *37*(3), 589–600. doi:10.100710803-006-0189-8 PMID:16900403

Munkhaugen, E. K., Gjevik, E., Pripp, A. H., Sponheim, E., & Diseth, T. H. (2017). School refusal behaviour: Are children and adolescents with autism spectrum disorder at a higher risk? *Research in Autism Spectrum Disorders*, *41*, 31–38. doi:10.1016/j.rasd.2017.07.001

National Research Council. (2001). *Educating children with autism*. National Academies Press.

Neisser, U. (1982). Memory: What are the important questions. *Memory observed: Remembering in natural contexts*, 3-19.

Norrholm, S. D., Jovanovic, T., Gerardi, M., Breazeale, K. G., Price, M., Davis, M., ... Tuerk, P. W. (2016). Baseline psychophysiological and cortisol reactivity as a predictor of PTSD treatment outcome in virtual reality exposure therapy. *Behaviour Research and Therapy*, *82*, 28–37. doi:10.1016/j.brat.2016.05.002 PMID:27183343

North, M., & North, S. (1994). Virtual environments and psychological disorders. *Electronic Journal of Virtual Culture*, *2*(4), 37–42.

North, M., & North, S. (1994). Relative effectiveness of virtual environment desensitization and imaginal desensitization in the treatment of aerophobia. *Electronic Journal of Virtual Culture*, *2*(4), 37–42.

Parsons, S. (2016). Authenticity in Virtual Reality for assessment and intervention in autism: A conceptual review. *Educational Research Review*, *19*, 138–157. doi:10.1016/j.edurev.2016.08.001

Parsons, T. D., Carlew, A. R., Magtoto, J., & Stonecipher, K. (2017). The potential of function-led virtual environments for ecologically valid measures of executive function in experimental and clinical neuropsychology. *Neuropsychological Rehabilitation*, *27*(5), 777–807. doi:10.1080/09602011.2015.1109524 PMID:26558491

Prensky, M. (2003). Digital game-based learning. *Computers in Entertainment*, *1*(1), 21–21. doi:10.1145/950566.950596

Rizzo, A., & Koenig, S. T. (2017). Is clinical virtual reality ready for primetime? *Neuropsychology*, *31*(8), 877–899. doi:10.1037/neu0000405 PMID:29376669

Rizzo, A, & Rothbaum, B. O. (2002). Ethical issues for the use of virtual reality in the psychological sciences. *Ethical issues in clinical neuropsychology*, 243.

Schrooten, I., Scholte, R. H., & Didden, R. (2017). Bullying Among Youth with Autism Spectrum Disorders. Handbook of Social Skills and Autism Spectrum Disorder, (1), 45.

Sohlberg, M. M., & Mateer, C. A. (2017). *Cognitive rehabilitation: An integrative neuropsychological approach*. Guilford Publications.

Stokes, T. F., & Baer, D. M. (1977). An implicit technology of generalization. *Journal of Applied Behavior Analysis*, *10*(2), 349–367. doi:10.1901/jaba.1977.10-349 PMID:16795561

Strain, P. S., Schwartz, I. S., & Bovey, E. H. (2008). Social competence interventions for young children with autism. *Social competence of young children: Risk, disability, and intervention*, 253-272.

Strickland, D. (2001, August). Virtual reality and multimedia applications for mental health assessment and treatment. *ACM SIGGRAPH 2001 Conference*.

Strickland, D., Marcus, L. M., Mesibov, G. B., & Hogan, K. (1996). Brief report: Two case studies using virtual reality as a learning tool for autistic children. *Journal of Autism and Developmental Disorders*, *26*(6), 651–659. doi:10.1007/BF02172354 PMID:8986851

Wang, P., & Spillane, A. (2009). Evidence-based social skills interventions for children with autism: A meta-analysis. *Education and Training in Developmental Disabilities*, 318–342.

Wang, S. Y., Cui, Y., & Parrila, R. (2011). Examining the effectiveness of peer-mediated and video-modeling social skills interventions for children with autism spectrum disorders: A meta-analysis in single-case research using HLM. *Research in Autism Spectrum Disorders*, *5*(1), 562–569. doi:10.1016/j.rasd.2010.06.023

Williford, J. S., Hodges, L. F., North, M. M., & North, S. M. (1993). Relative effectiveness of virtual environment desensitization and imaginal desensitization in the treatment of acrophobia. In *Graphics interface* (pp. 162–162). Canadian Information Processing Society.

Wood, J. J., Drahota, A., Sze, K., Har, K., Chiu, A., & Langer, D. A. (2009). Cognitive behavioral therapy for anxiety in children with autism spectrum disorders: A randomized, controlled trial. *Journal of Child Psychology and Psychiatry, and Allied Disciplines*, *50*(3), 224–234. doi:10.1111/j.1469-7610.2008.01948.x PMID:19309326

Xu, G., Strathearn, L., Liu, B., & Bao, W. (2018). Prevalence of Autism Spectrum Disorder Among US Children and Adolescents, 2014-2016. *Journal of the American Medical Association*, *319*(1), 81–82. doi:10.1001/jama.2017.17812 PMID:29297068

Zarr, M. (1994). Computer-aided psychotherapy: Machine helping therapist. *Psychiatric Annals*, *24*(1), 42–46. doi:10.3928/0048-5713-19940101-13

## KEY TERMS AND DEFINITIONS

**Anxiety Disorders:** A group of mental disorders characterized by significant feelings of anxiety towards specific environments or stimuli.

**Autism Spectrum Disorder:** A spectrum of mental conditions with two types of symptoms: problems in social communication and interaction as well as restricted and repetitive behavior, interests, or activities.

**Cave Automatic Virtual Environments:** Immersive virtual reality environment where projector images are directed to the wall of a room.

**Evidence-Based Interventions:** Practices or programs that have been peer-reviewed and had their effectiveness documented via empirical evidence.

**Head-Mounted Displays:** A display device worn on the head that has a small display in front of each eye.

**Hierarchal Rehearsal:** Rehearsal of skills starting with easier tasks, followed by a gradual increase in difficulty.

**In-Vivo Exposure Therapy:** Systematic and rapid exposure to feared situations in order to get rid of anxiety.

**Maladaptive Behavior:** Behaviors ranging from nail-biting and separation difficulties to self-harm, developed to escape from challenges and conflicts instead of adapting one's behavior to them.

**Socio-Economic Costs:** Direct and indirect economic burden on the society.

**Transfer of Knowledge:** Knowledge transfer is the practical problem of performing skills and knowledge learned in one context or situation to another context or situation.

**Vive Base-Station Area:** Vive base stations beam infrared signals to the headset and controllers in order to perform room-scale tracking of the users within an area of approximately 5 square meters.

# Chapter 11
# Autism Spectrum Disorder (ASD) and Attention-Deficit/Hyperactivity Disorder (ADHD) Children:
## From Users to Creators of Virtual Reality Learning Content

**Giuliana Guazzaroni**
*Università Politecnica delle Marche, Italy*

## ABSTRACT

*Autism spectrum disorder (ASD) is a serious neurological disorder. Using virtual reality (VR), researchers are exploring alternative solutions to treat ASD. Recent experiences show that VR can be a motivating platform to safely practice social and communication skills for children with ASD. It is also seen as an effective method to build empathy and help improve the general understanding of the condition. This study will focus on using and experimenting different 360-degree immersive learning environments for ASD and attention-deficit/hyperactivity disorder (ADHD) pupils and their schoolmates. The chapter will report on a few ASD students who use VR facilities to communicate, learn, improve self-awareness, autobiographical memory, and reduce school pressure, and a few ADHD students who enjoy a VR environment to improve concentration and self-esteem. Both the ASD students and the ADHD ones decided, during the trial, to become VR creators building their own content, with the help of a facilitator.*

## INTRODUCTION

Virtual reality (VR) plays an important role for autism spectrum disorder (ASD) children, and it represents a growing area of research. The term VR is reasonably broad (Newbutt et al., 2016). In fact, VR may be described as a simulation of the real world based on computer graphics, including virtual environment simulations, collaborative virtual environments, immersive virtual environments, virtual

DOI: 10.4018/978-1-5225-7168-1.ch011

worlds, 3D immersive graphics, head-mounted displays, 360-degree movies and photos etc. (Newbutt et al., 2016; Bellani et al., 2011; Guazzaroni, 2017; Radu, 2014). VR may represent a simulation of the reality based on computer graphics or immersive movies. These experiences can be multipurpose for educators, therapists, families to offer a safe and repeatable environment during treatment or learning (Newbutt et al., 2016). Moreover, VR simulates and recreates the real world, or it rebuilds a completely new reality which can be repeated as often as required (Bellani et al., 2011). Using 360-degree cameras, it is possible to offer real world immersive experiences. In other words, immersive movies can be watched using a head-mounted display. The real world is repeated in a way to enhance communication with the autistic student. The ASD is a developmental disorder characterized by core deficits in: social interaction, communication, and repetitive or stereotypic behavior. The causes of autism are largely unknown as different factors are involved. The degree of impairment may vary depending on the single individual. It is crucial to develop tools for neurocognitive rehabilitation enabling children with ASD to improve their ability to perform daily activities. In this context, VR represents a very promising tool (Bellani, 2011; Casas et al., 2012; Parsons & Cobb, 2011). VR potential benefits may support the learning process of autistic children, as VR seems to be particularly useful to enhance the daily life social behaviors (Parsons & Mitchell, 2002). In the last decade, there has been a rapid advance in the use of VR. Recently the level of sophistication has strongly increased, and more and more educators are introducing VR facilities to teach students with special needs. For example, ASD schoolchildren can learn and practice important skills such as eye pointing and gaze fixation. Perhaps because of the seriousness of the disorder, and the lack of effective treatments, VR has received more application in ASD children than in pupils affected by Attention-Deficit/Hyperactivity Disorder (ADHD), although both groups of individuals (ASDs and ADHDs) would appear to benefit from many of the same technology features. Recently VR has renewed, because of affordable head–mounted display (e.g. Google Cardboard viewer). For ASD and ADHD schoolboys and girls an immersive virtual scenario can be an attractive learning environment because it releases their pressure. There is a lot less physical inflection involved in current VR animation or in a 360-degree movie than within real human interactions, and for ASD individuals this simplification can help reduce confusion, and communicate in an effective. VR offers the potential to create a training and treatment environment, immersive and dynamic, allowing "sophisticated interaction, behavioral tracking, and performance recording" (Rizzo & Kim, 2005). VR has a seemingly endless number of real world applications. It is increasingly clear that this technology is not strictly used by gaming enthusiasts. VR is rapidly evolving into an effective tool for education, medical diagnosing and treatment. Highly effective VR technological solutions and useful practices have developed for medical professionals, researchers and educators. This chapter examines the use of different 360-degree immersive learning environments especially for ASD pupils, and their schoolmates. In particular, the chapter will report of a few ASD students that use VR facilities to communicate, to learn, to improve self-awareness, autobiographic memory and to reduce their school pressure level; of a few ADHD students that enjoys a VR environment to improve concentration, self-esteem and to learn in a pleasant way. On the other hand, their classmates experience VR immersive videos to develop empathy, friendship and understanding of the children with special needs. Both the ASD students and the ADHD ones decided, during the trial, to become VR creators building their own didactic content, with the help of a facilitator.

## BACKGROUND: ASD / ADHD INDIVIDUALS AND VR

### VR Technology Advancement and New Potential for Students With Special Needs

Thanks to new advance in technology, VR has recently become more affordable to many consumers. New 360-degree cameras and cheap VR headsets, like Google Cardboard, have offered the possibility to create low-cost learning content. Google Cardboard is a VR platform developed by Google. Named for its foldout cardboard viewer, the platform is a low-cost system to encourage interest and development in VR applications. Cardboard users can either build their own viewer from low-cost components using specifications published by Google, or purchase one. To use the VR platform, people run Cardboard compatible applications on their phone; place the phone into the back of the viewer, and view content through the lenses. Google engineers created the platform and introduced it in 2014. The Cardboard software development kit (SDK) is available for the Android and iOS operating systems. To create VR experiences different tools are available, useful applications for Android and iOS and special 3D or 360-degree cameras. In 2018, Facebook has released a special viewer, called Oculus Go. This is an all-in-one VR headset, which can be used with no phone to drop in. The student can simply put on the headset and dive into virtual realms, without using a smartphone to connect. A 360-degree camera is an omnidirectional camera with a 360-degree field of view that covers the entire sphere. Omnidirectional cameras are crucial for Google Cardboard or Oculus Go users, or other VR headset where large visual field coverage is needed. Moreover, omnidirectional cameras are important in areas where large visual field extent is needed, such as in panoramic photography and robotics (Frossard & Khasanova, 2017). In education 360-degree cameras are revolutionary to create tailor-made learning objects to be offered in VR head-mounted display or interactive whiteboard (IWB). For special needs children, VR tailor-made learning objects may offer the opportunity to observe real world repeated, on-demand, in a way educators/facilitators can communicate with an autistic student. Help to learn basic skills or avoid anxiety due to the real world routine. For ADHD individuals, 360-degree immersive environments present unique opportunities to learn without anxiety, as a special simulated reality is offered, to help basic cognitive process and to attract student's attention without any distractions. VR technologies, in fact, enable rehabilitation techniques to provide users the opportunity to interact in a safe environment, without the threats that exist in a real setting (Bashiri et al., 2017).

### VR and ASD Individuals

VR technology offers a three-dimensional, 360-degree virtual space and real-time virtual environment, which can be used as a training platform for autistic individuals. A VR environment may facilitate learning and the rehearsal of actions and responses in different settings (Parsons & Cobb, 2011). VR may be a help to autistic children in the classroom as it offers the possibility to be turned into real life scenarios. The challenges autistic individuals face in filtering external stimuli can lead to anything from mild anxiety to panic attacks. The pain associated with such overwhelming experiences of the outside world can result in restricted and repetitive behaviors, fear of change, and general retraction. VR environments propose a safe setting to practice realizable situations in the real world. An immersive virtual scenario can be an attractive learning environment for ASD individuals because it can take the pressure off. There is less physical inflection in VR animation or in virtual worlds than within real interactions as body language and facial expressions are simplified in avatars. Programmers may see this characteristic as a lack, but for ASD people this simplification can reduce their confusion. A virtual environment is a recreated world where human mistakes do not have consequences (Catren, 2017). VR has emerged as a very promising tool, it 'offers the potential to create systematic human testing, training, and treatment environments that allow for the precise control of complex, immersive, dynamic 3D stimulus presentations, within which sophisticated interaction, behavioral tracking, and performance recording is possible'. A VR environment may be used as a simulator of the real world, it can present materials that 'assess and rehabilitate' human performance using specific stimuli not easily manageable in real situations. Therefore, VR is a very promising tool for stimulus control, real-time performance feedback, error-free learning, self-guided exploration, safe testing and gaming (Rizzo & Kim, 2005).

## Social Skills Training for ASD Individuals

Parsons and Mitchell (2002) have pointed out the difficulties of people with ASDs in the social domain. Consequently, social behaviors should be taught. In this context, VR is an ideal tool to practice 'behaviors' in role-play situations. VR offers a 'safe environment for rule learning and repetition of tasks' (Parsons & Mitchell, 2002). For an impaired student, VR can be seen as a protected environment to learn and to repeat lessons. For ASD pupils, VR is a kind of dematerialized place to find out without distractions. An environment at the same time immersive and flexible, ideal to practice social skills. According to Howlin (1997), people with ASDs or with Asperger syndrome (AS) experience intense difficulties in the social domain. The consequence is that, these people live 'social exclusion' and concrete difficulties in friendship. Acceptance by other schoolmates and peers should be promoted and heartily taught by educators and therapists. Generally, all children learn social interaction without effort. On the other hand, individuals diagnosed with an ASD show three impairments in: 1. Communication 2. Socialization and 3. Imagination. Some people present normal to high IQ levels but they remain impaired in social understanding (Parsons & Michell, 2002). The literature is progressively recognizing the potential benefits of VR in supporting learning, especially related to social and life skills compared to other approaches (Bellani et al., 2011; Parsons & Cobb, 2011; Kandalaft et al., 2013; Guazzaroni, 2017). According to Kandalaft et al. (2013), transition into adulthood is a challenging time for people with ASDs. In fact, social impairments 'interfere with the process of building relationships [...] participating and integrating into the community'. In this context, VR technology eliminates the need for real world in social skills training, thus reducing this source of anxiety for the autistic children. Consequently, VR environments allow a 'safe and non-threatening practice' of social skills. Moreover, a virtual environment setting offers many advantages. It is 'stable, familiar and predictable, and can be adapted to suit individual needs'. Educational tasks can be repeated and practiced in an agreeable way. The repetition of the task may facilitate the effective learning of social skills (Parsons & Mitchell, 2002). The consequence is that virtual worlds are increasingly being used in psychological rehabilitation in children, and in educational practice (Herrera et al., 2008). One of the most important characteristics of ASD individuals is the difficulty with social interaction and communication with other people. Most researches focused on 'understanding the brain mechanisms underlying the deficits in social cognition and language associated with ASD. However, recent empirical and theoretical work has begun to reveal increasing evidence for altered self-representation, or intrapersonal cognition in ASD. In fact, children with autism present a developmental delay in the self-recognition ability (Uddin, 2011). Individuals with ASD have a different sense of self, difficulties in maintaining a stable self-concept and in adapting their self-concept to changing environments. The ability to differentiate between self and others is also impaired in autism. The effects of this atypical sense of self are seeable in the difficulties ASD individuals experience in social skills and communication (Lyons & Fitzgerald, 2013).

## VR and ADHD Individuals

The ADHD is a disorder characterized by a "persistent pattern of inattention and/or hyperactivity/ impulsivity" that occurs at school or in other social settings. ADHD has been recently treated using VR technology and/or other medical aid, for example the behavior therapy. The recent advancement of technology enables ADHDs to use optimal VR environments to practice real situations (Lee et al., 2001). According to the American Psychiatric Association, ADHD is a disorder that occurs in childhood. It is characterized by attention deficiency, hyperactivity, and impulsivity. Absence of self-confidence, relationship personality disorder, and incompatibility with social environment. As VR can reproduce everyday routine (for example everyday life in a classroom) by using this facility, ADHD students can interact in a virtual world and behave as they would in the real one. Educators may develop various environments to make ADHD children to be treated and helped to learn how to behave in specific social scenarios (Lee et al., 2001). The application of VR has recently emerged in educational and training areas, entertainment and medicine. Immersive VR, desktop VR, projective VR, and CAVE (C-Automatic Virtual Environment) are, according to Bashiri et al. (2017), the most used types of VR. The power of this technology is the possibility to build life-like environment for learning and for controlling problematic situations in the real life world. Numerous studies confirmed the benefits of VR in ADHD individuals' cognitive performance. Many authors pointed out the potential of VR in the assessment and training of attention without distractions (Bashiri et al., 2017; Mühlberger et al., 2016; Rapport et al., 2000). An increasing number of researchers believe that VR technology is ready for the assessment of ADHD. In fact, VR has become increasingly realistic and immersive. Thus, the results from a VR assessment better predict behavior in real world settings (Kulman, 2018).

## Experiential Learning

VR technology may offer a valid support for education. According to Aiello et al. (2012), VR facilities may enhance a sensomotorial activity in learning. VR lets students enter a possible virtual world. Sastry and Boyd (1998) say that a virtual environment offers a high level of presence when students can 'select, move and manipulate objects naturally'. Consequently, performing in a virtual environment makes users feel present in that VR setting. Simulations appear to be real creating a cognitive-sensory mechanism known as 'sense of presence' (Riva et al., 2009). Immersive VR environments offer a great variety of experiences students cannot normally practice at school. VR improvement can be found in head-mounted devices used by fighter pilots. The original aim was to place people in environments that contain the information they needed in order to interact in a natural way. 'As a result of total immersion in a virtual world, participants report a very real sense of being in another place'. This phenomenon is known as 'cognitive presence' and is joined together with the 'conviction that a virtual world is a valid, though different, form of reality'. The first VR systems were designed to simplify the interface for airplane pilots. According to some authors, VR is immersive and the interface has been completely removed. In fact, the users wear the computer and they can easily interact with the virtual environment. The subject-object distinction that exists between individuals and information in computers disappears when the learner use VR environments. Consequently immersive virtual worlds experience is a first-person experience. 'First-person experiences are therefore natural, non-reflective, and predominant in our everyday interactions with the world [...] The interface creates a boundary around the computer and its information, and establishes the distinction between us – subject – and it – object'. VR environments allow users to immerse in a virtual world without interfaces. The experiences in VR offer the same quality as experiences in the real world (Winn, 1993). VR should be designed in such a way that users would find it difficult to tell the difference from what is real and what is not (Guazzaroni, 2017). The experiential learning refers to learning through direct experiences of knowledge. Experiential learning is impossible in most cases, but VR technologies may allow direct interaction with virtual environments and objects. Experiential learning using VR is possible based on the experiment results, which showed that the enhanced vividness and interactivity of VR technologies allow the users to closely recognize virtual experiences as direct experiences, and that the learning effect is enhanced. It was also determined that experiential learning in a virtual environment is identical to an experience in reality (Maraj et al. 2017). Through experimentation and analysis, it was determined that the enhanced vividness and interactivity in a virtual environment allows the user to recognize the experience as being closer to a direct experience, and partially enhances the learning effect (Kwon et al., in press). A VR environment may be also seen as a complex system emerging from the interaction and sharing of knowledge, motivation and characteristics of the setting (Aiello et al., 2012). Implementing a VR learning experience involves the exploration of unusual pedagogical and technological boundaries. On the other hand, VR technology is immersive and users need headsets to block out the external world and literally immerse themselves in a digital realm. In VR, the concept of immersion is referred to user's involvement in the virtual environment. It causes a lack of awareness of time and of the real world, as well as a sense of immersion. The spatial immersion in the virtual world is a perception of being physically present in a non-physical world that provides a very absorbing environment (Freina & Ott, 2015). VR allows first-person experience in virtual worlds or the possibility to visit special views, for instance, war settings or other places a special need student could not visit. First-person non-symbolic experiences are natural and predominant in everyday interaction; using a VR headset user can experience a 'natural semantic' of the world or complex system (Guazzaroni, 2017).

## The Constructivist Learning Theory

Learning is a function of how people construct meaning starting from his or her own experience. Piaget (1998) suggests that students learn by expanding their knowledge by experiences, which are necessary for learning. The Constructivist learning theory says that all knowledge is constructed from a base of prior knowledge. Therefore, children learn best when they are allowed to construct a personal understanding based on experiencing things and reflecting on those experiences. VR environments seem to offer an ideal setting to create tailor made experiences, particularly for special needs students. According to Aiello et al. (2012), 'the constructivism paradigm also opens new perspectives for teaching through the use of VR technologies, considering the impossibility of separating the learning process from their context in which, through the action, the interactions essential for cognitive processes are realized'. Learning is an active and constructive process by which learners are not passive receivers of information. On the other hand, learners are active creators of their own knowledge, starting from their previous knowledge and in a continual interaction with the surroundings. In this learning environment, the new experiences are not added to those already experienced, but are actively revised and reorganized through an effective feedback and the constant configuration, consciously and unconsciously. The new knowledge and its own meaning is linked to the context in which it takes place. It represents a new model of education that renounces the traditional communication of information, and 'instead enhances sensorimotor interaction with the environment for effective knowledge construction'. As in the real world, VR offers 'total body involvement', which allows students to see the world through sensorimotor learning based on concrete experience and active experimentation (Aiello et al., 2012). A VR learning environment lets students to be transported to other places, to be fully immersed in experiences, and to feel a sense of presence. VR presents the opportunity to learn in a real situation, offering the users a sense of exploration and involvement. It is a concrete and immersive experience, based on an active learning paradigm. VR tools like Google Cardboard have the potential to enhance classroom by providing concrete knowledge, based on real experience, authentic and engaging learning (Oigara, 2018). Moreover, using VR technology in education means opening to informal learning environments. Furthermore, these technologies can favorite the transition from the 'Learning work' to the 'Learning adventure'. In other words, a positive class atmosphere where students' activities are aimed to satisfy a personal desire of acquiring knowledge (Leo et al., 2010). The constructivist teaching method has been used in special education settings. It is quite effective for those students who have special needs like ASD. Some of these students cannot be taught using traditional methods and a teacher is a guide for a learning journey and actively participates in the learning process with the students, encouraging to make progress. Constructivism means to discard standardized curricula in favor of a personalized course of study based on what the student already knows. Winterbottom and Blake (2008) have described a method for design based on constructivism. They have distilled five useful values:

1. **Atomic Simplicity:** This is the guiding principle of hypermedia systems (e.g. Wikis); complexity arises from the ways simple atomic parts are connected together to return a rich and interesting dynamic experience.
2. **Multiplicity:** There are many ways to an end, and not one single process. Learners can construct their knowledge and universe in myriad ways.
3. **Practical Exploration:** Learning and constructing knowledge are active and attractive tasks. Errors can be used to provide feedback; they are treated as an integral part of the exploration activity.
4. **Control:** People control their learning process by an active construction of their knowledge. Guidance is offered in the form of artefacts, advice and tutorials.
5. **Reflective Process:** The process of constructing knowledge requires acting with reflection in order to build effective connections between bits of knowledge. Support for iterative process is a way to foster reflections and communication with learners.

These five distinct values pointed out by Winterbottom and Blake (2008) may result very useful in the process of constructing knowledge and communicate with ASD and ADHD learners. In fact, especially for ASD individuals, the traditional learning tools may appear very difficult and inadequate. For this reason, VR technology and specific learning tasks based on constructivism principles have been disposed for ASDs and ADHDs in this scientific research.

## MAIN FOCUS OF THE CHAPTER: METHOD

### Participants

A total of 25 students participated in the experiment. Mean age of participants was 12.03 years. A first group of 17 participants (9 male, 8 female) were in the class inclusion immersive grouping, to become aware of their classmates with ASD or ADHD. A second group, of 8 participants (7 male, 1 female) were in the VR learning immersive grouping (from users to creators of VR content). The female of this second grouping is the main protagonist of the experimentation; she had a previous clinical diagnosis of ASD. Other 2 male individuals had a previous clinical diagnosis of ASD. 3 male students had a clinical diagnosis of ADHD, and 2 male individuals had a diagnosis of other intellectual disabilities. The two groups were selected to experiment a proper VR learning environment and to encourage special needs students' inclusion. None of them had used VR before.

### Procedures

The experiment was conducted in a school located in Tolentino (Istituto Comprensivo Giovanni Lucatelli), Italy during the school year 2017/2018. A few of the experiment processes were recorded, a questionnaire and an achievement assessment were conducted during the experiment. The ASD female individual was the main protagonist of the trial. At the beginning, the first grouping of 17 participants was involved. They had just started the first year of the secondary school and two individuals with ASD were inserted in their class group. A special lesson was prepared to help this first group of students to welcome the two ASD learners. Using Google Cardboard displays the 17 classmates could live as an ASD individual using a special immersive application. After this immersive session they were asked to complete a questionnaire to test if the VR facilities aided them, or not, to better understand their autistic classmates. Based on real experiences, in consultation with ASD individuals, The National Autistic Society created a series of immersive movies to give a flavor of how overwhelming an everyday surround, like a shopping center or an underground station, can be to an autistic person experiencing too much information (Autism TMI Virtual Reality Experience). These films are a powerful tool to help people truly understand ASD. Two immersive videos are shown to the class inclusion immersive grouping, using cardboard goggles. In the first immersive video the spectator was an active part of the video. The watcher was literally the main character panting while he/she was waiting for his/her mother purchasing a ticket in a vending machine. The child was prey of social anxiety and expressed his/her frustration. The second video is entitled 'The Party', it allowed the students of the class inclusion group to enter the world of an autistic teenager, Layla, who was at a surprise birthday celebration. The watcher could hear her thoughts about what she was experiencing and how it was affecting her. Layla shared the sensory overload and her bad response to an overwhelming situation. The drama provided audience with a mighty first person perspective on the challenges that social situations may present to ASD individuals. 'The visual and auditory effects in the film were based on scientific research about the kinds of symptoms seen in autistic individuals, such as difficulties with processing faces, and hypersensitivity to lights, loud noises and strong odours'. 'The Party' is a virtual experience of autism created by The Guardian (The Guardian, 2017). The two VR videos were offered to the 17 students using Google Cardboard viewers, after the VR sessions the 17 pupils answered a questionnaire. The questionnaire was composed by three questions:

**Question 1:** Does the virtual reality glasses let you experience, in first person, the problems related to an ASD child's anxiety in a real situations?

**Question 2:** Does the virtual reality experience let you understand the behavior of your ASD classmates in everyday situations?

**Question 3:** Does experiencing in first person the social anxiety of an ASD child let you increase your awareness, sympathy and sense of friendship towards your classmates?

Most of the students said that they lived the experience as if they really were autistic people and, after the vision, they could truly improve their understanding of an ASD individual. Consequently, they could cooperate, interact and study with their special classmates during the school year. To reinforce the interest in the VR environment, special immersive materials were showed to the first group of 17 students. They particularly enjoyed the virtual immersion. They could swim with sharks, live like lions, fly like eagles, observe an erupting volcano etc. The result of the test was the following: 15 out of 17 students (88,23%) believed that the VR environment let them experience, in first person, the problems related to an ASD child's anxiety in a real situations; 1 out of 17 (5,8%) affirmed that he/she is not sure if the VR environment let him/ her experience, in first person, the problems related to an ASD child's anxiety in a real situation; 1 out of 17 (5,8%) declared that he/she could not experience, in first-person, the problems related to an ASD child's anxiety using the Google Cardboard. All the students (100%) said that the VR experience let them understand the behavior of their ASD classmates in everyday situations. Moreover, everybody (100%) believed that experiencing, in first-person, the social anxiety of an ASD child let them increase their awareness and sense of friendship for their autistic classmates. Most of the parents of the 17 pupils welcomed this immersive activity and, when interviewed, they were aware of their sons and daughters' human understanding. They felt a great deal of fellow feeling for the special companions. During another VR sessions the 17 students affirmed that the VR environment was really immersive and very realistic too. After the VR sessions, all of them declared that they could not distinguish an immersive environment experience from something happened in the real world. Their feelings and their emotions were barely the same: 'Sometimes, autistic people become overloaded by everything around them. That can make the outside world feel like a terrifying place. And for their families, all the looks, judgements and tuts make it feel like a lonely and isolated place' (The National Autistic Society, 2016). The VR sessions were reinforced by a few special lessons. Here all students wrote a letter for the autistic students. In the text, they introduced themselves, described their interests and hobbies and asked a question. The autistic students prepared their letters as well, after reading those of their schoolmates. Apart from letters, the students' photos were distributed to the special needs students. They had to combine photos and letters to get to know classmates. At the end of the activity, the ice was broken and all the students knew something more of the others. In a separate VR session, the ASD female strongly refused to watch and live the immersive VR environment presented to the first group. The hypothesis was that she was not interested in VR if a facilitator showed her things she could not experience (e.g. Wild animals, big cities, exotic settings etc.), but she was involved when someone showed her something she really liked (e.g. Mongolfiera, balloons, firework etc.). On the other hand, both the two male ASD individuals were likely to immerse in unexperienced VR environments (e.g. Wild life settings, volcanoes national park, space exploration etc.). In a second phase, some VR settings were presented to the ASD female student. She was asked what she was watching through the Google Cardboard. The student did not answer, she only watched inside the viewer. She remained silent; it was not clear whether she was interested or not in exploring the content. Familiar and unfamiliar images were showed to her. During a session, she watched a mountain landscape with snow, a hilly landscape, a big city, a balloon, the taking off of a hot-air balloon etc. Later, the facilitator observed that she wanted to understand how a VR immersive environment worked. In fact, after watching, she opened the cardboard and tried to take pictures. She was not a passive consumer of VR educational content she appeared interested in creating something for her needs. An educator observed that she was interested in understanding how to create digital objects for the cardboard viewer. The headseat is an object that intrigued her but she did not ask questions and did not react to verbalization. She believed rather she could take 360-degree pictures with her viewer and seemed to want to create her own immersive content. The challenge was accepted and a series of immersive photos and videos were recorded and edited for Google Cardboard by students, educators and other experts. The verbalization and subsequent writing of the new immersive experiences were limited to simple exchanges or sequences. Therefore, specific VR 360-degrees videos were disposed for this learner. She was always one of the main character involved in the VR environment and consequently she could enjoy the learning experiences. She really appreciated the self-produced content. She knew what she saw, she could describe something based on her personal events. She could create videos, VR experiences and enjoyed them later, she could show her schoolmates, who remained in the classroom, her special activities (e.g. Laboratories for special needs students, swimming lessons etc.). When she watched, she danced and moved everywhere. She watched 360-degrees videos in every direction. She really appreciated the VR simulation. From this moment on the student, from a passive user of VR content, became an active creator who prepared his/her own material for subsequent verbalizations or other educational activities. Particularly, from a first observation, it seemed that the VR viewer improved eye contact and concentration time period in a specific task. Some special students called the Goggle Cardboard "the photo on the eyes" and asked "let's have a picture on the eyes!". A similar VR section was proposed to other school boys with hyperactivity and concentration problems. The vision was combined with topics relating to Art History. They could visit and interact in an Egyptian museum and in Stonehenge. Subsequently, the VR sessions were extended to other special needs students with problems related to autism, hyperactivity, and a micro-brain pupil etc. They appreciated and started an interesting immersive lesson. The 3 male individuals with ADHD were both users and creators of VR content. They helped teachers and facilitators in creating 360-degrees videos to be shared with the other schoolmates. The VR learning laboratory was active once a week for special needs students, while their classmates could enjoy the VR immersion during playtime or in specific lessons devoted to inclusion. In the following VR sessions, when the teacher offered the ASD female a VR viewer, showing content out of her experience, she strongly refused it. On the other hand, she asked to watch 360-degree videos recorded during her activities, such as the laboratories in which she participated or field trips. The already lived experience of the ASD female were filmed and showed different times using a viewer. The reasons were that the autistic girl could define the already lived experience, watch it again (e.g. How to prepare biscuits), reworking it, divide it in logical sequences, elaborate again the content, become aware of herself and of her behavior, improve her autobiographic memory. The girl presented a severe functional impairment in communication and needed substantial support, severe deficits in verbal and nonverbal communication, and difficulty coping with change. She had problems in social cues and she was very anxious in social interactions, particularly with unfamiliar individuals. Consequently, the impairments in social communication negatively influenced peer relationship and school assignment (Didehbani et al., 2016). In fact, impairments in communication is one of the most salient limitations of children with autism. Generally, they have difficulties in initiating and in responding to social interactions. Recently, after the melioration of the use of technology in the education of autistic children, practice sessions using VR technology have positively influenced communication skills in children with autism. VR is recognized to be effective in order to improve communication with ASD individuals (Halabi et al., 2017). Several sections of VR with the autistic girl showed that tailor made contents created pleasant experiences. She began to dance and her expression relaxed, anxiety decreased as well as the tendency to oppose the different didactic activities offered by her educators. She danced and asked to watch videos where she was the protagonist (e.g. A visit to the museum). Direct observations by her teachers and assistants confirmed that the activity was particularly appreciated. Also the choice of music was really important for the rhythm and playfulness of the VR experience (VR sessions were recorded). The special education teacher who had been with her for four years, observed amazed that the proposed activity was particularly appreciated by the student. She smiled, looked satisfied, scampered, sang and danced. In general, this ASD student showed disagreement and rejection for every educational or ludic activity. She strongly opposed every proposal and shouted or cried. When she finally started working, the activity time did not exceed 15 minutes. On the contrary, the VR videos attracted, calmed the strong anxiety and cheered the girl. Educators helped her to create VR perception proposals that were within her range. The recorded 360-degree videos were shown in virtual environments. Here her experiences were repeated. For instance, a series of videos were recorded during her cooking performances, with other students, in order to establish a sort of communication with her. A psychologist observed that offering video via eyewear was a good way to establish a communication with an autistic subject. In fact, educators shared and rewatched with her what they wanted to teach and/or to communicate with her. The nature of VR environments is useful to maintain 'the ability to induce controlled stimuli (verbal or non-verbal) and also allow to monitor the behavior of the child within the virtual environment (VE) […] Therefore, VR based systems can prove to be effective as a medium of educating children with ASD in controlled interactive environments' (Halabi et al., 2017). Individuals with ASD have great difficulties in building a self-narrative. If autobiographical material is not provided, the narrative is confused and vague. In fact, research evidence points out deficits in narrative abilities in ASD individuals (Lyons & Fitzgerald, 2013). According to Uddin (2011), the ability to remember events that happened in the past is problematic in autism, there are 'difficulties in accessing specific autobiographical memories'. The use of VR 360-degrees videos offered to this student and containing her own experience, appeared very promising to stimulate her autobiographical memory. Sometimes, the girl was unquiet and does spite (e.g. Overturn the flour during cooking session), in the 360-degrees videos she could watch herself, with what effects for her self-awareness? Could her ameliorate her vague autobiographical memory with the help of a VR environment? During a VR session, the autistic girl asked to watch again her experiences at the kitchen laboratory and her trip at the Carriage and Opera Museums, an ADHD student was present. One after the other, they watched and verbalized the experiences, the girl could reactivate her memory and verbalized a simple story about the observations made at the museum. During the vision she moved, twirled and danced. The ADHD individual was not particularly interested in watching at his performances during the Labs. On the contrary, he wanted to explore new worlds and territories. He plunged into the depths of the sea, tried to catch sharks, greeted the people he saw in the VR space, and flied in a helicopter over a volcano. He explored new perspectives while the girl refused or was not interested in things she could not experience directly. She retraced the trip to Macerata (Museums and Lyrical arena). Her autobiographical memory seemed to improve and became less vague. During a particularly stressful day, the ASD girl saw the VR sessions she created in the swimming pool, her anxious and continues cry turned into a nice smile. But above all, she reinforced her motivation to come back the next day to attend her swimming course. Previously, he said: 'pool no, no'. In a subsequent VR session, two students were involved. A male pupil suffering from microcephaly and an ASD male student. The first one appreciated the VR vision of cooking laboratories, where he could observe himself and his peers. Later he watched other VR unexperienced environments (Volcanos, sharks etc.). His attention was stimulated and his anxiety subsided. His strong anxiety manifested itself with continuous monologues and a need to talk compulsively. He watched his field trip and different cooking sessions. He touched the floor and other objects imagining touching the objects he watched in the viewer. He tried to verbalize his VR experiences helped by an educator. The ASD male individual, appreciated the cooking laboratories, his school trip and, while watching the VR experience, he verbalized the names of his peers. He enjoyed not only the 360-degrees videos containing episodes of his real life, but also unexperienced settings (the savannah with lions, giraffes, eagles etc.). In the unknown wild environment, his movements were slower and he could barely name the things he saw. Nevertheless, he turned around cautiously to explore the savannah and the lions. His relationship with the facilitators that helped him during his VR sessions, completely changed after the VR experiences. In the following months, when he saw the VR participants he ran to hug them, to greet them warmly and to ask for new adventures with what he called 'eye picture'. This ASD individual had a special attitude for taking his own pictures and for using Google Maps, to explore familiar places of his town. He was particularly interested in taking 360-degrees pictures of his flat, his family and his ceramic lessons in a school laboratory or his horse riding lessons. He appeared very creative and he showed to his best schoolmates his 360-degrees photos. A VR session was offered to a schoolchild with a severe development impairment. He watched the videos, he seemed passive and he needed someone to hold the viewer, he smiled but he could not verbalize what he watched in the VR environment. A common trait was that all the students that had participated to VR session, changed their affective relationship with the educators and facilitators and asked for more explorations.

## Materials: Technology and VR Environment

Specific 360-degrees videos were recorded during a kitchen laboratory, a pottery laboratory, a garden laboratory, some swimming lessons, horse riding lessons, a field trip, a visit to the Carriage Museum and Opera Museum in Macerata (Italy), to create particular VR learning content. The VR experiences were developed using a minimal software and a portable hardware, which included: a 360-degrees video camera (Samsung Gear 360 2017); a mobile 360 video editing tool called: V360; a few interactive storytelling tools to create VR stories; YouTube to upload private VR videos, Google Cardboard viewer to enjoy VR content, and a few smartphones (Samsung S6). Using this equipment a series of VR material was produced:

1. VR videos regarding cooking activities.
2. VR content relating to pottery.
3. VR videos of swimming and horseback riding lessons.
4. VR material regarding museums, trips, outing, vegetable garden etc.

The stories related to these series were enriched by a special selection of music, thus students could move or dance while watching. The technological equipment offered to students was minimal and easy to use.

## Materials: Intervention Method

The materials were developed to provide a realistic and dynamic VR experience to engage in, practice communication, stimulate self-recognition, self-awareness, autobiographical memory or improve soft skills for ASD and ADHD individuals. Soft skills are a combination of social skills, communication skills and emotional intelligence that enable people to perform well, and achieve their goals with complementing hard skills. The Collins English Dictionary defines the term soft skills as 'desirable qualities [...] that do not depend on acquired knowledge: they include common sense, the ability to deal with people, and a positive flexible attitude'. Social scenarios were selected recording real laboratory lessons or other experiences (e.g. Field trip) to emphasize the learning objective of the VR session in different contexts, such as visiting a new place or learning how to do biscuits or other artefact (e.g. Pottery). These scenarios were selected from real world social situations and were introduced and discussed with learners. A coach facilitated each session with participants in real life. The VR sessions occurred at school in a comfortable classroom as studies have emphasized (Newbutt et al., 2016), the positive effects of VR sessions for people with ASD or ADHD will be better realized if they are placed in easy settings like school or home. The VR content were developed to stimulate self-awareness. In fact, research points out that ASD individuals' self-awareness is weak and it appeared to be impaired in autism. 'In particular, the recognition of a separate existence of other people seems to be delayed in children with autism' (Lyons & Fitzgerald, 2013). Moreover, recent work has revealed 'evidence for altered self-representation, or intrapersonal cognition in ASD (Uddin, 2011). On the other hand, children with ADHD show deficits in multiple areas of their lives, one is low self-esteem and low perceptions of self-competence (Rizzo, 2011). Consequently, the proposed VR content for both ASD and ADHD was self produced and self recorded. Very often 360-degrees videos offered in the VR space, contained the students themselves during their daily activities (e.g. Swimming). VR offers the potential to create a simulated setting to test and train children and, used in a proper way, VR can help to rehabilitate human performances under a range of stimuli (Rizzo & Kim, 2005). Different authors affirmed the advantages of VR in cognitive performance such as deficits in attention for ADHD. VR, here, is positively used to train attention without distractions (Bashiri et al., 2017). For example, an ADHD student can visit repeatedly a cultural heritage place, like Stonehenge. Reading the same notions in a traditional book or listening to the teacher's lesson is difficult and sometimes it is impossible for an ADHD. VR immersion provides an absorbing environment to explore and interact with. In addition to this, creating new learning contents is stimulating and rehabilitating for ADHD individuals. They can show their achievements to the rest of their classmates using a IWB or a cardboard viewer. The self-esteem and personal relationships of ADHDs improve.

## Issues, Controversies, Problems

According to some authors (Uddin, 2011), it is unmistakable that self-related cognition in ASDs is altered. Young people with autism present a developmental delay in the acquisition of self-recognition. A critical aspect of self-related cognition is the ability to remember events happened in the past. Autistic individuals present difficulties in accessing peculiar autobiographical memories. It was pointed out that adult ASDs 'generated fewer specific memories than age, gender, and IQ-matched controls. In addition, individuals with ASD extracted less meaning from their memories than adult controls'. It was suggested that it is a 'failure in using experiences to update the self' (Uddin, 2011; Crane et al., 2009). The autobiographical memory in children with autism is marked by errors of omission, and it seems

*Figure 1. A VR learning session with school children*

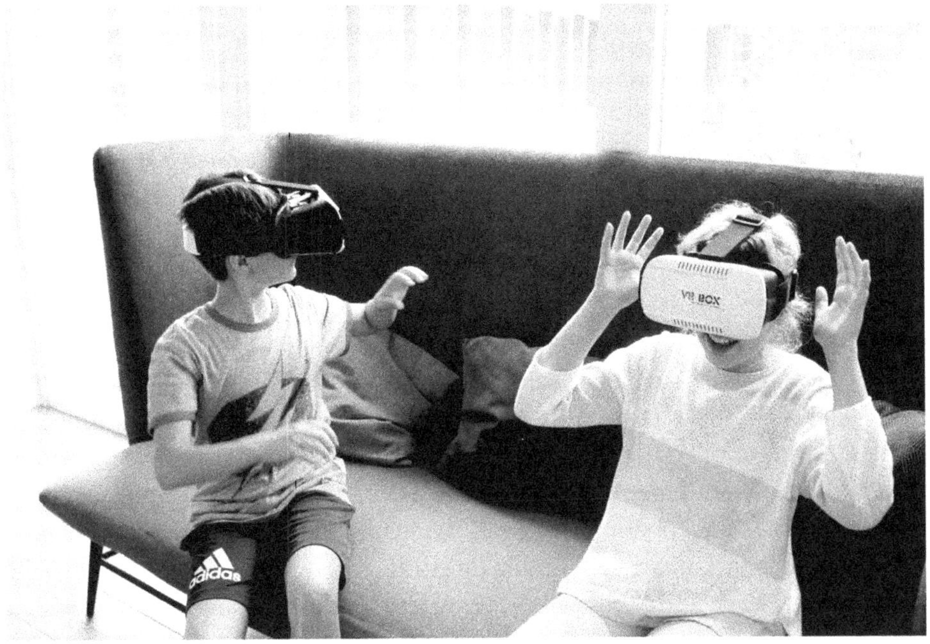

poor especially for early-life events. The components that compose the autobiographic memory system are impaired in autism (Uddin, 2011; Lyons & Fitzgerald, 2013). During the above described trials, the involved autistic children had difficulties to remember and verbalize what did they do in their recent past. But when they saw again and again their didactic experiences using the Google cardboard, they could remember and verbalize their own school life experiences. Directions for future research should emphasize this aspect of the VR content. Research literature shows that the self-awareness or the self-other awareness is delayed and impaired in children with autism 'including gaze following, abnormal response to sound and deficits in attention, showing of objects, responding and orienting to own name, looking at other's face, pretend play, protodeclarative pointing and gaze monitoring, empathy and imitation, joint-attention behavior, affect and personal relatedness' (Lyons & Fitzgerald, 2013). Nevertheless, during VR sessions ASDs students could improve their self-other awareness. In fact, they could see again and again their laboratories and name all their schoolmates after some exercises. The autistic female of the trial was the main character of the 360-degrees movies and she could ameliorate her gaze following, looking at other's face, gaze monitoring, and her self-awareness during the VR sessions. One of the most relevant characteristics of autism is the lack of empathy and emotional engagement with others. ASD individuals cannot interpret emotions in the right way, they cannot process their own emotions and have difficulties with the emotional engagement with other people; they are generally focused on their own concerns (Lyons & Fitzgerald, 2013). The VR immersion of the experimentation was based on the repetition of educational experiences and it included different actors. The ASD students during the sessions could communicate with a facilitator and develop an improved awareness of the lived environment and of the other peers. The educators, during the immersion, tried to transmit emotions and behaviors appropriate to the context (soft skills). Individuals with ASD have difficulties in constructing a self-narrative. In fact, if the autobiographic memory is inadequate, the narrative is disoriented and vague. The VR sessions and the associated didactic activities during the experimentation were devoted to improve the communication and the building of basic narrative skills using 360-degrees videos and sequences. The results show the effectiveness of immersive VR in motivating and engaging the autistic students. One-to-one repetitive interactions prolonged attention and engage reinforcement strategies. Regarding the involved ADHD students, their inattention was contrasted by immersive VR sessions. Specifically, the creation of 360-degree films motivated these students by offering considerable reinforcement in the study of the subjects involved (e.g. Art History). VR technology can contribute greatly to the treatment of ADHD individuals. In fact, the pupils involved in the experimentation could improve their behavior and performances at school. ADHD is associated with a wide range of social, emotional and cognitive difficulties. This aggregation of 'negative experiences has an impact on various factors, such as the individual's self-perceptions of competence and self-esteem, which in turn may advocate maladaptive coping strategies and interfere with treatment' (Rizzo, 2011). The activities presented during VR lessons ameliorated the self-esteem of ADHDs. These peers could build useful materials for themselves or for their schoolmates with the result they could succeed in a field and improve the image they had of themselves. Moreover, they had the possibility to act as the main character of a movie created to help peer learning. They changed their minds and start thinking of themselves as creators of learning content and not plain passive users. They could choose what they want to represent using an immersive environment. They started to consider themselves as active creators of nice objects and improve their self-awareness and self-esteem. ADHD is one of the most ordinary psychiatric disorders in childhood. This condition presents significant difficulties in education, social performance, and personal relationships. Given the importance of rehabilitation for these people, the use of VR technology is helpful (Bashiri et al., 2017). One ADHD student, during the VR sessions, presented some side effects of VR. Bashiri et al.(2017) wrote that side effects range from 'headaches, seizures, nausea, fatigue, drowsiness, disorientation, apathy, and dizziness. These symptoms are related to cybersickness or virtual reality sickness, which can endanger health and safety, as well as the effectiveness of VR'. Scientists have confirmed that VR headsets might cause motion sickness or VR sickness. VR viewer industry and software developers have worked hard to prevent it because they fear this will be a leading deterrent to mass adoption of VR (Mason, 2017).

## SOLUTIONS AND RECOMMENDATIONS

Studies have pointed out that 'cybersickness is a barrier to the use of training or rehabilitation tools in virtual reality environments'. Nevertheless, only one student out of 25 suffered cybersickness. Cybersickness can be prevented by knowing its causes. Different measures may be taken to fix or manage VR's side effects. Studies have indicated various methods to prevent cybersickness, including a correct calibration of VR technology and a meticulous customization to students' needs, offering a more natural user interface (UI). Kemeny et al. (2017) have proposed technics advancing a number of different ways to reduce cybersickness while navigating in virtual environments. An example is to reduce the field of view (FOV) or the immersion level. In order to avoid special needs students to suffer VR sickness, a good rule is to start with seated VR experiences first and offer standing ones later. Only after the pupil feels comfortable with the viewer. Another recommendation is to increase VR exposure time slowly. Studies say that women are more susceptible than men are, as are those with a history of headache (Murphy,

2015). In order to develop a positive interaction in a virtual environment, it is crucial to understand how a person perceives himself/herself in a real or in a VR environment. This knowledge will be more important when VR technology will become available to a large number of students (Tambovtsev, 2016).

## FUTURE RESEARCH DIRECTIONS

VR technology represents a crucial opportunity for teachers to introduce new experiences to their students, both those with special needs and those without. In this chapter 25 students aged about 12 years old participated in a trial. After the immersive VR experimentation for special needs and those without, during school year 2017/2018, some interesting trends emerged. VR facilities represent an emerging tendency in education. Google Cardboard, for instance, is an economic platform to offer an immersive educational experience. Using VR environments is useful to suggest different perspectives to different individuals. An inauthentic learning content may be changed in an authentic one (Wu et al., 2013). Moreover, VR technology allows first-person experience in virtual worlds. First-person non-symbolic experiences are natural in everyday life. VR promotes a learning environment that allows students to learn from non-symbolic first-person experience (Winn, 1993). Most of the learning scenarios are unexplored and the possibilities are still unknown, as students and teachers may expand their physical world. Consequently, the potential for the future of education are enormous (Guazzaroni, 2017). The role of VR technology for students with special needs represents a growing area of research, expecially in the field of ASD and ADHD. In recent years different efforts have been devoted to support the notion that VR learning environments may furnish a useful and attractive place for people with ASD to live an immersion and develop specific skills encouraging communication needs and integration (Newbutt et al., 2016). One of the most important characteristics of ASD individuals is difficulty with social interaction, self-recognition and poor autobiographical memory (Uddin, 2011; Lyons & Fitzgerald, 2013). In the experience described in this chapter, the use of proper VR technology and the creation of tailor made material, in the education of autistic children have positively influenced communication skills, self-recognition and autobiographical memory. Nevertheless, more studies and practices are needed in this field in order to largely adopt VR artifacts for these individuals. VR technology is also positive for ADHD people. VR, here, is constructively used to train attention without distractions (Bashiri et al., 2017). In fact, VR immersion provides an absorbing environment to explore and interact with. In addition to this, creating new learning objects is very stimulating and rehabilitating for ADHD individuals. The self-esteem and personal relationships improve. The educational material should be created by learners and facilitators to provide a realistic and dynamic VR experience to engage in, practice communication, stimulate self-recognition, self-awareness, autobiographical memory and to improve soft skills for ASDs, ADHDs and/or other special needs students. The crucial goal is to enable people to perform well and to develop desiderable qualities using VR learning environments in a proper way.

## CONCLUSION

The way students engage and learn has changed and technology plays a central role. Thanks to new advance in technology, VR has recently become more affordable to many users. New 360-degree cameras, VR web based platforms and cheap VR headsets, like Google Cardboard, have offered the possibility to create low-cost sophisticated learning objects. In the future, the classroom learning experience will shift towards more active student involvement in their learning. In this context, VR environments may promote collaboration, and more closely real-life working conditions, building student confidence and preparing them for a future with even more advanced technologies. Digitization has changed the traditional classroom teaching providing high-tech learning environment. Schools are using both technology enhanced and traditional teaching methods to ameliorate the learning and teaching experience for students, both for those with special needs and those without, and educators as well. VR learning environments, in combination with traditional teaching, will improve practical project based learning. Moreover, technology enhanced learning combined with extracurricular activities will see holistic personality development of children (Temurnikar, 2018). VR technology is a decisive opportunity for teachers to introduce new experiences to students. In this chapter 25 students were involved in experimenting different 360-degree immersive learning environments for ASDs, ADHDs and their schoolmates. The results were positive and the educators considered the research as a starting point for further developments. The most important results are: 1. Develop empathy, friendship and understanding of special needs students; 2. Reduce school pressure; 3. ASDs use VR facilities to communicate, learn, improve self-awareness and memory; 4. ADHDs enjoy VR facilities to improve concentration and self-esteem; 5. Students become VR creators to build own didactic content. In conclusion, implementing a VR experience involves the exploration of unusual pedagogical and technological boundaries. VR offers a total physical involvement of the learner, that may see the world and its complexity through complete immersion and active experimentation.

## REFERENCES

Aiello, P., D'Elia, F., Di Tore, S., & Sibilio, M. (2012). A constructivist approach to virtual reality for experiential learning. *E-Learning and Digital Media*, *9*(3), 317–324. doi:10.2304/elea.2012.9.3.317

American Psychiatric Association. (2013). *Diagnostic and statistical manual of mental disorders: DSM-5*. Washington, DC: American Psychiatric Publishing.

Bashiri, A., Ghazisaeedi, M., & Shahmoradi, L. (2017). The opportunities of virtual reality in the rehabilitation of children with attention deficit hyperactivity disorder: A literature review. *Korean Journal of Pediatrics*, *60*(11), 337–343. doi:10.3345/kjp.2017.60.11.337 PMID:29234356

Bellani, M., Fornasari, L., Chittaro, L., & Brambilla, P. (2011). Virtual reality in autism: State of the art. *Epidemiology and Psychiatric Sciences*, *20*(3), 235–238. doi:10.1017/S2045796011000448 PMID:21922965

Blake, E. H., & Winterbottom, C. (2008). Constructivism, virtual reality and tools to support design. In *Proceedings of the 7th ACM conference on Designing interactive systems*, (pp. 230-239), New York, NY: ACM.

Casas, X., Herrera, G., Coma, I., & Fernández, M. (2012). A kinect-based augmented reality system for individuals with autism spectrum disorders. In *Proceedings of the International Conference on Computer Graphics Theory and Applications and International Conference on Information Visualization Theory and Applications* (vol. 1, pp. 440-446). GRAPP.

Catren, N. R. (2017). *Virtual reality may be a help to autistic children in the classroom*. Retrieved March 5, 2018, from http://www.independent.co.uk/news/science/virtual-reality-may-be-a-help-to-autistic-children-in-the-classroom-a7676391.html

*Collins English dictionary*. (2014). Glasgow, UK: HarperCollins Publishers.

Crane, L., Goddard, L., & Pring, L. (2009). Specific and general autobiographical knowledge in adults with autism spectrum disorders: The role of personal goals. *Memory (Hove, England)*, *17*(5), 557–576. doi:10.1080/09658210902960211 PMID:19499459

Didehbani, N., Allen, T., Kandalaft, M., Krawczyk, D., & Chapman, S. (2016). Virtual reality social cognition training for children with high functioning autism. *Computers in Human Behavior*, *62*, 703–711. doi:10.1016/j.chb.2016.04.033

Freina, L., & Ott, M. (2015). A literature review on immersive virtual reality in education: state of the art and perspectives. In *The International Scientific Conference eLearning and Software for Education* (vol. 1, pp. 133-141). Bucharest, RO: eLSE.

Frossard, P., & Khasanova, R. (2017). Graph-based classification of omnidirectional images. *Proceedings of the 2017 IEEE International Conference on Computer Vision Workshop*, 860-869.

Guazzaroni, G. (2017). The impact of augmented reality and virtual reality study material in the future of learning: a teamwork experience. In G. Kurubacak & H. Altinpulluk (Eds.), *Mobile Technologies and Augmented Reality in Open Education* (pp. 77–94). Hershey, PA: IGI Global. doi:10.4018/978-1-5225-2110-5.ch004

Halabi, O., El-Seoud, S. A., Alja'am, J. M., Alpona, H., Al-Hemadi, M., & Al-Hassan, D. (2017). Immersive virtual reality in improving communication skills in children with autism. *International Journal of Interactive Mobile Technologies*, *2*(11). Retrieved from http://online-journals.org/index.php/i-jim/article/view/6555/4365

Herrera, G., Alcantud, F., Jordan, R., Blanquer, A., Labajo, G., & De Pablo, C. (2008). Development of symbolic play through the use of virtual reality tools in children with autistic spectrum disorders: Two case studies. *Autism*, *12*(2), 143–157. doi:10.1177/1362361307086657 PMID:18308764

Howlin, P. (1997). *Autism: Preparing for Adulthood*. London: Routledge. doi:10.4324/9780203426913

Kandalaft, M. R., Didehbani, N., Krawczyk, D. C., Allen, T. T., & Chapman, S. B. (2013). Virtual reality social cognition training for young adults with high-functioning autism. *Journal of Autism and Developmental Disorders*, *43*(1), 34–44. doi:10.100710803-012-1544-6 PMID:22570145

Kemeny, A., George, P., & Mérienne, F. (2017). New VR Navigation Techniques to Reduce Cybersickness. *Electronic Imaging, The Engineering Reality of Virtual Reality*, *6*, 48-53. Retrieved April, 29 2018, from http://www.ingentaconnect.com/contentone/ist/ei/2017/00002017/00000003/art00009?crawler=true&mimetype=application/pdf

Kulman, R. (2018). *Virtual Reality (VR) assessment of ADHD*. Retrieved March, 5 2018, from http://learningworksforkids.com/2018/01/virtual-reality-vr-assessment-adhd

Kwon, C. (in press). Verification of the possibility and effectiveness of experiential learning using HMD-based immersive VR technologies. *Virtual Reality (Waltham Cross)*.

Lee, J. M., Cho, B. H., Ku, J. H., Kim, J. S., Lee, J. H., Kim, I. Y., & Kim, S. I. (2001). A study on the system for treatment of ADHD using virtual reality. In *Engineering in Medicine and Biology Society. Proceedings of the 23rd Annual International Conference of the IEEE* (*vol. 4*, pp. 3754-3757). Istanbul: IEEE. 10.1109/IEMBS.2001.1019654

Leo, T., Manganello, F., & Chen, N. S. (2010). From the learning work to the learning adventure. *Proceedings of EDEN 2010*.

Lyons, V., & Fitzgerald, M. (2013). Atypical sense of self in autism spectrum disorders: a neuro-cognitive perspective. In M. Fitzgerald (Ed.), *Recent Advances in Autism Spectrum Disorders* (vol. 1). INTECH Open Access Publisher. Retrieved April 9, 2018, from https://mts.intechopen.com/books/recent-advances-in-autism-spectrum-disorders-volume-i/atypical-sense-of-self-in-autism-spectrum-disorders-a-neuro-cognitive-perspective

Maraj, C. S., Martinez, S. G., Badillo-Urquiola, K. A., Stevens, J. A., & Maxwell, D. B. (2016). Preliminary review of a virtual world usability questionnaire. In S. Lackey & R. Shumaker (Eds.), Lecture Notes in Computer Science: Vol. 9740. *Virtual, Augmented and Mixed Reality. VAMR 2016* (pp. 35–46). Cham: Springer. doi:10.1007/978-3-319-39907-2_4

Mason, B. (2017). *Virtual reality has a motion sickness problem*. Retrieved April 29, 2018, from https://www.sciencenews.org/article/virtual-reality-has-motion-sickness-problem

Mühlberger, A., Jekel, K., Probst, T., Schecklmann, M., Conzelmann, A., Andreatta, M., ... Romanos, M. (2016). The influence of methylphenidate on hyperactivity and attention deficits in children with ADHD: A virtual classroom test. *Journal of Attention Disorders*. doi:10.1177/1087054716647480 PMID:27178061

Murphy, K. (2015). *Feeling woozy? It may be cyber sickness*. Retrieved April 29, 2018, from https://well.blogs.nytimes.com/2015/11/14/feeling-woozy-it-may-be-cyber-sickness

Newbutt, N., Sung, C., Kuo, H. J., Leahy, M. J., Lin, C. C., & Tong, B. (2016). Brief report: A pilot study of the use of a virtual reality headset in autism populations. *Journal of Autism and Developmental Disorders*, 1–11. PMID:27272115

Oigara, J. N. (2018). Integrating virtual reality tools into classroom instruction. In J. Keengwe (Ed.), *Handbook of Research on Mobile Technology, Constructivism, and Meaningful Learning* (pp. 147–159). Hershey, PA: IGI Global. doi:10.4018/978-1-5225-3949-0.ch008

Parsons, S., & Cobb, S. (2011). State-of-the art of virtual reality technologies for children on the autism spectrum. *European Journal of Special Needs Education*, *26*(3), 355–366. doi:10.1080/08856257.2011.593831

Parsons, S., & Mitchell, P. (2002). The potential of virtual reality in social skills training for people with autisitic spectrum disorders. *Journal of Intellectual Disability Research*, *46*(5), 430–443. doi:10.1046/j.1365-2788.2002.00425.x PMID:12031025

Piaget, J. (1998). *The origin of intelligence in the child. Jean Piaget: Selected Works*. London: Routledge.

Radu, I. (2014). Augmented reality in education: A meta-review and cross-media analysis. *Personal and Ubiquitous Computing*, *18*(6), 1533–1543. doi:10.100700779-013-0747-y

Rapport, M. D., Chung, K. M., Shore, G., Denney, C. B., & Isaacs, P. (2000). Upgrading the science and technology of assessment and diagnosis: Laboratory and clinic-based assessment of children with ADHD. *Journal of Clinical Child Psychology*, *29*(4), 555–568. doi:10.1207/S15374424JCCP2904_8 PMID:11126633

Riva, G., Waterworth, J. A., Waterworth, E. L., & Mantovani, F. (2009). From intention to action: The role of presence. *New Ideas in Psychology*, 1–14.

Rizzo, A., & Kim, G. J. (2005). A SWOT analysis of the field of virtual reality rehabilitation and therapy. *Presence (Cambridge, Mass.)*, *14*(2), 119–146. doi:10.1162/1054746053967094

Rizzo, P. (2011). *Accuracy of self-perceptions in children and adults with ADHD* (Unpublished doctoral dissertation). University of Zurich, Switzerland. Retrieved April, 7 2018, from http://www.zora.uzh.ch/id/eprint/52775/1/RizzoFinales_Manuskript_dez_2011.pdf

Sastry, L., & Boyd, D. R. S. (1998). Virtual environments for engineering applications. *Virtual Reality (Waltham Cross)*, *3*(4), 226–234. doi:10.1007/BF01408704

Tambovtsev, D., Floksy, N., & Peshé, O. (2016). *How to Avoid the Effect of Motion Sickness in VR*. Retrieved March 9, 2018, from https://vrscout.com/news/avoid-motion-sickness-developing-for-vr

Temurnikar, A. (2018). *New age classrooms are the future of education (Interview)*. Retrieved May 5, 2018, from http://bweducation.businessworld.in/article/New-Age-Classrooms-are-the-Future-of-Education-/10-04-2018-146020/

The Guardian. (2017). *The Party: a virtual experience of autism – 360 video*. Retrieved March 9, 2018, from https://www.theguardian.com/technology/2017/oct/07/the-party-a-virtual-experience-of-autism-360-video

The National Autistic Society. (2016). *Too much information*. Retrieved March, 9 2018, from http://www.autism.org.uk/vr

Uddin, L. Q. (2011). The self in autism: An emerging view from neuroimaging. *Neurocase*, *17*(3), 201–208. doi:10.1080/13554794.2010.509320 PMID:21207316

Winn, W. (1993). A conceptual basis for educational applications of virtual reality. In Human Interface Technology Laboratory. Washington Technology Center, University of Washington.

Wu, H. K., Lee, S. W.-L., Chang, H. Y., & Liang, J. C. (2013). Current status, opportunities and challenges of augmented reality in education. *Computers & Education*, *62*, 41–49. doi:10.1016/j.compedu.2012.10.024

## ADDITIONAL READING


Azuma, R. T. (1997). A survey of augmented reality. *Presence (Cambridge, Mass.)*, *6*(4), 355–385. doi:10.1162/pres.1997.6.4.355

Bethel, D. M. (1973). *Makiguchi the Value Creator: Revolutionary Japanese Educator and Founder of Soka Gakkai*. New York, Tokyo: John Weatherhill.

Billinghurst, M. (2002). Augmented reality in education. In *New Horizons for Learning*. Seattle, WA: Technology in Education.

Botella, C., Fernández-Álvarez, J., Guillén, V., García-Palacios, A., & Baños, R. (2017). Recent Progress in Virtual Reality Exposure Therapy for Phobias: A Systematic Review. *Current Psychiatry Reports*, *19*(7), 42. doi:10.100711920-017-0788-4 PMID:28540594

Bronack, S. C. (2011). The role of immersive media in online education. *Journal of Continuing Higher Education*, *59*(2), 113–117. doi:10.1080/07377363.2011.583186

Burke, S. L., Bresnahan, T., Li, T., Epnere, K., Rizzo, A., Partin, M., ... Trimmer, M. (2018). Using Virtual interactive Training Agents (ViTA) with adults with autism and other developmental disabilities. *Journal of Autism and Developmental Disorders*, *48*(3), 905–912. doi:10.100710803-017-3374-z PMID:29168090

Damasio, A. R. (2010). *L'Autre moi-même – Les nouvelles cartes du cerveau, de la conscience et des emotions*. Paris, F: Odile Jacob.

De Bono, E. (1995). *Six thinking hats*. Boston, USA: Little Brown and Company.

Dewey, J. (1966, first published 1916). Democracy and education: an introduction to the philosophy of education. New York, USA: Free Press.

El Sayed, N. A. M., Zayed, H. H., & Sharawy, M. I. (2011). ARSC: Augmented reality student card. An augmented reality solution for the education field. *Computers & Education*, *56*(4), 1045–1061. doi:10.1016/j.compedu.2010.10.019

Freeman, D., Reeve, S., Robinson, A., Ehlers, A., Clark, D., Spanlang, B., & Slater, M. (2017). Virtual reality in the assessment, understanding, and treatment of mental health disorders. *Psychological Medicine*, *47*(14), 2393–2400. doi:10.1017/S003329171700040X PMID:28325167

Gardner, H. (2006). *Five minds for the future*. Boston, USA: Harvard Business School Press.

Guazzaroni, G. (2012). *Experiential mapping of museum augmented places. Using mobile devices for learning*. Saarbrücken, D: LAP.

Guazzaroni, G. (2012). Emotional mapping of museum augmented places (EMMAP). In M. Pieri (Ed.) Mobile Learning. Esperienze e Riflessioni "Made in Italy". Bari, IT: Progedit.

Guazzaroni, G. (2012, December). Emotional mapping of museum augmented places. In Archeomatica (3), 44-46.

Guazzaroni, G. (2013, October). Street poetry in augmented reality. In S. Leone (Ed.), *Synergic Integration of Formal and Informal E-Learning Environments for Adult Lifelong Learners*. Hershey, PA: IGI Global.

Guazzaroni, G. (2013, October). The ritual and the rhythm: interacting with augmented reality, visual poetry and storytelling across the streets of scattered L'Aquila. In eLearning Papers on Design for Learning Spaces and Innovative Classrooms (34).

Guazzaroni, G. (2013). Emotional mapping of the archaeologist game. In M. Lytras, P. Ordoñez De Pablos and F.J. García-Peñalvo (Eds.), Advanced Human-Computer Interaction: Computers in Human Behavior, Elsevier, 29 (2) 335-344. doi:10.1016/j.chb.2012.06.008

Guazzaroni, G. (2015). Realtà aumentata un'opportunità di apprendimento. In L. Salvucci (Ed.), Strumenti per la Didattica della Matematica. Ricerche, esperienze, buone pratiche (pp. 145-152). Milano, IT: Franco Angeli.

Guazzaroni, G. (2018). Walking eight. Archaeology of the next future. In M. G. Ullate (Ed.), *Proceedings of Cultural Management and Governance for European Pilgrimage Routes and Religious Tourism and Thermal Tourism – Cultour plus – Cori. IT.*

Guazzaroni, G., & Compagno, M. (2013). AR moulded-objects performing Giuseppe Verdi's 200th birthday. *Archeomatica*, *4*, 38–41.

Guazzaroni, G., & Leo, T. (2011). Emotional mapping of a place of interest using mobile devices for learning. In I. Arnedillo Sánchez, & P. Isaías (Eds.), *Proceedings of IADIS International Conference on Mobile Learning* (pp. 277-281). Avila, E. March 10-13 2011.

Huang, K., Liu, T., Graf, S., & Lin, Y. (2008). Embedding mobile technology to outdoor natural science learning based on the 7e learning cycle. In J. Luca, & E. Weippl (Eds.), *Proceedings of World Conference on Educational Multimedia, Hypermedia and Telecommunications* (pp. 2082-2086). Chesapeake, VA.

Kiyokawa, K., Billinghurst, M., Hayes, S., & Gupta, A., Sannohe & Y., Kato, H. (2002). Communication behaviors of co-located users in collaborative AR interfaces. In *Proceedings of the IEEE and ACM International Symposium on Mixed and Augmented Reality* (pp. 139-148). Los Alamitos, CA: IEEE Press. 10.1109/ISMAR.2002.1115083

Klopfer, E., & Squire, K. (2008). Environmental detectives: The development of an augmented reality platform for environmental simulations. *Educational Technology Research and Development*, *56*(2), 203–228. doi:10.100711423-007-9037-6

Lave, J., & Wenger, E. (1991). *Situated Learning: Legitimate Peripheral Participation*. Cambridge, UK: Cambridge University Press. doi:10.1017/CBO9780511815355

Leone, S., & Guazzaroni, G. (2010). Pedagogical sustainability of interoperable formal and informal learning environments. In F. Lazarinis, S. Green, & E. Pearson (Eds.), *Developing and Utilizing E-Learning Applications*. Hershey, PA: IGI Global. doi:10.4018/978-1-61692-791-2.ch001

Leone, S., Guazzaroni, G., Carletti, L., & Leo, T. (2010). The increasing need of validation of non-formal and informal learning. The case of the community of practice "webm.org". In *Proceeding of IADIS International Conference on Cognition and Exploratory Learning in Digital Age*. CELDA 2010. Timisoara, RO.

Schank, R. C. (1995). What we learn when we learn by doing. In *Technical Report No. 60*. Northwestern University, Institute for Learning Sciences.

Schmid Mast, M., Kleinlogel, E. P., Tur, B., & Bachmann, M. (2018). The future of interpersonal skills development: Immersive virtual reality training with virtual humans. *Human Resource Development Quarterly*, *29*(2), 125–141. doi:10.1002/hrdq.21307

Squire, K., & Klopfer, E. (2007). Augmented reality simulations on handheld computers. *Journal of the Learning Sciences*, *16*(3), 371–413. doi:10.1080/10508400701413435

## KEY TERMS AND DEFINITIONS

**Attention-Deficit/Hyperactivity Disorder (ADHD):** A brain disorder characterized by an ongoing pattern of inattention and/or hyperactivity-impulsivity that interferes with functioning or development.

**Augmented Reality (AR):** The possibility to overlay computer graphics or computer audio onto the real world and augment, in this way, human perceptions.

**Autism Spectrum Disorder (ASD):** A developmental disorder that affects communication and behavior.

**Immersive Learning Environment:** A virtual environment where students can connect, interact, find 360-degree learning objects, and complete educational tasks wearing a special head-mounted display.

**Learning Adventure:** The adventure of learning is directed to satisfy a personal desire of acquiring knowledge, and it is aimed at providing expertise in some specific domain.

**Learning Environment:** A digital space where students can connect, interact, find learning content, and complete educational tasks.

**Virtual Reality (VR):** The possibility to immerse in a completely virtual world using special goggles to visualize computer graphics or computer sound.

# Chapter 12
# From Chat Therapy to Virtual Reality (VR):
## The Case of Idego – Digital Psychology

**Simone Barbato**
*Idego – Psicologia Digitale s.r.l., Italy*

**Lorenzo Di Natale**
*Idego – Psicologia Digitale s.r.l., Italy*

## ABSTRACT

*This chapter aims to highlight some aspects linked with the psychological interventions adaptability to the virtual setting, focusing on advantages, limits, and the effectiveness criteria of an online intervention, and of the virtual reality (VR) applications in the clinical psychology field. First of all, the authors will examine the characteristics of the web-based setting and of the online psychological counseling service, underling opportunities and risks of text talk-based chat therapy and the issues dealing with the role of the therapist. This will be followed by the analysis of Twende! Project, an online psychological counseling service created by the Italian company Idego – Digital Psychology s.r.l. The chapter will conclude with the presentation of VR systems as an e-therapy tool, considering their application scopes in order to treat mental disorders and showing their adaptability and operational effectiveness in several clinical psychology areas.*

## INTRODUCTION

The coming of computers and social networks has radically changed the traditional communication system – regarding human interaction and the way in which its premises are conceived -, which is becoming more accessible, fast and efficient. This is developing unprecedented opportunities to create psychological areas suitable to cultivate human relations. Until the new communication technologies appearance (Baldini & Balestrini, 2005), the social interaction norms (punctuation, sequence, canons, codes) have become stratified over the centuries without special modifications. The new means of communications

DOI: 10.4018/978-1-5225-7168-1.ch012

have also led to the denaturalisation of the social relation, expanding human biological limitations and sense organs.

Among the effects of the technological development, the authors observe the transformation of several kind of works. In the psychological field, beyond the questions raised by the information technology development (Tonioni, 2013), there are an increasing number of innovative tools and resources in medicine and clinical psychology area of interests.

In fact, there is an aspect, linked both to the market and to the society more in general, that may renovate deeply the profession of the psychologists with unexplored possibilities: this is the communication technologies use in order to provide psychological services.

Currently, the arrival of new software and devices consists in a new opportunity to apply the cybertherapy in an economic way, reaching several patients and improving living conditions and mental health.

In this sector, the Digital Psychology as research area considers how human beings behaviour and psychological moods are influenced by the new media; moreover, it examines the way in which the technology may be designed in order to integrate the human beings strengths and weaknesses (Riva, 2014). In the incoming future, this branch of psychology will play an increasingly central role with the aim of knowing and knowing to plan the technologies so that they support the psychological well-being.

In order to explore these issues, this work will present a review of the recent advances in applying the new media in the psychological and psychotherapeutic field and it will underline some aspects linked to the clinical psychology adaptability to the different virtual settings. The Authors primary aim in this area of research is to update the psychological culture, in order to deal with the psychological disease considering the most recent transformation of the social, cultural and economic fabric.

In the next years, Virtual Reality Apps and software will be more and more frequent for what concerns telemedicine and mental health.

The adaptability of psychological interventions to the web mediated setting will be analysed, in particular examining its application fields, its advantages and disadvantages and also the standards of evidence of a web-based intervention.

The Authors will advance the idea that the Virtual Reality (VR) systems represent a credible, realistic and efficient outlook in the clinical psychology field.

It will be presented the case of IDEGO – Digital Psychology, an Italian social reality, established by the Authors of this chapter, which has fostered several projects in the areas of interest of e-Health, online psychological counselling, Virtual Reality, in order to support the practice of psychologists, psychotherapists and other professionals, working in the fields of mental health, psychotherapeutic practice, psychiatric rehabilitation and sport psychology. These issues will be explored by the on field experience of the Authors in this sector, offering causes for reflection about the best practices at the base of the web-based interventions planning. In this context, the Authors will first present the planning methodology of *Twende! Online Counselling*, an online psychological counselling service, using the web and the chat as tools to reach the new generations through the Psychology. This will be followed by a real case of a VR system for the therapy of psychosis, created by the Authors in collaboration with the Tor Vergata University of Rome: *"Tor Vergata Virtual Reality Rehub"*.

## BACKGROUND

The new generations, increasingly involved in the social networks, such as Facebook, YouTube, Instagram, and in the sharing activities, are the uncontested protagonists of the web. The term "digital natives" was coined by the American author Mark Prensky in 2001 and describes young people, especially under 25 years old, who have grown up surrounding by and using interactive displays. This has spread a debate into the academic world: their habits have become object of study for researchers and experts (Prensky, 2001, pp. 1-6; Ito, Bittanti, & Cody, 2010; Lenhart, Purcell, & Smith, 2010), who are analysing how the technology affects the brain of the new generations. In this regard, the hypothesis of the cognitive organization changing is sure plausible (Riva, 2014). In fact, the digital revolution seems to have produced a real anthropological transformation and the digital natives are its absolute protagonists. The idea that the new generations possess a new form of intelligence has managed to represent a scientific hypothesis in various academic environments (Rivoltella, 2012). The configuration of an 'updated' cognitive profile would be dictated by the need to develop new functional skills for the technologies with which digital natives interact since their first years of life. Digital intelligence "is presented as the product of the intersection and co-evolution of some cultural and technological characteristics of society, [as for example] the affirmation of the digital revolution we have witnessed over the last thirty years and the proactive adaptation to these changes in the cognitive capacity of the human species" (Ferri, 2011).

Research on attention and the internet (Boot, Kramer, Simons, Fabiani, & Gratton, 2008, pp. 387-398; Johnson et al., 2007, pp. 630-638; Grace-Martin, 2001, pp. 95-107) have had significant developments, both in terms of learning potential that seem to be favored by the web, and in reference to the risks that it could provoke, such as the increase in distractibility and the decrease in concentration (Tonioni, 2013). The configuration of the written text on the web is very different from the traditional reading and resembles a constant distraction: attention is dispersed by the continuous stimuli occurring on the screen (Tonioni, 2013). As an illustration, when a person reads something on the web, he or she tends to 'jump' everywhere searching information that can capture his or her interest: it seems to fail the linear method of contents assimilation typical of the classic reading, line by line, from left to right, from top to bottom (Tapscott, 2008).

Furthermore, the appearance of computers and the Internet has greatly influenced the memorisation process: thanks to a simple and fast click, or with a touch, it is possible to obtain easily all the required information and storing them may be superfluous and a waste of time. The web is a sort of knowledge library at hand, which offers the opportunity for all to retrieve information and ideas in a moment (Tonioni, 2013).

The possibility to deposit information on external supports has made memory increasingly depending on digital tools. "The multiplication of objects with internal memory [...]emphasizes immensely the unloading of personal memory" (Simone, 2012). According to this, it has passed from "a modality of knowledge based on linearity to one in which the simultaneity of stimuli and elaboration prevailed" (Simone, 2012). This represents a gradual transition from a knowledge that was learnt mainly through books, and therefore thanks to the alphabetical vision, to a knowledge that is acquired also through non-alphabetical vision or through listening, and then through videos or codes based on the images.

The interaction with digital devices is increasingly precocious and has become an integral part of the identity of the new generations and not simply a hobby. In the crisis of the techno-liquid society (Bauman, 2000), virtual identity and the control that can be easily carried out on it, modeling it as everyone prefers, are another aspects that shoul be examined. In a moment of instability and reorganization, the virtual world provides the adolescent with several expressive possibilities, including also risks, which would be more difficult in real life (Pravettoni, 2002).

Digital communication has also played an important role in the transformation of the family structure, removing to parents part of their credibility (Cantelmi, 2013). The digital natives, in fact, can freely access a large amount of information that allows them, without controls or censorship, to be faced with new ideas, new people, new educational models - often conflicting with each other or against the tide - which in the past would not be accessible. Digital natives are ‘children orphans of teachers’ and they build their own knowledge thanks to technological means (Cantelmi, 2013).

A new way of expressing suffering and unease comes from a new model of mind. Japanese Hikikomori (Hashimoto, 2015) represent a prime example of this phenomenon: a new form of social isolation, which mainly affects children, consisting in the total seclusion from society; Hikikomori have profiles on several social networks, avatars, meet other Hikikomori virtually, sharing and playing with them (role-playing games), but they are all alone behind a computer and this is the only form of relationship that they can support.

Having regard to these phenomena, the Experts have carry out studies and researches. In particular, Digital Psychology has fostered a significant literature, inclusive of a rising theoretical position, as can be evidenced by the introduction of the notion of ‘cyberdependence’ or ‘cyberaddiction’ (internet addiction disorder and smartphone addiction for example) in the DSM -V, the latest version of the Statistical and Diagnostic Manual of Mental Disorders.

In respect of these new mental diseases, on one side, cybertherapy has developed successfully. On the other hand, the spread of these techno-mediated services has been opened a discussion about the therapeutic efficacy and on the scientific validity of such practices (Grohol, 1993): for instance, the debate concerns the possibility for the therapist, who makes use of the new technological means, to access the unconscious of the patient; the consequences of absence of non-verbal cues.

The debate on the feasibility of e-therapy, in particular dealing with the online psychological interventions, has been characterized for a long time by the aversion of a part of the international academic world. Clinical activities were considered unsuitable for the virtual context and the attitude of the first ten years of research in this sector was oriented towards forms of web-mediated psychological counseling (Grohol, 2010, pp. 3-20). In the last five years, however, international research has radically changed course thanks to an increasing number of studies demonstrating the effectiveness of internet therapy. Consequently, the application areas and the online practices tools have multiplied; furthermore, they also include other services in addition to *text talk* and the psychotherapy on Skype, taking advantage from the potentialities of the new technologies.

From the early 2000s, it has been developed a new course of the research: it is in this period, in fact, that it has been produced the guidelines for the use of VR in the therapeutic field (Botella et al., 2004), deepening characteristics and potentialities of technology within it.

## CHARACTERISTICS OF THE WEB-BASED SETTING AND ONLINE PSYCHOLOGICAL INTERVENTION

The analysis of the psychological aspects that occur on the web and of the online psychological support are traditional objects of research in Digital Psychology. In fact, the psychology – web link has deep roots: the online psychological self-help groups were born in 1982, by the idea of the current president of the International Society for Mental Health Online (ISMHO), Martha Ainsworth; while the service *Ask Uncle Ezra* was the first academic experiment in 1986 to support the Cornell University students.

In the early 1990s, the psychologist Jonh Grohol, after having tragically lost a friend due to an untreated depression, began to answer to questions on mental health via web. He also coined the term e-therapy, which refers to every web-mediated psychotherapeutic intervention, and founded *Psych Central*, a website that still exists, with a huge team of psychotherapists and over 230 psychological support chats. Grohol has always maintained that e-therapy represents an important opportunity to introduce many people, in need of assistance, to the psychotherapeutic relationship benefits: the web-based therapy aims to promote and support the traditional psychological practice, without replacing it.

Dunaway (2000), in his work *Assessing the Potential of Online Psychotherapy*, believed that e-therapy should have been an additional tool of mental health services able to reach more consumers, so as to bring them closer to traditional therapy. The preliminary studies carried out in those years indicated how e-therapy was already expanding market opportunities for psychotherapy and counselling, making these services accessible to sections of the population that could not otherwise have accessed it: according to the article of Dunaway (2000), disabled persons agoraphobics, people who live in badly connected centers or who have preconceptions about traditional treatment.

The e-therapy does not serve the purpose of treating or diagnosing mental disorders, because it has objective limits, such as distance and the lack of non-verbal cues; for this reason, it remains on a different level compared to the face-to-face therapy (Martinez, 2010).

Many of the characteristic aspects of online therapies are still subject of discussion, especially those related to the virtual setting and ethical-deontological issues. However, the Authors maintain that an in-depth analysis of the phenomenon under consideration is significant and necessary, in order to examine its implications about the psychological intervention assumptions: the aspects of the relationship on which the intervention is based; the advantages and the risks of these practices; the main elements of effectiveness of the intervention models.

### Chat Therapy: Opportunities and Risks

In the area of synchronous communication (video call, chat and instant messaging tools), patient and psychologist use a remote communication device at the same time, interacting with each other simultaneously. Compared to asynchronous communication tools (e-mail and message boards), in which the person can take hours - or even weeks - to answer back, synchronous communication requires the presence of both interlocutors.

For what concerns temporality, instant messaging is halfway between asynchronous communication, on the one hand, and video calling and face-to-face on the other. Compared to them, the chat, by level of presence and spontaneity, represents an intermediate channel of communication, and consequently an interesting field of investigation. The Authors have the purpose of presenting the risks and opportunities of instant messaging as a clinical tool of psychological intervention.

According to the scientific literature (Cantelmi & Grifo, 2002; Calderoni, 2013; Fisher & Fried, 2003, pp. 103-111; Kraus, Zack, & Stricker, 2004; Onken & Shoham, 2014, pp. 3-12), the main risks in carrying out these practices consist in:

- **The Absence of Visual and Auditory Contact:** The web-based communication deprives the person from the body, who becomes *disembodied* (Riva, 2014), and complicates the process of understanding emotions. The aesthetic presentation and the visual-auditory feedback are missing; in particular, this last element permits to provide personal and relational information in order to allow the identification of possible misunderstandings;
- **Privacy and Confidentiality:** The therapeutic relationship must be able to guarantee the data protection of the patient;
- **E-Skills (Computer-Related Skills):** The lack of textual communication training for the therapist could have relevant repercussions on the whole process, reducing considerably its quality and effectiveness;
- **Patient-Therapist Distance:** The distance between the patient and the therapist can also extend over several thousand kilometers and, in this case, it is difficult to respond effectively and quickly when a crisis happens; therefore the identification of the user is particularly significant. The therapist should also consider the risk that the online intervention could contrast with the avoidance coping of the patient;
- **Disinhibition Effect:** On one side, this disinhibition reveals quickly personal and secret information, emotions, fears and wishes of the user; but, on the other, it can lead to manifestation of hostility through anger, criticisms and rude language, causing anxiety and recriminations (Calderoni, 2013; Suler, 2004).

The potential advantages of online psychological intervention via chat are:

- **Non-Clinical Problems:** The computer offers the possibility to interact with people with non-clinical problems, who should request a psychological consultation without the fear of being considered wrong; the consultation via PC is also on average less expensive;
- **Ease of Access:** The absence of geographical restrictions permits to people, who have difficulty sustaining traditional therapy, to communicate easily with the therapist (for examples people physical or psychic mobility problems or who live in badly connected places);
- **Reflection:** Writing allows to slow down the communication process; composing and rereading a message increases self-awareness and introspection. Writing, the patient focuses more on his emotions, promoting the associations and speeding up his intuition. In this way, while the patient is writing, he has an opportunity to exchange views: this forms a sort of diary of thoughts and feelings that can be consulted until the next online intervention session;
- **Disinhibition Effect:** As mentioned above, this is both a risk and an advantage of the chat therapy. Through the computer, people tend to open up and provide personal information more easily, making the psychotherapeutic relationship more deep in a short time. The protective shield improves the self-disclosure, speeding up the clinical interview. Moreover, the so called phenomenon *"stranger on the train"* must be considered in this context: the most personal and open conversations are more likely to happen between two people whom may never interact again (Wallace, 2000).

## Text Talk: A Psychoeducational and Therapeutic Language

Chat is a more controlled therapeutic tool than other forms of distance counselling: typing and re-reading the message implies lower levels of emotional activation. The communication process is therefore slowed down and - at the expense of spontaneity - reflection, associations, elaboration and intuition are improved (Calderoni, 2013). The absence of the body reduces the risk of rejection and promotes the loss of the inhibition; people feel more protected and therefore, in some cases, paradoxically closer. Furthermore, the synchronicity allows scheduling sessions in 'appointments': this can encourage the definition of a more structured setting, favoring a feeling of intimacy, presence and interpersonal exchange. The presence of pauses in the conversation, arriving late or not showing-up for sessions are important elements that can have deep psychological meanings.

These elements make instant messaging an interesting tool for the experts, especially for the first contact with the patient, in order to overcome his psychological and cultural barriers (Calderoni, 2013).

First of all, the quality of the textual relationship depends on the writing skills of the psychologist. Those who write unwillingly or have poor knowledge language can hardly involve anyone in a online textual chat: misunderstandings and conflicts become more frequent. The psychologist has to understand exactly what the user is trying to say; otherwise, the patients could, in fact, project their own expectations, anxieties and fantasies onto the messages of the interlocutor (Kraus et al., 2004). The disparity in writing skills between interlocutors (expert-patient) can be problematic. It is important that, as would happen in a clinical work f-2-f, the psychologist knows how to modify his writing techniques (also basic elements of grammar and sentence composition) to interact more effectively and emphatically with the patient (Speyer & Zack, 2009).

## STANDARDS OF EVIDENCE FOR AN INTERVENTION BASED ON TEXT TALK

As mentioned above, web-mediated communication presents several characteristics that differentiate it from traditional communication. The protective shield can help the user to provide personal information more easily, favouring self-disclosure: the screen is a sort of shield, behind which the fear of being judged or misunderstood disappear (Attril, 2012, pp. 855-872).

The web-mediated setting involves the lack of the condition of physicality: the absence of the body and of the typical signals of the interaction f-2-f makes the feelings difficult and could provoke misunderstandings in the communicative exchange (Riva, 2014). At the same time, the textual analysis of the message can reveal to the psychologist important information about the personality elements of the patients. The expressions, the vocabulary used, the structure of the sentences, the organization of the text present a profile of the user potentialities, through which the expert can recognize the nuances of his cognitive style. From this point of view, each virtual message represents a short self-presentation, a personal portrait.

Calderoni (2013) stresses the importance of the digital skills of the therapist, who must be able to use completely the new means of communication: typing on the keyboard very slowly, making frequent texting mistakes, or arranging the text in a chaotic and disorganized way contrast with the regular flow of a chat conversation. The risk is to slow down the communication or to text unintelligible messages: in both cases this decreases the quality and effectiveness of the chat therapy (Calderoni, 2013).

Online counseling requires unique attitudes that go beyond those required for traditional counselling. In order to promote the effectiveness of psychological counselling, a series of measures can help the consultant to re-propose his personality and communication style in the online relationship, compensating in part the absence of non-verbal cues. The Authors have identified some examples:

- **Closeness and Contact:** The lack of personal contact must be compensated with the quality of the textual relationship and the expression of words that offer a perception of understanding and presence. For example, answering in chat, the therapist should text the name of the patient or emoticons, aiming to replace the nod of the head and to give to the user the feeling of contact and closeness that the virtual setting could weaken (Reynolds, Smith, Birnholtz, & Hancock, 2013);
- **Text Message:** The therapist should recognize the verbs and nouns that are most used in the digital message by the user, to understand which are the main terms to be proposed and around which developing the interview and which are the prevalent sensory channels (visual, auditory, tactile-kinesthetic: VAK) in order to get in tune with the specific modes of relationship expressed by the user. Moreover, the therapist should observe the nouns that can be considered as nominalized predicates (Rooksby, 2003; Calderoni, 2013);
- **Text-based Empathy:** The therapist should establish an alliance with the user, showing empathy through the text talk. In this regard, the consultant should text descriptions of what he is feeling in that moment, in order to help the user understand the meaning of the written words. Calderoni (2013) gives an example: *"While I am writing, I stuck for a moment in wonder at what you are telling me."*;
- **Presence in the Cyberspace:** Considering the absence of non-verbal cues, the therapist could type "I am listening to you" (Rooksby, 2003). The advisor should listen to the narration of the patient into feeling him of being understood with an open and serene attitude;

Font and punctuation. The font and the punctuation are very significant. Changing the font size used in typing, as well as using punctuation (for example *"!!!"* to mark an exclamation), could encourage the expression of the emotional experiences. The correct use of punctuation, emoticons, uppercase is effective also in focusing on a specific passage or excerpt of the interview. Disambiguating a sentence texting a smile, expressing hesitation with dots, underlining a concept through punctuation (*"Do you want to look your best????"*) or the use of uppercase (*"Let's start with YOU"*) are some examples. On the other hand, the improper or excessive use of these methods could undermine the quality of the interview. Emotional bracketing (putting the [emotions] in brackets) is another possible useful technique (Murphy & Mitchel, 1998, pp. 377-386).

The misunderstandings occurring online (Calderoni, 2013) represent a focusing topic in this field.

Considering the absence of the body language and expressions, the somatic markers - such as the rapid heartbeat – are lacking. Consequently, it can happens that an online written sentence, extrapolated from a context and without considering the facial expression, can assume opposite meanings in the mind of the user, depending on his emotional mood, personality, his expectations or beliefs. According to Lee (1996), a fragile person could not correctly evaluate the different reading possibilities of the web communication, taking into account only the meanings that he wants to understand. In this case, the protective shield plays the role of a persecutor, becoming a projective mirror and the counselor should adopt some important precautions for the purpose of counteracting these risks, typing for instance emoticons (crasis of the words *"emotion"* with *"icon"*). The text talk is "halfway between the phone and the letter", having the characteristics of both written and oral communication (Lee, 1996, pp. 275-296).

## TWENDE! PROJECT: BEGINNING AND IMPLEMENTATION

In order to provide the Reader with a useful case study in this field and with the aim of enhancing the comparison between the several fragmented approaches and experiences of online counselling, it will be presented the case of Twende! Created by IDEGO - Digital Psychology, Twende! project was born, in June 2016, an online psychological counseling service for young adults, carried out by qualified professionals, conceived and designed with the aim of intervene on different psychological, geographical, cultural and social barriers that hinder personal investment in mental health as well as the establishment of an aid relationship.

### Twende!: Implementation

Considering the limits and the boundaries of the virtual environment, and of instant messaging in particular, Twende! service is not proposed as a replacement of the psychological traditional tools, but as an integration. Twende!, in fact, relies on the peculiarities of chat as an instrument which offers the interlocutor a degree of intermediate presence / absence, a favorable space for the first contacts for all those who are not yet ready to bear the costs (psychological and social) of the *vis à vis* conversation, especially in a psychological culture such as the Italian one, in which stigma and labeling are still present for those who use professional services. Twende! is therefore not aimed at taking charge of the users in chat, but rather at welcoming, clarifying doubts or psychological uncertainties, exploring the initial issues brought by the user and, finally, at orientating towards the more structured and traditional path. The Service, allocated to the web domain www.idego.it, includes 4 free meetings of 60 minutes textual advice. Sessions are held exclusively by instant chat (synchronous communication) in which the text talk is the only content. The number of meetings was identified by theoretical studies as a sufficient path length, thanks to which it is possible to understand the reason for the request of the service and collect precious information. Although 4 meetings can be considered a long time, it should be regarded that the 50-60 minutes of 'typing' interview corresponds in quantitative terms to a third of what can be orally dealt. This does not in fact detract from the effectiveness of the tool. Specifically, the 'quality' of the contents remains unchanged: protected from the shield (the screen), it is not rare that the time duration of the interview may even be reduced compared to f-2-f (Barak, 2007, pp. 971-984).

### The Deontological Aspects

All the Psychologists belonging to Twende! are required to respect the professional ethical code below:

- To provide their services independently, on the basis of what the Italian Code of Deontology establishes;
- To be recognizable on the website so it is possible to verify their identity and the place where they live, the information relating to the enrolment in the Italian Professional Register, the professional titles and the educational route;

- To process the personal data of the beneficiaries in compliance with the Privacy Policy, with a view to guaranteeing security and confidentiality. This is why the Professionals of Twende! use Gmail accounts to text via e-mail (asynchronous communication) with the Beneficiary of the Service (reservation time shift, cancellations, time changes, other communications), while Telegram (synchronous communication) is used to carrying out the 4 text advisory sessions. Aiming for security in data processing, psychologists make use of an e-mail dedicated to the service, protect their Gmail account with a password, log in exclusively to carry out the professional activity, provide for the cancellation of all personal information about the user and the related conversations after 90 days from the end of the counseling period.
- To manage possible emergency situation.

On the other side, the Users:

- Are identified by completing a form and sending a copy of their own ID card at the end of the first session;
- Are aware of the nature of the services offered and the legislation on privacy policy.

The Platform Twende! also:

- Guarantees hardware and software systems that provide efficient and up-to-date data protection systems;
- Provides all the information necessary to the user about the main features of the service;
- Allows the user to have sight the italian Code of Deontology and the guidelines in reference to distance psychological services.

## Selection, Supervision and Training

As previously discussed, online psychological interventions require more skills for the therapist, compared to traditional methods. Therefore, for a high quality Service, a top selection process of the applications appears appropriate. Twende! Project recruitment process provides an evaluation of the curriculum vitae, one simulated online psychological counseling - designed to verify the acquaintance with new media, the writing and textual quality of interventions - and a *final vis-a-vis* interview through Skype.

The associated Professionals have to respect several guidelines referring to both online practices and the Italian existing legislation on this matter.

Finally, the psychologists of Twende! meet regularly once a month in groups to share their professional experiences, improve the quality of interventions and structure the best practices related to text talk performance.

## Some Results

During the first 12 months of activation of the Service, 1021 requests were received, of which 64% (of the Users) had never addressed a psychologist before. Il 77% of them are female, showing that woman in Italy are more sensitive to the issue of the psychological well-being.

One of the most significant data is the fragmentation of the requests: 50% came from Provincial Capitals. The aggregate requests of Milan, Rome and Naples do not exceed 19%. This data probably reflects how a part of Users face psychological pathways to a greater extent where there is a lack of services and direct connection infrastructures. 14% of people state they have turned to the Service not knowing who else to turn to, 19.2% because they consider it convenient and 19.7% because it is free.

About the average age, this is higher than expected: 30.3 years old. 17% are employed, 18% unemployed and 28% are students.

On the basis of the age and the key words expressed in the requests received, we can see that the greatest disorder concerns not so much the period of university study, but the subsequent phase of entry into employment, characterized feelings of uncertainty.

A significant data relates to the reasons for which online counseling is required: 38% concern anxiety issues; then, relationship, family, food and mood issues.

Moreover, the dropout of the Users is particularly considerable: almost 50%. This value seems to counteract the high number of requests received: the free Service it is appealing, but on the other side, reduces the individual investment in the pathway.

In this regard, however, it should be noted that about 2/3 of the dropout occurred entirely between the sending of the request for counseling and the first session (these Users never arrived at the first meeting). On the other hand, the dropout probability drops exponentially with the carrying on of the sessions; but once the textual relationship has been established, there is a high probability that the User will continue.

The continuation over the 4 free sessions takes place in 12% of cases, which corresponds to about 23% of the completed psychological pathways.

## VIRTUAL REALITY IN CLINICAL PSYCOLOGY: APPLICATION SCOPES

In the clinical psychology area of interest, the Virtual Reality (VR) systems qualify as effective tools, easily adaptable to several psychotherapeutic approaches: a behavioral psychologist can use VR technology to activate a fear response in a patient affected by phobic disorders; a cognitive one to evaluate dysfunctional behavior; while a psychodynamic psychologist can use virtual environments (VE) in order to elicit an emotional response.

One of the main advantage of the VR therapeutic applications is the possibility of manipulating many of the variables of the immersive setting. *In virtuo* (in the virtual) exposure practices, compared to *in vivo* practices, permit to control and repeat the intervention protocols, modifying them on the basis of the patient needs; the stimuli can be presented gradually.

By providing users with a highly realistic, engaging, safe and controllable simulation, they are able to develop skills, confidence, mental and psychophysical preparation to face real-world tasks (Smith & Steel 2001). This helps to work on dysfunctional beliefs in a situation similar to that in vivo, but checking the whole trial. A tailor-made intervention, within which the therapist can control the exposure conditions, so as to establish the level of difficulty each time. VR thus becomes an *"experiential interface"* (Wann & Mon-Williams, 1996, pp. 829-847): knowledge is produced by "experiencing" and reflecting on it.

VR environments guarantee the patient compliance and engagement, confidentiality, privacy and data protection, encouraging the patient to undergo the therapy (Wiederhold & Wiederhold, 2001; Vincelli & Riva, 2007, pp. 67-92).

In clinical psychology, VR finds space in several application fields. It must be considered, however, that VR systems are tools, rather than a true and proper therapy. This implies the necessity of a direct supervision as well as of specific training paths for the therapists, underling the predominance of the clinical aspect on this instrument.

## Anxiety Disorders

The treatment of anxiety disorders based on the cognitive-behavioral intervention of stimulus exposure, together with a re-elaboration of the stimuli, is particularly effective when the counselor uses VR application (Riva, 2007, pp. 18-23). On the basis of this intervention, there is the concept of Systematic Desensitization (SD), developed by Joseph Wolpe (1972): a consolidated method widely used in behavioral therapy. It consists in exposing the patient gradually to the phobic stimulus (Andrews et al., 2003), with the aim of associating anxiety with an antagonistic response, such as muscle relaxation, to break the link between anxious response and anxiogenic stimulus.

Owing to the improvement of the new technological means, Virtual Reality Exposure Therapy (VRET) has been conceived, whose effectiveness has been confirmed by several international publications starting from 2000 (Pull, 2005, pp. 7-14; Riva, 2005, pp. 220-240; Wiederhold & Wiederhold, 2006, pp. 451-458) and numerous researches, for instance the study on Social Anxiety Disorder (Klinger et al., 2006) and the other one on the treatment for reducing fear of public speaking (North, North, & Coble, 2002, pp. 59-70).

Compared to imaginative and in vivo exposure, in virtuo exposure has several advantages: on one side, it is more immersive and, on the other, the therapist has greater control of the fundamental variables of the phobic stimulus. From this point of view, it would become possible to integrate the cognitive behavioral therapy protocols: Experential Cognitive Therapy (ECT), as Riva (1999) defined it.

## Post-Traumatic Stress Disorder (PTSD)

According to the cognitive-behavioral protocols, the trauma-exposure is based on two principles (Bisson & Andrew, 2009):

- The habit, to reduce anxiety after prolonged exposure;
- The information processing, which allows the re-evaluation of old information and the incorporation of a new, alternative and functional memory of trauma.

Also in this case, the exposure can be carried out in vivo or in an imaginative form. Through VR it is possible to act on the responses (emotional and physiological) elicited in the presence of the feared stimuli, both internal and external (Powers & Emmelkamp, 2008). The VR also compensates for one of the typical symptoms of PTSD, that is the loss of memory of traumatic experiences. On the other hand, these systems permit the possibility of reconstructing controlled situations that would be otherwise extremely expensive, or impossible, to reproduce in vivo.

An intervention protocol presented by Difede and Hoffman (2002) was successfully used on survivors the events of 11 September 2001, with the aim of increasing emotional involvement and treating the memory of traumatic events, associated with a not directly reachable emotional pain. This methodology has been re-elaborated in a study published by Wiederhold and Wiederhold (2006), which showed that VR can also be used for the early care of this disorder, not only for the patients who have already a clinical PTSD diagnosis.

## Obsessive-Compulsive Disorder (OCD)

VR technology is used also as a way of treatment of Obsessive-Compulsive Disorder, involving the vicarious exposure to stimuli linked to contamination, in order to prevent the compulsive ritual. Lack and Storch (2008) have observed how vicarious exposure can play an important role within a behavioral protocol.

The working group of Kim (2010) has instead used VR to obtain an assessment of compulsive control behaviors with the aim of creating an interactive measure of the OCD control behaviors.

## Autism

Strickland et al. (1996) in the United States have carried out studies using VR in order to verify the effectiveness of virtual environments in encouraging the learning in autistic children. The patients were able to learn and repeat tasks such as the recognition and verbalization of colors, objects and moving scenes (Strickland, Marcus, Mesibov, & Hogan, 1996, pp. 651-659). In this context, the main advantage of VR technology is the possibility of creating a personalized and individualized task, respecting the needs of the child. The Experts hope that this experience could be applied in future to the real life context, for example when the child goes to school and meet the new classmates: if the child follows a VR training, he may be less fearful towards the surrounding world, so intricate and full of stimuli, often unknown, that can cause an autistic withdrawal.

## Eating Behavior Disorders

In recent years there have been several experiments of VR linked to the treatment of eating disorders. The real world and the virtual reality induce comparable reactions, and once the patient has learned to control his emotions and reactions in the virtual environment, the impact with real life turns out to be more manageable and less problematic (Erzegovesi & Gorini, 2003).

One of the most promising Italian projects in the field of the treatment of eating disorders using VR systems is that undertaken by the clinic Villa Santa Chiara in the province of Verona: Dr. Marco Vicentini has adopted an integrated protocol, designed by Professor Giuseppe Riva, which provides the possibility of integrating cognitive-behavioral psychotherapeutic treatment with VR sessions; accompanying the patient in virtual reality, the therapist evaluates the emotions, actions and choices, leading him to re-structure and correct the distortion of the image of himself and his body.

## Neuropsychological Rehabilitation

The use of VR puts the persons in front of complex, interactive and easily generalizing stimuli of everyday life: the close equivalence of human reactions in the real world and in the virtual reality makes these devices suitable for learning and rehabilitation, as active interaction with reality is considered the most important element in a physical and cognitive rehabilitation process. The patient in the virtual environment performs actions with directly observable effects. This of active participation makes the rehabilitation considerably more effective from both a qualitative and quantitative point of view. Normally the human learning processes are preponderant in the perceptive-motor field; while, when the same actions are carried out in the virtual world, also the symbolic intelligence is used, that is the combination of logical and forecasting abilities. The rehabilitation interventions involving VR technology have already been developed to promote functional recovery after strokes, heart attacks, of Alzheimer disease, Parkinson disease, sclerosis and other disabilities (Lange, Flynn, Chang, Profitt, & Rizzo, 2010, pp. 345-352).

## Schizophrenia: The Experience Tor Vergata University of Rome

The Authors Lorenzo Di Natale and Simone Barbato have designed the so called "ReHub Project", the aim of creating a protocol of Cognitive, Semantic, Metacognitive and Socio-relational rehabilitation through Virtual Reality for Psychotic Disorders. In collaboration with the Degree Course in Psychiatric Rehabilitation Techniques of the Tor Vergata University of Rome and thanks to the technical contribution of Rainbow CGI srl, the Authors intend to demonstrate the effectiveness of this integrated methodology, that can also reduce time and costs of the therapy, as well as representing a strengthening of the traditional tools. The demonstration of these project has been presented at the 21th National Congress of the Italian Society of Psychopathology (22-25 February 2017) (Niolu et al., 2017).

The choice of this rehabilitative protocol has its roots in the most recent literature, from which emerge the potential, still largely unexplored, of VR technology as an innovative, stimulating, dynamic and multitasking rehabilitation tool. From 1957 to today, the studies in this area have assessed scientific of the effectiveness both in the psychiatric patient's evaluation, diagnosis and treatment planning.

The use of the VR puts the person in front of complex, interactive and stimuli easily generalizing to everyday life, enhancing learning through the use of multiple perceptive components, still preserving its gradual approach. Several studies have demonstrated the efficacy of this technique in the treatment of phobias, post-traumatic stress disorder, attention deficit disorder in children and anxiety treatment (Gregg, Barrowclough, & Haddock, 2007, pp. 494-510).

The patient feels "present", physically immersed, in a safe world and with whom he interacts, forwarding stimuli and receiving immediate feedback to manage. The literature also addresses the issue of the "Humanization" effect (Ku et al., 2006, pp. 531-539): the virtual reality avatar is perceived as human, consistent with true aspects of communication, socio-relational interaction and management of daily-functional tasks.

The control of VR variables makes it possible to create a "controlled", "safe" and "harmless" environment - without negative repercussions on real life, such as feelings of failure or emotional frustration -, enhancing the learning of social skills (Kim et al., 2010, pp. 86-93). A recent study, dealing with the simulation of a job interview, underlines that the protagonists, through an exercise, have felt the experiment as a good, positive and stimulating experience, proving an improvement in self-confidence and the necessary conversational skills to carry out a job interview (Smith et al., 2014, pp. 2450-2463).

The most recent developments of the VR offer the possibility to immerse the patient in increasingly complex scenarios, to make it feeling a deep mental state of engagement (Htc Vive, joystick, gloves and other devices), to foresee a large number of factors and controllable variables, to reproduce in an elastic and flexible way infinite situations. An innovative tool with a strong emotional impact, which produces learning (Riva, 2014) and which is preparing to completely redesign many areas of medical-health intervention.

## The Project

The key points of this treatment concern metacognitive and social aspects, in relation to the psychotic patient cognitive spheres. Several studies in the literature show that the use of VR promotes and stimulates these processes such as attention, executive functions, memory, spatial orientation, motor skills. The VR can represent in this sense an enhancement, or an overcoming, of the classic Computerized Cognitive Remediation therapy:

- To integrate the activation of multiple cognitive areas;
- To promote benefits on other social processes;
- To guarantee a highly usable, simple and understandable experience.

Moreover, the literature highlights that, during the cognitive tasks and the conversations held in a virtual environment, people have shown less difficulty implementing the therapy (Rus-Calafell, Gutiérrez-Maldonado, & Ribas-Sabaté, 2013, pp. 81-89).

This project aims to research and experiment a stimulating and effective methodology that, applied to a target of patients in the psychotic field, can reduce time and costs of therapy, as well as confirm all the other therapeutic-rehabilitative benefits. While remaining in the safe and controlled environment of the hospital, the patient will have the opportunity to experiment different life scenarios (super market, open places, bus stop, etc.) and exercise different tasks.

In addition to cognitive, emotional and social skills, the entire protocol is aimed at reinforcing the patient semantic capabilities, a core variable for the treatment. In this sense, the VR allows the patient to overcome the boundaries of the hospital structure and offers an infinite number of expressive possibilities.

In the rehabilitative path, cognitive intervention is one of the most validated and effective approaches; in this framework of neuropsychological interpretation, the key to understand the semantic network, thought as a connection system linking mental and cognitive functions (from memory to language and meta cognitive aspects), plays an important role in psychotic disorders, as evidenced by the last decades of literature.

The program is supported by a cognitive approach, but its main core is the rehabilitation of the other two central poles in psychosis: the metacognitive and the socio-relational aspects. The present rehabilitation VR protocol, therefore, fully exploiting the functionalities expressed by the most recent media, allows a new model of intervention, able to combine the three nuclear aspects and related to the social functioning of the patients; thanks to the integration of the treatment it will be possible to open an important perspective of therapeutic interest and innovation with respect to the Italian and foreign experiences on the use of the VR in psychiatry.

## The Rehabilitation Protocol

The structure of the Semantic, Metacognitive and Socio-relational Cognitive Rehabilitation Protocol via Virtual Reality systems provides:

- Cognitive and functional evaluation before and after treatment;
- 24 sessions of Cognitive Individual Computerized Remediation;

- 8 sessions of Cognitive Semantic, Metacognitive and Socio-relational Rehabilitation through Virtual Reality (as indicated in the Table 1).

The Rehabilitation modules by means of VR provides:

- A module a session;
- 30 minutes immersion, per module, through VR;
- Each session-module will have an introductory colloquial part and a final restitution (estimated time for a complete session: about 60 minutes).
- The course will be divided as follows, on the basis of the most common deficits in psychosis:

Within the Protocol, the 8 VR scenarios are designed to reproduce environmental and social situations that stimulate the person as it would happen in the reality, controlling the sense-perceptive stimulation as well as the possibility of modulating quality, intensity, frequency and duration of the intervening variables, while ensuring high levels of interactivity through specific hardware such as data gloves (gloves for interaction with the virtual world) or joysticks. In this way, tide up the room, waiting for the bus, shopping at the supermarket in VR, the patient will have the opportunity to know and experiment objects and situations, learning how to use and control them through direct experience in real time.

Schizophrenia spectrum disorders and obsessive compulsive disorder produce severe deficits in cognitive functions, which are most commonly expressed in: difficulty in understanding, poor concentration, difficulty in expressing thoughts, difficulty in integrating thoughts and emotions-behavior, communication difficulties, difficulties in decision-making processes.

ReHub aims to work on these deficits through different tasks on the basis of the immersive context: the purpose is to promote at the same time the ability to maintain the attention throughout the duration of the Task without being distracted by other stimuli, to maintain the sequence of the task without losing sight of the delivery, to exercise the attention divided appropriately, to self-correct, to organize their behavior and their real and virtual material, to cease, finally, persevering behavior, within the hospital regime.

By encouraging the learning of new strategies in a context of probable and daily immersive situations, the VR will allow the patient to hoard the therapeutic experience, lasting the learning path and reducing the number and frequency of relapses.

*Table 1.*

| Module | Cognitive | Socio-Relational | Matacognitive |
|---|---|---|---|
| 1 | 2 semantic exercises | Active Listening | Attribution of Style |
| 2 | 2 semantic exercises | Active Proposal | Infer Conclusions |
| 3 | 2 semantic exercises | Deny Requests | Belief Changing |
| 4 | 2 semantic exercises | Express pleasant feelings | Self-Confidence |
| 5 | 2 semantic exercises | Express unpleasant feelings | Mood |
| 6 | 2 semantic exercises | Share fear to someone | Empathy |
| 7 | 2 semantic exercises | Apologize | Theory of Mind |
| 8 | 2 semantic exercises | Keeping apart from Stressful Situation | Stigma |

## CONCLUSION

Many technological tools represent a valid and effective integration to the traditional methods used by psychologists and psychotherapists. Today, the need for an improvement of the psychological culture is becoming increasingly urgent. It appears necessary to use these technological instruments with scientific awareness, so that they can be really effective: this is the case of the web, for example, that can be used to intercept and treat social anxiety. In addition, the Authors call for more and more up-to-date therapeutic tools in order to face the real life situation dealing with young people, who, regardless of psychopathological aspects, are digital natives.

VR is a technological medium that, as highlighted in the course of the discussion, has proven to be a valid, credible and effective tool in many fields of experimental psychology and clinical treatment. This is also evidenced by the constant development of research and empirical studies in these areas, encouraged both by the scientific community itself and by the reduction in size and costs of the new generation technological devices.

One of the fundamental questions posed by the use of VR in the clinic concerns whether these applications can be considered as an independent intervention method or as an effective tool to be included in a wider protocol (Riva, 2007). The prevalent orientation of the scientific community claims the prevalence of the clinical aspect on the tool: numerous reviews and meta-analyzes (Wiederhold & Weiderhold, 2006) demonstrate the effectiveness of VR systems in the treatment of various psychological disorders, observing how the experimental and clinical protocols depend on the theoretical orientation and on the presence of a therapist. The intervention focuses, in fact, on the relationship, both therapeutic and rehabilitative, which remains a relevant aspect of each innovative protocol.

In this sense, VR, as well as the web, is not a substitute for the traditional methods available to the therapist, but rather represents an integration. This concretizes a limit to its own application.

A further limitation is connected to the fact that a large number of people are not yet able to the use properly the computerized systems and the technological devices. A first challenge to be won is, therefore, to develop understandable interfaces, even for professionals who do not have a technological background.

In this regard, it should be added that most of the virtual environments available are closed source: they can not be modified, preventing the content from being customized according to the patient needs.

Finally, the lack of reference standards is another obstacle to the use of these instruments, because in most cases they are media, hardware and software, designed to fulfill a specific purpose and suitable for a given context, becoming this problematic when widely used on a large scale.

In conclusion, the research and development work carried out by the authors within the so-called 'emotional technologies' stems from the idea that the mental health professional has the duty, as well as the task, to deepen and study the advantages and limitations that each new instrument should bring to its field of investigation.

## REFERENCES

Andrews, G., Creamer, M., Crino, R., Hunt, C., Lampe, L., & Page, A. (2003). *Trattamento dei disturbi d'ansia, Guida per il clinico e manuali per chi soffre del disturbo*. Turin, Italy: Centro Scientifico Editore.

Attril, A. (2012). Self-disclosure online. In Encyclopedia of Cyber Behaviour (pp. 855-872). Oxford, UK: Encyclopedia of Cyber Behaviour. doi:10.4018/978-1-4666-0315-8.ch071

Baldini, M., & Balestrini, N. (2005). *La parola nella galassia elettronica*. Milan, Italy: Armando Editore.

Barak, A. (2007). Emotional support and suicide prevention through the Internet: A field project report. *Computers in Human Behavior*, *23*(2), 971–984. doi:10.1016/j.chb.2005.08.001

Bauman, Z. (2000). *Liquid Modernity*. Cambridge, UK: Polity Press.

Bisson, J., & Andrew, M. (2009). Psychological treatments of post-traumatic stress disorder (PTSD). *The Cochrane Library*. Retrieved from http://www.thecochranelibrary.com

Boot, W. R., Kramer, A. F., Simons, D. J., Fabiani, M., & Gratton, G. (2008). The effects of video game playing on attention, memory, and executive control. *Acta Psychologica*, *129*(3), 387–398. doi:10.1016/j.actpsy.2008.09.005 PMID:18929349

Botella, C., Quero, S., Baños, R. M., Perpiña, C., García Palacios, A., & Riva, G. (2004). Virtual Reality and psychotherapy. *Studies in Health Technology and Informatics*, *99*, 37–54. PMID:15295145

Calderoni, A. (2013). *Psicologia digitale*. Rome, Italy: Ecomind.

Cantelmi, T. (2013). *Tecnoliquidità. La psicologia ai tempi di internet: La mente tecno-liquida*. Milan, Italy: San Paolo.

Cantelmi, T., & Grifo, L. (2003). *La mente virtuale*. Milan, Italy: San Paolo.

Difende, J., & Hoffman, H. G. (2002). Virtual reality exposure therapy for World Trade Center Post-traumatic Stress Disorder: A case report. *Cyberpsychology & Behavior: The Impact of the Internet. Multimedia and Virtual Reality on Behavior and Society*, *5*(6), 529–535.

Dunaway, M. O. (2000). Assessing the potential of online psychotherapy. *The Psychiatric Times*, (17): 10.

Erzegovesi, S., & Gorini, A. (2003). *Bella come sei. Vincere la Bulimia*. Milan, Italy: San Paolo.

Ferri, P. (2011). *Nativi digitali*. Milan, Italy: Pearson.

Fisher, C., & Fried, A. (2003). Internet-mediated psychological services and the American Psychological Association ethics code. *Psychoterapy: Theory, Research, Practise. Training (New York, N.Y.)*, (40): 103–111.

Grace-Martin, M., & Gay, G. (2001). Web Browsing, Mobile Computing and Academic Performance. *Journal of Educational Technology & Society*, *4*, 95–107.

Gregg, L., Barrowclough, C., & Haddock, G. (2007). Reasons for increased substance use in psychosis. *Clinical Psychology Review*, *27*(4), 494–510. doi:10.1016/j.cpr.2006.09.004 PMID:17240501

Grohol, J. (1993). *Best Practices in eTherapy. Definition and scope of e-therapy*. Retrieved from http://psychcentral.com/best/best3.htm

Grohol, J. (2010). From Netscape to Twitter: Fifteen Years of Mental Health Online. In A. Brunet & F. Herbert (Eds.), *Internet Use in the Aftermath of Trauma* (pp. 3–20). Amsterdam: Ios Press.

Hashimoto, A. (2015). *The Long Defeat Cultural Trauma, Memory and Identity in Japan*. New York, NY: Oxford University Press. doi:10.1093/acprof:oso/9780190239152.001.0001

Ito, M., Bittanti, S., & Cody, M. (2010). *Hanging out, messing around and geeking out*. Retrieved from https://mitpress.mit.edu/sites/default/files/titles/free_download/9780262013369_Hanging_Out.pdf

Johnson, K. A., Kelly, S. P., Bellgrove, M. A., Barry, E., Cox, M., ... Gill, M. (2007). Response variability in attention deficit hyperactivity disorder: Evidence for neuropsychological heterogeneity. *Neuropsychologia*, *45*(4), 630–638. doi:10.1016/j.neuropsychologia.2006.03.034 PMID:17157885

Kim, K., Kim, S. I., Cha, K. R., Park, J., Rosenthal, M. Z., Kim, J. J., ... Kim, C. H. (2010). Development of a computer-based behavioral assessment of checking behavior in obsessive-compulsive disorder. *Comprehensive Psychiatry*, *51*(1), 86–93. doi:10.1016/j.comppsych.2008.12.001 PMID:19932831

Klinger, E., Legeron, P., Roy, S., Chemin, I., Lauer, F., & Nugues, P. (2006). Virtual reality exposure in the treatment of social phobia. In G. Riva., C. Botella, P. Legeron & G. Optale (Eds.), Cybertherapy: Internet and Virtual Reality as Assessment and Rehabilitation Tools for Clinical Psychology and Neuroscience. Amsterdam: IOS Press.

Kraus, R., Zack, J., & Stricker, G. (2004). *On line Counseling: a Handbook For Mental Health Professionals*. San Diego, CA: Elsevier.

Ku, J., Jang, H. J., Kim, K. U., Park, S. H., Kim, J. J., Kim, C. H., ... Kim, S. I. (2006). Pilot study for assessing the behaviors of patients with schizophrenia towards a virtual avatar. *Cyberpsychology & Behavior*, *9*(5), 531–539. doi:10.1089/cpb.2006.9.531 PMID:17034319

Lack, C. W., & Storch, E. A. (2008). The use of computers in the assessment and treatment of obsessive-compulsive disorder. *Computers in Human Behavior*, *24*(3), 917–929. doi:10.1016/j.chb.2007.02.010

Lange, B. S., Flynn, S. M., Chang, K., Profitt, R., & Rizzo, A. (2010). Development of an interaction game-based rehabilitation tool for dynamic balance training. *Topics in Stroke Rehabilitation*, *17*(5), 345–352. doi:10.1310/tsr1705-345 PMID:21131259

Lee, J. (1996). Charting the codes of cyberspace: a rethoric of electronic mail. In R. Strate, R. Jacobson, & S. Gibson (Eds.), *Communication and cyberspace: Social interaction in an electronic environment* (pp. 275–296). Hampton Press.

Lenhart, A., Purcell, K., & Smith, A. (2010). Social Media & Mobile Internet Use among Teens and Young Adults. *Pew Internet & American Life Project*. Retrieved from http://www.pewinternet.org/files/oldmedia/Files/Reports/2010/PIP_Social_Media_and_Young_Adults_Report_Final_with_toplines.pdf

Martinez, L. (2010). *Getting there*. Bloomington, IN: Xlibris Corporation.

Murphy, L., & Mitchell, D. (1998). When writing help to heal: E-mail as therapy. *British Journal of Guidance & Counselling*, (3): 377–386.

Niolu, C., De Lorenzo, V., Stella, G., Di Lorenzo, G., Mastrofini, F., Modugno, L., ... Siracusano, A. (2017). Tor Vergata Virtual Reality Rehub. *Proceedings of the 21th National Congress of the Italian Society of Psychopathology*.

North, M. M., North, S. M., & Coble, J. R. (1997). Virtual reality therapy: An effective treatment for psychological disorders. *Studies in Health Technology and Informatics*, *44*, 59–70. PMID:10175343

Onken, L., & Shoham, V. (2014). Tecnhology and the Stage Model of Behavioral Intervention Development. In L. Marsch, S. Lord, & J. Dallery (Eds.), *Behavioral Healthcare and Technology. Using Science-Based Innovations to Trasform Practise* (pp. 3–12). Oxford, UK: Oxford Press. doi:10.1093/med/9780199314027.003.0001

Powers, M. B., & Emmelkamp, P. M. (2008). Virtual reality exposure therapy for anxiety disorders: A meta-analysis. *Journal of Anxiety Disorders*, *22*(3), 561–569. doi:10.1016/j.janxdis.2007.04.006 PMID:17544252

Pravettoni, G. (2002). *Web Psychology*. Milan, Italy: Guerini e Associati.

Prensky, M. (2001). Digital natives, digital immigrants. *On the Horizon*, (5): 1–6.

Pull, C. B. (2005). Current status of virtual reality exposure therapy in anxiety disorders. *Current Opinion in Psychiatry*, *18*(1), 7–14. PMID:16639177

Reynolds, L., Smith, M. E., Birnholtz, J. P., & Hancock, J. T. (2013). Butler lies from both sides: Actions and perceptions of unavailability management in texting. *Proceedings of the 2013 2nd ACM Conference on Computer Supported Cooperative Work*. 10.1145/2441776.2441862

Riva, G. (1999). Virtual reality as communication tool: A sociocognitive analysis. *Presence (Cambridge, Mass.)*, *8*(4), 462–468. doi:10.1162/105474699566341

Riva, G. (2005). Virtual Reality in Psychotherapy [Review]. *Cyberpsychology & Behavior*, *8*(3), 220–240. doi:10.1089/cpb.2005.8.220 PMID:15971972

Riva, G. (2007). Cyberterapia: Ambienti Reali, Emozioni Virtuali. *Psicologia Contemporanea*, *201*(3), 18–23.

Riva, G. (2014). *Nativi digitali. Crescere e apprendere nel mondo dei nuovi media*. Bologna, Italy: Il Mulino.

Rivoltella, P. C. (2012). *Neurodidattica. Insegnare al cervello che apprende*. Milan, Italy: Raffaello Cortina.

Roobsky, E. (2003). *E-mail and Ethics. Style and ethical relations in computer-mediated communication*. London: Routledge.

Rus-Calafell, M., Gutiérrez-Maldonado, J., & Ribas-Sabaté, J. (2013). A virtual reality-integrated program for improving social skills in patients with schizophrenia: A pilot study. *Journal of Behavior Therapy and Experimental Psychiatry*, *45*(1), 81–89. doi:10.1016/j.jbtep.2013.09.002 PMID:24063993

Simone, R. (2012). *Presi nella rete. La mente ai tempi del web*. Milan, Italy: Garzanti.

Smith, M. J., Ginger, E. J., Wright, K., Wright, M. A., Taylor, J. L., Humm, L. B., ... Fleming, M. F. (2014). Virtual reality job interview training in adults with autism spectrum disorder. *Journal of Autism and Developmental Disorders*, *44*(10), 2450–2463. doi:10.100710803-014-2113-y PMID:24803366

Smith, M. J., & Steel, M. J. (2001). *The use of virtual simulation for dismounted infantry training*. Shrivenham, UK: Cranfield University - Royal Militar College of Science.

Speyer, C., & Zack, J. (2010). *Online Counseling: Beyond the Pros and the Cons*. Retrieved from https://www.easna.org/wp-content/uploads/2010/08/WS2B-E-counselingBeyondthatProsandCons-Handout.pdf

Strickland, D., Marcus, L. M., Mesibov, G. B., & Hogan, K. (1996). Two case studies using virtual reality as a learning tool for autistic children. *Journal of Autism and Developmental Disorders*, *26*(6), 651–659. doi:10.1007/BF02172354 PMID:8986851

Suler, J. (2001). *The psychology of cyberspace*. Retrieved from http://users.rider.edu/suler/psycyher.html

Tapscott, D. (2008). *Grown up digital. How the net generation is changing your World*. New York, NY: Mac Graw Hill- Professional.

Tonioni, F. (2013). *Psicopatologia web-mediata. Dipendenza da internet e nuovi fenomeni dissociativi*. Milan, Italy: Springer. doi:10.1007/978-88-470-2817-3

Vincelli, F., & Riva, G. (2007). La Realtà Virtuale come supporto alla psicoterapia cognitivo-comportamentale. In F. Vincelli, G. Riva, & E. Molinari (Eds.), *La realtà virtuale in psicologia clinica* (pp. 67–92). Milan, Italy: Mc Graw-Hill.

Wallace, P. M. (2000). *La psicologia di Internet*. Milan, Italy: Cortina Editore.

Wann, J., & Mon-Williams, M. (1996). What does virtual reality NEED? Human factors issues in the design of three-dimensional computer environments. *International Journal of Human-Computer Studies*, *44*(6), 829–847. doi:10.1006/ijhc.1996.0035

Wiederhold, B. K., & Wiederhold, M. D. (2001). Virtual reality technology in the treatment of anxiety disorders. In M. Akay & A. Marsh (Eds.), *Information Technologies in Medicine*. London: John Wiley & Sons. doi:10.1002/0471206458.ch2

Wiederhold B. K., & Wiederhold, M. D. (2006). Virtual Reality as a Tool in Early Interventions. *Human Dimensions in Military Operations: Military Leaders' Strategies for Addressing Stress and Psychological Support*, 451-458.

## KEY TERMS AND DEFINITIONS

**Chat Therapy:** The provision of psychological services through remote communication technologies employing instant messaging tools.

**Digital Native:** Coined by Mark Prensky in 2001, the new generations characteristic of being immersed in the web-based technologies.

**Immersivity:** The peculiarity of VR systems of simulating reality in such a way as to make the user feeling the illusion of being part of it.

**Medium-Transparency:** The property of the digital tool of creating an immersive reality without being aware of the presence of the technological device itself.

**Non-Verbal Cues:** Visual signs typical of the face-to-face communication associating with the words. Body language, tone, gestures, facial expressions.

**Protective Shield:** The function of promoting the self-disclosure of a person in the web-based communication.

**Virtual Reality:** A web-generated tridimensional environment, which is immersive, interactive, and experienced through the use of special technological devices.

# Chapter 13
# Uses of Virtual Reality (VR) for Chronic Pain

**Bradley Chi**
*Zucker School of Medicine at Hofstra/Northwell, USA*

**Brian Chau**
*Loma Linda University Health, USA*

**Phillip Ta**
*Loma Linda University Health, USA*

## ABSTRACT

*Chronic pain affects many people worldwide with significant individual impact and societal cost. One such area involves the psychiatric co-morbidities associated with chronic pain. Despite its prevalence, the underlying mechanism of chronic pain is not fully understood although evidence suggests the importance of biologic, psychologic, and social factors in the perception of pain. Virtual reality has the potential to be a powerful therapeutic option for chronic pain. This may be due to its impact on attention, emotion, and potentially central nervous system plasticity. Virtual reality therapy has been used successfully for a variety of chronic pain conditions showing its potential. It has also been safely used in pediatric populations. However, the major current limitation is quality of evidence; therefore, future studies should aim to address this issue.*

## INTRODUCTION

Chronic pain is highly prevalent worldwide but our current understanding of the condition, its influences, and its consequences are not fully understood. Despite this, clinicians and scientists have recognized multiple factors influencing chronic pain including biological, psychological, and social factors (Katz, Rosenbloom, & Fashler, 2015). As understanding of this complex subject has improved, alternative therapeutic methods have been developed to target the various factors believed to play a role in the chronic pain experience. This chapter presents the relationship between chronic pain and mental health, outlines the mechanisms underlying chronic pain and virtual reality (VR) therapy, and then reviews the expanding role of VR in the treatment of chronic pain.

DOI: 10.4018/978-1-5225-7168-1.ch013

## BACKGROUND

While acute pain has an intuitive role in human adaptation, the role of chronic pain is ill-defined and maladaptive. Initially, biologically-driven theories of chronic pain, such as the gate-control theory, were used to explain chronic pain (Ehde, Dillworth, & Turner, 2014; Melzack & Wall, 1965). Shortly thereafter, researchers began to realize the complexity and multi-faceted issues involved with chronic pain. Observations of the psychologic and social effects of chronic pain became apparent. This led psychologists to apply behavioral and cognitive therapy to these patients (Ehde et al., 2014; Fordyce & Company, 1977). With the success of these therapies, recognition of chronic pain has evolved to encompass the variety of areas it can impact patients' lives. One way to capture this complexity is describing chronic pain as a perceptual phenomenon, therefore encompassing the biologic, psychologic, and social influences and impacts (Songer, 2005).

Before the next section discusses the biologic component, the following will touch on the equally important psychologic and social aspects. Chronic pain is highly correlated with negative emotions such as depression, anxiety, anger, isolation, and demoralization (Gatchel, Peng, Peters, Fuchs, & Turk, 2007). This can lead to the psychologic impacts described later but can also impact the relationship between patient and healthcare system. These negative emotions impact motivation for treatment and compliance with therapies (Gatchel et al., 2007). Furthermore, patients suffering from chronic pain often deal with repeated failures of treatment, which can lead to frustration and irritation with the healthcare system (Gatchel et al., 2007). This emotional distress is compounded by rejection from the medical system as healthcare providers may label these patients as "complainers" or "symptom magnifiers" (Gatchel et al., 2007). Therefore, the psychosocial components of chronic pain described below should be viewed holistically, keeping mindful of their interconnected relationships.

Evidence that chronic pain is highly comorbid with mental health conditions is strong. In particular, comorbidity with mood disorders and anxiety disorders are prevalent. Large surveys recording 12-month prevalence of comorbid chronic pain and mood disorders are as high as 17.5%, with major depression being the most common comorbid condition (Demyttenaere et al., 2007; Von Korff et al., 2005). In a survey of Canadian patients with chronic pain, over 80% had symptoms of depression, as measured by the Beck Depression Inventory, of which over half were moderate to extremely severe levels (Choinière et al., 2010). Additionally, over one third expressed suicidal ideation. Similarly, these surveys found significant correlations between chronic pain and almost all anxiety disorders. The highest odds ratios were for generalized anxiety disorder (OR 2.6-2.7) and post-traumatic stress disorder (OR 2.6) (Demyttenaere et al., 2007; Von Korff et al., 2005). Patients with chronic pain are also at increased risk of suicidal ideation and death (Hassett, Aquino, & Ilgen, 2014). While some of this is attributed to the psychiatric comorbidities, current evidence supports chronic pain as an independent risk factor for suicide(Ilgen et al., 2013). In addition to these comorbidities, patients suffering from chronic pain are associated with other challenges, including financial, functional, occupational, and psychosocial. A large survey of people suffering from chronic pain, two-thirds had sleep disruption, half had difficulty walking and with household chores, and one-third had a dependent lifestyle (Breivik, Collett, Ventafridda, Cohen, & Gallacher, 2006). Other significant findings included difficulty with sexual relations (40%) and feeling inadequate as a spouse or partner (20%) (Breivik et al., 2006). All of which shows the wide-ranging impact chronic pain has on people's lives.

Further evidence of the link between chronic pain and comorbid psychiatric disorders is the efficacy found with psychological-based approaches such as cognitive behavioral therapy (CBT), meditation, operant conditioning, and insight-cased approaches (Turk, Swanson, & Tunks, 2008). Of these, the most robust evidence is for CBT which was been shown in multiple studies to result in small to moderate improvements in pain intensity, pain disability, mood, and catastrophizing (Ehde et al., 2014). A 2012 Cochrane review of studies comparing CBT to treatment as usual or wait-list control conditions for patients with chronic pain found mild improvements in the four outcomes mentioned above, but at 6 months follow up, only improvement in mood persisted. When comparing CBT to active control, the review found mild improvement of pain disability and catastrophizing persisting to 6 months follow up, but no improvement in pain intensity or mood (Williams, Eccleston, & Morley, 2012). Multiple other randomized control trials (RCT) focused on specific pain conditions such as migraine headache, orofacial pain, fibromyalgia, and arthritis. In totality, the studies support the conclusion that CBT is effective as treatment for chronic pain with the treatment effect being mild to moderate improvement in pain and mood (Ehde et al., 2014). Again, these findings support a strong link between chronic pain and mental health.

## MAIN FOCUS OF THE CHAPTER

### Theories of Pain

In its evolutionary role, pain is in an important adaptive defense mechanism that allows humans to protect themselves from potential dangers (Melzack & Wall, 1965). Despite this, maladaptive pain is now a common problem significantly impacting millions of people worldwide. A basic understanding of how the body perceives pain is important to discuss the potential mechanisms explaining the role of VR in pain reduction. While the current understanding of pain is complex and incomplete, the following section aims to outline our current understanding of the mechanisms governing pain. Pain can be viewed as a sensation and/or a perception. The sensation of pain refers to the biologic process of sensing pain (Turk & Okifuji, 2002). This differs from perception of pain, which refers to the brains processing and interpretation of pain sensation (Turk & Okifuji, 2002).

Initially, the sensation of pain requires stimuli activating peripheral pain receptors. When activated, these receptors transmit signals through the peripheral nervous system (PNS) back to the central nervous system (CNS), specifically the spinal cord. Within the spinal cord, these signals are transmitted along pain-specific neural tracts up to the brain stem and cortex where the pain is interpreted and enters our consciousness. Two main types of fibers carry the pain signal from receptor to CNS: a-delta and c fibers. This is an important distinction as the fibers carry different types of pain (Gold, Belmont, & Thomas, 2007). A-delta fibers allow rapid conduction along the nerve and therefore are ideal for carrying signals of acute pain, while c-fibers have limited conduction velocity making them useful for chronic pain (Gold et al., 2007). In addition to the ascending pain pathway described, there is also a descending pain modulatory pathway. This cortical pathway is part of a complex pain modulatory system in which multiple factors both peripherally and centrally affect an individual's perception of pain. All of this is important because of the synergistic relationship between understanding the pain pathway and development of therapeutic options. For example, attempts to understand the analgesic effect of opioid medications led to the discovery of mu opioid receptors at various levels of the nervous system (Akil, Mayer, & Liebeskind, 1976). Conversely, understanding of c-fibers allowed development of targeted medications such as NSAIDs and capsaicin cream, both of which reduce c-fiber activation (Gold et al., 2007; Heppelmann, Messlinger, Neiss, & Schmidt, 1990). Finally, the understanding of the pain pathway may help us explain potential mechanisms underlying the analgesic effects of VR therapy.

While the difference between pain sensation and perception is recognized, the mechanism controlling pain perception is not fully understood. This is significant because pain perception impacts people, not pain sensation. Throughout history, multiple theories have been proposed to explain the human pain perception system. These include the specificity theory, first described by Von Frey in 1895, which postulated that the perception of pain was simply a result of summation of sensory pain stimuli (Moayedi & Davis, 2013). The major flaw in this theory is the observation that identical stimuli can produce varying reactions ranging from painful to non-painful. For example, American soldiers returning from war expressed that they did not feel pain despite having severe wounds from battle (Melzack & Wall, 1965). Their lack of pain may be attributed to the relief of leaving the battlefield alive. This suggests that perception of pain is influenced by one's circumstances and not only a product of specific stimuli. Another proposal by J.P. Nafe in 1929, called the pattern theory, surmised that nerve fibers were non-specific, and that pain was a product of intense activation of any nerve fiber given the appropriate stimulus (Moayedi & Davis, 2013). Given our current understanding of specific nerve fiber types and their differences, this theory no longer holds.

While a multitude of other theories have been proposed, arguably the most influential, is called the gate control theory (GCT), popularized by Melzack and Wall in 1965 (Melzack & Wall, 1965). This theory postulates that there is a "gate control system" that modulates the communication between PNS and CNS. They identified the substantia gelatinosa (SG) as the area likely to act as this gate keeper (Melzack & Wall, 1965). The SG is between the afferent nerve fibers coming from the periphery and central transmission cells (T) located in the dorsal horn of the spinal cord that transmit to the brain (Melzack & Wall, 1965). The SG opens or closes the "gates", modifying the communication of T cells with the brain (Melzack & Wall, 1965). Opening or closing by the SG is dictated by a variety of inputs. Most important for discussion in this chapter is the belief that external factors play a role altering the effects of the gate control system, which rectifies some of the flaws present in the other theories. The three major factors described are: (1) Activity prior to stimulation, (2) Stimulus-evoked activity, and (3) Balance of fiber types (Melzack & Wall, 1965). Each of these factors regulate the extent to which the gate opens and closes, which in turn, changes how one perceives the stimulus. Activity prior to stimulation refers to an individual's environment and circumstances such as emotional state. This is consistent with the observation that people experience identical stimuli in different ways depending on the situation and past experiences. This also suggests that in addition to peripheral to central transmission of signal, there is modification of signal that is centrally mediated. Melzack and Wall's GCT spurred a change in research focus and solidified the idea that the CNS actively plays a role in pain perception.

As more evidence arose, certain limitations to the GCT revealed themselves and therefore Melzack described the body-self neuromatrix theory of pain (BSNT) in 1999 (Melzack, 2001, 1999). This theory aims to correct the limitations of the GCT in explaining phantom limb pain (PLP), or other chronic pain conditions without peripheral stimulus. Additionally, the theory further elevates the role and importance of the brain in modulating pain perception. Neuromatrix is the term given by Melzack to describe a neural network of neurons connecting the thalamus, cortex, and limbic system (Melzack, 2001, 1999). This network is formed through genetics and an individual's sensory influences, resulting in a personalized neurosignature (Melzack, 2001, 1999). The neuromatrix is influenced by external inputs such as sensory stimuli, but also hormonal imbalances, emotional stress, and psychologic distress (Melzack, 2001, 1999). Overall, the BSNT suggests that the brain plays the central role in pain perception and that a vast array of factors have the potential to modulate its effects.

## Mechanisms of VR in Pain

One reason VR has promising potential for treatment of pain is that it can have effects on many of the areas previously mentioned. This differs from a pharmacologic agent that acts on specific signaling pathways. Despite this potential, the current understanding of the mechanisms explaining how VR diminishes pain is not well understood (Gold et al., 2007). The following section discusses the theories and evidence for how VR therapy can impact pain.

A popular theory is that VR decreases perception of pain by acting as a distraction. Studies measuring brain activity showed certain regions of the brain, such as the anterior cingulate cortex (ACC) and periaqueductal gray (PAG), had activity that correlated with performing tasks of distraction and pain perception (Bantick et al., 2002; Hoffman et al., 2006; Valet et al., 2004). The ACC and PAG are believed to communicate with each other and modulate multiple pathways involved with pain perception (Vogt, Sikes, & Vogt, 1993). These could therefore explain some of the effects of VR on pain. Another area that immersive VR can have a powerful effect on is one's emotions. Evidence suggests that emotions play an important role in modulating perception of pain, with certain emotions heightening pain perception while others dull pain perception (Neugebauer, Li, Bird, & Han, 2004). The major area within the brain that controls emotion is the limbic system, specifically the amygdala, and some studies have shown that the ACC and PAG interact with the amygdala (Gold et al., 2007). As described in the BSNT, perception of pain is controlled through an extremely complex network that requires further understanding. Based on our current knowledge, the effects of VR on pain may be, but are not limited to, its effects on attention and emotion. These findings partially explain the acute pain relief found with VR therapy but cannot explain long-term benefits.

The following section outlines potential explanations for sustained pain relief with VR therapy. In the previous paragraph, the power of VR to create a virtual experience was alluded to. Part of what makes this so powerful is the ability to create an illusion of ownership of one's body. To understand body ownership, it is important to define body schema and body image—two concepts that combine to form body ownership. In brief, body schema refers to one's representation of body position while body image refers to one's external representation of the body (Gallagher & Cole, 1995). For example, controlling the movement of one's body during a coordinated dance would rely on body schema while commenting on one's attractiveness would involve body image. An early study that showed how body ownership could be manipulated is now known as the rubber hand illusion (RHI) (Botvinick & Cohen, 1998). In this experiment, researchers were able to fool subjects into thinking a rubber hand was their own hand by simultaneously stroking the subject's hand and the rubber hand (Botvinick & Cohen, 1998). Follow up studies found limitations in how the RHI could be achieved. One study altered the positioning of the rubber hand by turning it either 90 or 180 degrees (Ehrsson, Spence, & Passingham, 2004; Tsakiris & Haggard, 2005). In both instances, this stopped the RHI, demonstrating the importance of body schema on creating these ownership illusions. Another study replaced the rubber hand with inaccurate objects such as the opposite hand (Tsakiris & Haggard, 2005). Again, this modification ended the RHI, showing the importance of body image on forming ownership illusions (Costantini & Haggard, 2007). With further development, researchers have been able to create a full body illusion with virtual reality showing the power of VR in this realm (Slater, Spanlang, Sanchez-Vives, & Blanke, 2010). The power to create these illusions may form the foundation of VR therapies' effect on chronic pain.

One way for chronic changes to occur is adaptive changes of the CNS, also known as neuroplasticity. Traditionally, the CNS is thought of as rigid and unchanging, with distinct regions that perform specific functions (Ramachandran & Altschuler, 2009). Elimination of a distinct region would permanently remove its associated function. While largely true, more recent observations have demonstrated that some ability for neuroplastic change is available. An example is central remapping, which explains the phenomenon that amputees may feel tactile sensation in the phantom limb when touched on the face (Ramachandran, Stewart, & Rogers-Ramachandran, 1992). Normally, the sensory cortex of the brain processes sensory information from differing regions of the body along an organized map called a homunculus. In the sensory homunculus, the face is located adjacent to the upper limb (Ramachandran & Altschuler, 2009). The concept of remapping suggests that in amputees, there is a neuroplastic change that results in stimuli of the face activating the homunculus at both the face region and the adjacent upper limb region, allowing tactile sensation to be felt at both locations (Ramachandran, 1993; Yang et al., 1994). Similar CNS changes are also believed to play a role in certain chronic pain conditions such as PLP and complex regional pain syndrome (CRPS) (Ramachandran & Rogers-Ramachandran, 2000). Researchers have described this theory as "learned" paralysis or pain (Ramachandran & Altschuler, 2009). For example, patients with PLP often describe a paralyzed feeling of being unable to move a frozen arm. The learned theory explains that this is the brain's adaptive response to repetitive motor commands that do not result in visual arm movement (Ramachandran & Altschuler, 2009). As each additional motor command fails, the brain begins to believe that the amputated arm is indeed "paralyzed" (Ramachandran & Altschuler, 2009). While this malleability has significant clinical impact on patients, it also provides potential in therapy development as, in theory, reversing the maladaptive neuroplastic changes should also be possible (Ramachandran & Altschuler, 2009).

An early application of this phenomenon for chronic pain was in 1992 when Ramachandran described the use of mirror visual feedback or mirror therapy (MT) for PLP (Ramachandran & Altschuler, 2009). For amputees with PLP, MT involves viewing a reflection of one's healthy limb in a mirror, which creates the illusion of having a "normal" amputated limb. Multiple studies have validated the success of this type of therapy for PLP, which helps with both the learned paralysis and pain discussed previously (Chan et al., 2007; Darnall, 2009; Ramachandran, Rogers-Ramachandran, & Cobb, 1995). The concept behind learned pain is that an injury to a body limb leads to extreme sensitivity to pain such that any movement results in pain (Ramachandran & Altschuler, 2009). Overtime, the brain's adaptive response to any sensory stimuli from that area becomes exaggerated pain (Ramachandran & Altschuler, 2009). Therefore, this is very similar to learned paralysis, as a maladaptive neuroplastic response occurs dues to a disconnect between stimulus and expected result. While the mechanism explaining the effects of MT are not fully understood, there are three main mechanisms that likely contribute.

Firstly, MT rectifies the disconnect between stimulus and response. For example, a PLP using MT will see corresponding movement of the reflected limb to motor commands to move the phantom limb. This connects the stimulus (motor command) with the expected response (movement of limb) (Ramachandran & Altschuler, 2009). Similarly, for learned pain, a stimulus of any type causes pain. Using MT, the patient sees the reflection of a freely moving limb unrestricted by pain. Again, this connects the stimulus (movement of limb) with the healthy response (painless movement). In theory, this could result in CNS changes that reverse the maladaptive changes associated with the illness (Ramachandran

& Altschuler, 2009). Recent brain imaging studies support this hypothesis as one study of PLP patients treated with MT found significant reversal of cortical dysfunction in the primary somatosensory cortex (Foell, Bekrater-Bodmann, Diers, & Flor, 2014). Secondly, MT may facilitate rehabilitation through stimulation of mirror neurons. First described in 1992, mirror neurons are cells that activate through visualization of a stimulus causing a replicate action within the person (di Pellegrino, Fadiga, Fogassi, Gallese, & Rizzolatti, 1992). For example, seeing a pin violently prick a hand often causes one to pull back his or her own hand in fear of pain despite never being physically touched (Ramachandran & Altschuler, 2009). Therefore, through the visualization done in MT, it may be possible to train mirror neurons and improve rehabilitative efforts (Ramachandran & Altschuler, 2009). In both mechanisms, changes are adaptive and therefore one would expect results to take time. In practice, MT is frequently reported to work instantly therefore another mechanism must be present. One theory suggests that visual confirmation of a normal limb acts as a safeguard against unwarranted pain (Ramachandran & Altschuler, 2009). For example, after an individual undergoes an amputation, he/she is no longer able to visualize the limb and feel phantom pain. Using MT, they can visualize the reflected limb, showing the brain that the limb is intact and pain-free, thereby acting as visual confirmation that the limb is normal (Ramachandran & Altschuler, 2009). This allows the brain to override the sensory information coming from the phantom limb. This process would act acutely as simple visualization would immediately activate the illusion of a healthy limb.

A discussion of MT is relevant to this chapter because of the similarities between VR therapy and MT. Like MT, VR creates a visual environment that results in a type of body transfer illusion (Moseley, Gallace, & Spence, 2012). The net effect of which is likely reversal of maladaptive neuroplastic changes (Ramachandran & Altschuler, 2009; Ramachandran & Rogers-Ramachandran, 2000). Despite similarities, differences may impact the potential efficacy of VR therapy. Two potential advantages of MT are realism of the visual hand and realistic speed of hand movements (Ramachandran & Altschuler, 2009). Currently, it is not known how much these factors impact efficacy of therapy. Potential advantages to VR include increased interaction with the environment, ability to perform more actions/tasks, use for bilaterally affected patients, and personalization with software changes (Ramachandran & Altschuler, 2009). Additional research may help differentiate which factors are most important. In summary, current evidence suggests there are multiple factors contributing to the impact of VR therapy on chronic pain, including distraction and reversal of maladaptive CNS changes.

## Use of VR for Chronic Pain

While overall evidence for VR therapy for chronic pain is limited, early findings are promising and warrant further research and application. As alluded to earlier, VR is a computer technology that allows users to experience a simulated virtual environment. The VR devices available are increasingly diverse but two general types of devices are available: non-immersive and immersive VR devices. Non-immersive refers to an external display showing the VR environment. Immersive refers to use of a head mounted display, a device worn over the eyes that displays the virtual environment while completely blocking out the user's surroundings. Evidence for the efficacy of VR in acute pain is relatively abundant compared to chronic pain and immersive VR has been shown to be more efficacious than non-immersive VR for acute pain (Shahrbanian, Ma, Aghaei, Korner-bitensky, & Simmonds, 2012). Advantages of VR therapy such as decreased opioid consumption, minimal adverse effects, simple application, and customizability make it a promising technology for use in chronic pain. Given the broad array of conditions that can manifest with chronic pain, the following section will review the current evidence related to these conditions.

The most common causes of chronic pain are musculoskeletal such as lower back and joint pain. Multiple studies have demonstrated the use of VR therapy for these types of conditions. A pilot study of six patients found significant pain reduction in patients with chronic pain during VR sessions (Wiederhold, Gao, Sulea, & Wiederhold, 2014). Long-term effects were not measured. Based on subjective comments from patients, the authors concluded that the primary effect of VR in pain reduction was distraction from pain that occurred during the VR sessions. Similarly, a study of 30 pain clinic patients demonstrated significant pain reduction following a single VR session. While pain was reduced both during and immediately post-session, pain reduction was greater during the session (60%) than post-session (33%) (Jones, Moore, & Choo, 2016). Another study trialed self-administered VR therapy within the home environment for eight chronic pain patients. Combined findings did not reveal significant quantitative difference in pain scores pre-post sessions. Despite this result, a majority of patients were positive about the experience and reported subjective decrease in pain (Garrett, Taverner, & McDade, 2017). This study highlights the individualized effects of VR on patients as each patient has a unique response and impression of VR therapy.

As previously mentioned, PLP is a chronic pain condition that is common in amputee patients. Pain manifests in the amputated limb—the mechanism of which is not fully understood, but is believed to be due in part to maladaptive CNS neuroplasticity (Ramachandran & Rogers-Ramachandran, 2000). A review of the literature on use of VR therapy for PLP noted multiple studies supporting positive outcomes for patients suffering from PLP (Dunn, Yeo, Moghaddampour, Chau, & Humbert, 2017). Pain reduction, measured both quantitatively or qualitatively, was found across all studies and adverse effects were minimal (Dunn et al., 2017). While these findings are promising, the major limitation is their low quality. All studies were either case studies or case report studies suggesting the need for higher quality studies for better understanding. Additional challenges include differing protocols and prolonged benefit. Increase in technology and software innovation has allowed more limb control and immersion within the VR environment. This limits the ability to standardize protocols across study institutions. Finally, the eight studies identified in the review focused on immediate post-intervention changes in pain (Dunn et al., 2017). Given the chronic nature of PLP, further research to understand the long-term impact of VR is needed.

Some evidence suggests the potential for VR treatment of CRPS, another chronic pain syndrome. Pilot studies on four pediatric patients with CRPS demonstrated feasibility of VR for CRPS patients as well as markedly improved function and pain during VR sessions. Subjective feedback on sessions was positive (Won, Tataru, Cojocaru, Krane, Bailenson, & Niswonger, 2015). Another study involving 10 patients with CRPS trialed a virtual reality body swapping intervention (Jeon, Cho, & Lee, 2014). While there was no significant reduction in pain, patients did report significant improvement of body perception disturbance, a common complaint of CRPS patients (Jeon et al., 2014). Finally, two case reports of traditional treatment refractory CRPS patients treated with VR therapy demonstrated significant pain reduction with sustained benefit for multiple months (Chau, Phelan, Dunn, Yeo, Hata, 2016; Chi, Chau, Phelan, Ta, Hata, 2017). These studies suggest the potential for use of VR in treatment of CRPS. Additionally, current ongoing studies on this condition are active and promising.

In addition to multiple motor, sensory, and functional deficits, spinal cord injury (SCI) patients can present with persistent neuropathic pain. The literature in this area is limited but does suggest the potential for VR in reducing pain associated with SCI. An RCT investigating VR-augmented motor imagery found treatment reduced pain (Soler et al., 2010). Additionally, analgesic effects seen with combined VR and transcranial direct current stimulation treatment suggest a synergistic effect between treatments. This shows the potential for VR to augment other types of treatment. Another example is virtual reality hypnosis used for neuropathic pain in a SCI patient (Oneal, Patterson, Soltani, Teeley, & Jensen, 2008). While promising, more evidence is needed to verify the use of VR therapy in SCI-associated pain.

Another relatively common chronic pain condition, fibromyalgia, predominantly effects women. There are two studies that have assessed the use of VR for this condition. An initial case study found significant pain reduction in a fibromyalgia patient after 15 sessions of MT in conjunction with pain medication. The authors concluded that VR may be a useful adjunct to pharmacotherapy in treating fibromyalgia (Botella et al., 2013). In a 2013 study, VR therapy was used to supplement 10 sessions of group CBT for six patients suffering from fibromyalgia. Importantly, patients were followed 6-months post-treatment and outcomes including reduction in pain and depression, improved functional status, and increased positive affect persisted (Chirico et al., 2016). These studies suggest a potential role for VR in treatment of fibromyalgia, particularly as adjuncts to more traditional therapies such as medication or CBT.

Researchers have targeted VR for relief of cancer-related discomfort for many years. A patient's experience with cancer can involve chronic pain, chemotherapy side effects, procedural discomfort, and psychologic effects. The strongest evidence for VR in cancer therapy is reduction in side effects from chemotherapy, but literature also supports efficacy in acute pain reduction from cancer-related procedures, and improvement of psychologic symptoms such as anxiety (Chirico et al., 2016). Cancer is also an active area in the private sector with multiple startup companies offering VR for anxiety, pain, and other cancer-related complications.

## Use of VR in Pediatrics

Chronic pain is common in pediatric populations, often significantly impacting affected individuals (King et al., 2011). In the last few decades, rates of chronic pain have also increased in children making this an important issue (Bandell-Hoekstra et al., 2001; Sillanpää & Anttila, 1996). The following section addresses the current understanding of chronic pain in children compared to chronic pain in adults. The prevalence of chronic pain in pediatric populations ranges from 15-30% (Palermo, Eccleston, Lewandowski, Williams, & Morley, 2010; Perquin et al., 2000; Roth-Isigkeit, 2005; Stanford, Chambers, Biesanz, & Chen, 2008). Studies have shown that girls have higher rates and greater intensity of pain relative to boys, and in general, rates of chronic pain also rise with increasing age (King et al., 2011). While many conditions can cause chronic pain in children, the most common is headache, followed by abdominal pain, musculoskeletal pain, and a variety of other chronic pain conditions (King et al., 2011). Of these, headache is the most studied although there is growing literature on other chronic pain conditions. As with adults, children suffering from chronic pain experience psychologic effects with evidence suggesting a correlation between chronic pain and depression, anxiety, and decreased self-esteem (Rhee, 2000; Stanford et al., 2008). Additional impacts include negative effects on school performance, and family and social life. There is also evidence of lasting effects in a study which found young adolescents with chronic abdominal pain had significantly higher rates of anxiety as adults (Campo et al., 2001).

One obstacle to better understanding chronic pain in children relates to limitations in the literature on this subject. Studies have typically been focused on a single chronic pain condition (e.g. headache) making it difficult to generalize findings. However, some trends across multiple studies are present. Significant impacts on education include disruption in school attendance and school activity participation (Hershey, Powers, Bentti, & DeGrauw, 2000; Reid, Lang, & McGrath, 1997; Walker, Guite, Duke, Barnard, & Greene, 1998). Additionally, mothers of children with chronic pain reported significant impact on family quality of life, including restrictions on family social life and difficulty of family members to deal with the condition (Hunfeld et al., 2001). Studies looking at functional disability have used indices such as the Functional Disability Inventory, to represent a more complete picture of a child's functional ability (Walker & Greene, 1991). One study of children with chronic pain due to both headache and musculoskeletal causes found the intensity of pain to be highly correlated with functional disability (Kashikar-Zuck, Goldschneider, Powers, Vaught, & Hershey, 2001). Additionally, functional disability was highly correlated with depression (Kashikar-Zuck et al., 2001). These findings suggest that as with adults, chronic pain has significant effects on functionality and mental health in children. Interestingly, intensity of pain was not correlated with depression (Kashikar-Zuck et al., 2001). Therefore, assessing functional disability may be more useful than pain intensity when predicting the psychologic impact of chronic pain on patients. In addition, it highlights the importance of understanding external factors that affect functional disability and response to chronic pain.

One difference between the response of children and adults to chronic pain is the effect of coping mechanisms on functional disability (Kashikar-Zuck et al., 2001; Keefe et al., 2000). Studies of adults have shown that mature coping mechanisms are correlated with improved functionality while catastrophizing is correlated with diminished functionality (Keefe et al., 2000). Alternatively, in pediatric populations, evidence suggests there is no correlation between coping skills and functional disability (Kashikar-Zuck et al., 2001). The reason for this is not understood, but multiple theories have been proposed to explain the difference. One theory is that coping mechanisms mature with age, and therefore catastrophizing by children is simply a reflection of parental reactions to their condition or their limited life exposure (Kashikar-Zuck et al., 2001). A second theory is that the effect of catastrophizing actions requires consistency across a period of time and situations, which requires abstract thinking (Kashikar-Zuck et al., 2001). As children are less developed abstract thinkers, it would follow that the effect of catastrophizing is diminished. The importance of understanding coping mechanisms and other factors that may influence functionality in children with chronic pain lies in its clinical implications. As seen with coping mechanisms, there are differences in response between adult and pediatric populations. Thus, in developing treatment options, it is important to recognize these differences and create pediatric-specific therapies.

Given the psychologic impacts of chronic pain on children, psychotherapies have been used as part of the treatment plan. CBT and behavioral therapies are the most popular methods used (Fisher et al., 2014). A 2014 systematic review and meta-analysis of 35 RCT on the topic found sufficient evidence to support efficacy of psychotherapies on chronic pain, disability, and depression for certain conditions (Fisher et al., 2014). The strongest evidence is for reduction of pain in patients with headache following treatment, in which the number to treat was 2.72 at post-treatment and 2 at follow-up—meaning less than three children needed to be treated for one child to receive benefit (Fisher et al., 2014). Also, children with abdominal pain and musculoskeletal pain had significant improvements in pain and disability following treatment although only those suffering from musculoskeletal pain received reduction in depression (Fisher et al., 2014). When analyzing the entire cohort of chronic pain subjects, there was insufficient evidence to suggest psychologic interventions caused an effect on depression, anxiety, or sleep patterns (Fisher et al., 2014). In summary, current psychologic therapies are effective in reducing pain in children, but evidence is inconclusive in their effect on the psychologic co-morbidities of chronic pain. This emphasizes the need for research to better understand psychologic conditions associated with chronic pain, factors modulating them, and potential therapies.

VR therapy has been successfully used for pain in the pediatric population for almost two decades (Mahrer & Gold, 2009; Malloy & Milling, 2010). In fact, the first study demonstrating use of VR for treating pain was a case study in 2000 of two adolescents receiving burn wound care (Hoffman, Doctor, Patterson, Carrougher, & Furness, 2000). Since that time, while multiple studies of childhood acute pain have been completed, the only study addressing chronic pain is the small trial on CRPS mentioned previously (Won, Tataru, Cojocaru, Krane, Bailenson, & Niswonger, 2015). Evidence supporting use of VR therapy for acute pain in children is relatively strong with studies on both experimental and clinical acute pain. A set of studies assessed use of non-immersive VR to decrease experimenter-mediated cold pressor pain in children. They found that those who received VR therapy experienced greater pain reduction than those who did not (Dahlquist et al., 2007, 2010; Hoffman, Seibel, et al., 2006). Additionally, those treated with interactive VR reported less pain than those treated with non-interactive VR (Dahlquist et al., 2007). In a follow-up study, comparing immersive VR and non-immersive VR, adolescents treated with immersive VR reported greater reduction in pain (Dahlquist et al., 2010). These experimental pain studies provide strong evidence that VR therapy can reduce acute pain, as study conditions can be strictly controlled. However, they are limited, because of the inability to show clinical significance.

A variety of smaller studies have shown decreased pain in pediatric patients undergoing a variety of painful procedures. These include burn wounds dressing changes, intravenous placement, and port access (Gershon, Zimand, Pickering, Rothbaum, & Hodges, 2004; Gold, Kim, Kant, Joseph, & Rizzo, 2006; Gold & Mahrer, 2017; Hunter G. Hoffman et al., 2008; Kokinsky, Enska, Nilsson, & Finnstro, 2009). In summary, current evidence supports use of VR therapy for acute pain in children. As with adults, immersive VR is more effective than non-immersive VR although the benefits are maximized in older children (Won et al., 2017). Overall, the results with acute pain in children and chronic pain in adults illustrate the potential for VR therapy in pediatric chronic pain.

Finally, it is important to consider some of the unique challenges that pertain to use of VR for pediatric populations. While there are many similarities between adults and children with respect to VR, an important difference is the level of presence experienced within virtual environments. Presence refers to a subjective sensation that an individual feels engaged with a virtual world (Won et al., 2017). Children were found to have higher levels of presence using VR than adults, suggesting there is a difference in how people process virtual environments (Baumgartner, 2008; Sharar et al., 2007). Findings from brain imaging studies displayed greater activation in the prefrontal cortex of older adolescents and adults, as compared to young children (Baumgartner, 2008; Jäncke, Cheetham, & Baumgartner, 2009). The prefrontal cortex is known to be an area in the brain where executive functioning occurs and is needed to fully experience VR (Baumgartner, 2008; Jäncke et al., 2009). These findings are consistent with the difference in presence between children and adults, as young children are still developing executive function. Implications of this difference should be considered in studies involving children. For example, to ensure children separate real world from virtual world, more thorough debriefing following VR therapy may be useful (Won et al., 2017).

Another concern pertains to the safety of children using VR. Current evidence suggests that VR therapy has minor adverse effects (Won et al., 2017). Similar to VR use in adults, the primary complaint is motion sickness. Despite this, other potential safety considerations have been discussed. Developmental differences may be a potential concern, as children have more difficulty separating real and virtual as previously mentioned. This may manifest with the virtual environment as well as virtual avatars that possess special abilities (Won et al., 2017). Ensuring that children comprehend the differences may be useful in preventing unwanted effects. While increased immersion and interactivity are correlated with efficacy of VR therapy, they also increase the risk of collisions with surrounding objects (Won et al., 2017). Therefore, proper room setup and supervision should be part of any VR therapy session. Finally, VR devices offer social aspects that may prove beneficial for children suffering from chronic pain as these patients often have school and social disadvantages described earlier (Forgeron et al., 2010). Conversely, as with all social media devices, there is the possibility of social isolation which may be particularly detrimental during developmental years (Won et al., 2017). Despite these concerns, overall evidence suggests that VR therapy should be safe for use in children provided proper precautions are taken.

## CONCLUSION

The evidence for use of VR therapy in treatment of chronic pain is growing. VR has been used successfully for a variety of chronic pain conditions as stand-alone or adjunctive treatment. Some findings were consistent across studies and highlight advantages to using VR. For example, adverse effects were rare and limited to motion discomfort. VR was used on a wide range of patients differing in condition, functional status, and age (pediatric and geriatric populations) suggesting its broad applications. Furthermore, VR is relatively easy to use, portable, and is potentially customizable for individual patients. Cost of devices have been significantly decreasing in recent years, making VR an increasingly affordable option. Finally, as an adjunct to pain medications, VR has the potential to help alleviate our dependence on opioid medications. All these factors make VR therapy a promising treatment option for chronic pain and its comorbid psychiatric disorders.

## REFERENCES

Akil, H., Mayer, D. J., & Liebeskind, J. C. (1976). Antagonism of stimulation-produced analgesia by naloxone, a narcotic antagonist. *Science*, *191*(4230), 961–962. doi:10.1126cience.1251210 PMID:1251210

Bandell-Hoekstra, I. E. N. G., Abu-Saad, H. H., Passchier, J., Frederiks, C. M. A., Feron, F. J. M., & Knipschild, P. (2001). Prevalence and characteristics of headache in Dutch schoolchildren. *European Journal of Pain (London, England)*, *5*(2), 145–153. doi:10.1053/eujp.2001.0234 PMID:11465980

Bantick, S. J., Wise, R. G., Ploghaus, A., Clare, S., Smith, S. M., & Tracey, I. (2002). Imaging how attention modulates pain in humans using functional MRI. *Brain*, *125*(2), 310–319. doi:10.1093/brain/awf022 PMID:11844731

Baumgartner, T. (2008). Feeling present in arousing virtual reality worlds: Prefrontal brain regions differentially orchestrate presence experience in adults and children. *Frontiers in Human Neuroscience*, *2*. doi:10.3389/neuro.09.008.2008 PMID:18958209

Botella, C., Garcia-Palacios, A., Vizcaíno, Y., Herrero, R., Baños, R. M., & Belmonte, M. A. (2013). Virtual Reality in the Treatment of Fibromyalgia: A Pilot Study. *Cyberpsychology, Behavior, and Social Networking*, *16*(3), 215–223. doi:10.1089/cyber.2012.1572 PMID:23496678

Botvinick, M., & Cohen, J. (1998). Rubber hands "feel" touch that eyes see [8]. *Nature*, *391*(6669), 756. doi:10.1038/35784 PMID:9486643

Breivik, H., Collett, B., Ventafridda, V., Cohen, R., & Gallacher, D. (2006). Survey of chronic pain in Europe: Prevalence, impact on daily life, and treatment. *European Journal of Pain (London, England)*, *10*(4), 287. doi:10.1016/j.ejpain.2005.06.009 PMID:16095934

Campo, J. V., Di Lorenzo, C., Chiappetta, L., Bridge, J., Colborn, D. K., & Gartner, J. C. Jr. … Brent, D. (2001). Adult Outcomes of Pediatric Recurrent Abdominal Pain: Do They Just Grow Out of It? *Pediatrics*. doi:10.1542/peds.108.1.e1

Chan, B. L., Witt, R., Charrow, A. P., Magee, A., Howard, R., & Pasquina, P. F. … Tsao, J. W. (2007). Mirror Therapy for Phantom Limb Pain. *The New England Journal of Medicine*. doi:10.1056/NEJMc071927

Chau, B., Phelan, I., Dunn, J., Yeo, E., & Hata, J. H. S. (2016). *Complex Regional Pain Syndrome: A Case Report*. Academic Press.

Chi, B., Chau, B., Phelan, I., Ta, P., & Hata, J. H. S. (2017). *Successful Complex Regional Pain Syndrome Treatment with Immersive Virtual Reality: Case Report*. Academic Press.

Chirico, A., Lucidi, F., De Laurentiis, M., Milanese, C., Napoli, A., & Giordano, A. (2016). Virtual Reality in Health System: Beyond Entertainment. A Mini-Review on the Efficacy of VR During Cancer Treatment. *Journal of Cellular Physiology*, *231*(2), 275–287. doi:10.1002/jcp.25117 PMID:26238976

Choinière, M., Dion, D., Peng, P., Banner, R., Barton, P. M., Boulanger, A., … Ware, M. (2010). The Canadian STOP-PAIN project - Part 1: Who are the patients on the waitlists of multidisciplinary pain treatment facilities? *Canadian Journal of Anaesthesia = Journal Canadien d'anesthésie*. doi:10.100712630-010-9305-5

Costantini, M., & Haggard, P. (2007). The rubber hand illusion: Sensitivity and reference frame for body ownership. *Consciousness and Cognition*, *16*(2), 229–240. doi:10.1016/j.concog.2007.01.001 PMID:17317221

Dahlquist, L. M., McKenna, K. D., Jones, K. K., Dillinger, L., Weiss, K. E., & Ackerman, C. S. (2007). Active and Passive Distraction Using a Head-Mounted Display Helmet: Effects on Cold Pressor Pain in Children. *Health Psychology*, *26*(6), 794–801. doi:10.1037/0278-6133.26.6.794 PMID:18020853

Dahlquist, L. M., Weiss, K. E., Law, E. F., Sil, S., Herbert, L. J., & Horn, S. B. … Ackerman, C. S. (2010). Effects of videogame distraction and a virtual reality type head-mounted display helmet on cold pressor pain in young elementary school-aged children. *Journal of Pediatric Psychology*. doi:10.1093/jpepsy/jsp082

Darnall, B. D. (2009). Self-Delivered Home-Based Mirror Therapy for Lower Limb Phantom Pain. *American Journal of Physical Medicine & Rehabilitation*, *88*(1), 78–81. doi:10.1097/PHM.0b013e318191105b PMID:19096290

Demyttenaere, K., Bruffaerts, R., Lee, S., Posada-Villa, J. A., Kovess, V., & Angermeyer, M. … Von Korff, M. (2007). Mental disorders among persons with chronic back or neck pain: Results from the World Mental Health Surveys. *Pain*. doi:10.1016/j.pain.2007.01.022

di Pellegrino, G., Fadiga, L., Fogassi, L., Gallese, V., & Rizzolatti, G. (1992). Understanding motor events: A neurophysiological study. *Experimental Brain Research*, *91*(1), 176–180. doi:10.1007/BF00230027 PMID:1301372

Dunn, J., Yeo, E., Moghaddampour, P., Chau, B., & Humbert, S. (2017). Virtual and augmented reality in the treatment of phantom limb pain: A literature review. *NeuroRehabilitation*, *40*(4), 595–601. doi:10.3233/NRE-171447 PMID:28211829

Ehde, D. M., Dillworth, T. M., & Turner, J. A. (2014). Cognitive-Behavioral Therapy for Individuals With Chronic Pain. *The American Psychologist*, *69*(2), 153–166. doi:10.1037/a0035747 PMID:24547801

Ehrsson, H. H., Spence, C., & Passingham, R. E. (2004). That's my hand! Activity in premotor cortex reflects feeling of ownership of a limb. *Science*, *305*(5685), 875–877. doi:10.1126cience.1097011 PMID:15232072

Fisher, E., Heathcote, L., & Palermo, T. M. de C., Williams, A. C., Lau, J., & Eccleston, C. (2014). Systematic Review and Meta-Analysis of Psychological Therapies for Children With Chronic Pain. *Journal of Pediatric Psychology*. doi:10.1093/jpepsy/jsu008

Foell, J., Bekrater-Bodmann, R., Diers, M., & Flor, H. (2014). *Mirror therapy for phantom limb pain: Brain changes and the role of body representation*. European Journal of Pain. doi:10.1002/j.1532-2149.2013.00433.x

Fordyce, W. E., & Company, M. C. V. (1977). Behavioral methods for chronic pain and illness. *Pain*, *3*(3), 291–292. doi:10.1016/0304-3959(77)90029-X

Forgeron, P. A., King, S., Stinson, J. N., McGrath, P. J., MacDonald, A. J., & Chambers, C. T. (2010). Social functioning and peer relationships in children and adolescents with chronic pain: A systematic review. *Pain Research & Management*, *15*(1), 27–41. doi:10.1155/2010/820407 PMID:20195556

Gallagher, S., & Cole, J. (1995). Body image and body schema in a deafferented subject. *Journal of Mind and Behavior*.

Garrett, B., Taverner, T., & McDade, P. (2017). Virtual Reality as an Adjunct Home Therapy in Chronic Pain Management: An Exploratory Study. *JMIR Medical Informatics*, *5*(2), e11. doi:10.2196/medinform.7271 PMID:28495661

Gatchel, R. J., Peng, Y. B., Peters, M. L., Fuchs, P. N., & Turk, D. C. (2007). The Biopsychosocial Approach to Chronic Pain: Scientific Advances and Future Directions. *Psychological Bulletin*, *133*(4), 581–624. doi:10.1037/0033-2909.133.4.581 PMID:17592957

Gershon, J., Zimand, E., Pickering, M., Rothbaum, B. O., & Hodges, L. (2004). A pilot and feasibility study of virtual reality as a distraction for children with cancer. *Journal of the American Academy of Child and Adolescent Psychiatry*, *43*(10), 1243–1249. doi:10.1097/01.chi.0000135621.23145.05 PMID:15381891

Gold, J. I., Belmont, K. A., & Thomas, D. A. (2007). The Neurobiology of Virtual Reality Pain Attenuation. *Cyberpsychology & Behavior*, *10*(4), 536–544. doi:10.1089/cpb.2007.9993 PMID:17711362

Gold, J. I., Kim, S. H., Kant, A. J., Joseph, M. H., & Rizzo, A. "Skip." (2006). Effectiveness of Virtual Reality for Pediatric Pain Distraction during IV Placement. *Cyberpsychology & Behavior*. doi:10.1089/cpb.2006.9.207

Gold, J. I., & Mahrer, N. E. (2017). Is Virtual Reality Ready for Prime Time in the Medical Space? A Randomized Control Trial of Pediatric Virtual Reality for Acute Procedural Pain Management. *Journal of Pediatric Psychology*. doi:10.1093/jpepsy/jsx129 PMID:29053848

Hassett, A. L., Aquino, J. K., & Ilgen, M. A. (2014). The risk of suicide mortality in chronic pain patients. *Current Pain and Headache Reports*, *18*(8), 436. doi:10.100711916-014-0436-1 PMID:24952608

Heppelmann, B., Messlinger, K., Neiss, W. F., & Schmidt, R. F. (1990). Ultrastructural three-dimensional reconstruction of group III and group IV sensory nerve endings ("free nerve endings") in the knee joint capsule of the cat: Evidenence for multiple receptive sites. *The Journal of Comparative Neurology*, *292*(1), 103–116. doi:10.1002/cne.902920107 PMID:2312785

Hershey, A. D., Powers, S. W., Bentti, A. L., & DeGrauw, T. J. (2000). Effectiveness of amitriptyline in the prophylactic management of childhood headaches. *Headache*, *40*(7), 539–549. doi:10.1046/j.1526-4610.2000.00085.x PMID:10940092

Hoffman, H. G., Doctor, J. N., Patterson, D. R., Carrougher, G. J., & Furness, T. III. (2000). Virtual reality as an adjunctive pain control during burn wound care in adolescent patients. *Pain*, *85*(1), 305–309. doi:10.1016/S0304-3959(99)00275-4 PMID:10692634

Hoffman, H. G., Patterson, D. R., Seibel, E., Soltani, M., Jewett-Leahy, L., & Sharar, S. R. (2008). Virtual reality pain control during burn wound debridement in the hydrotank. *The Clinical Journal of Pain*, *24*(4), 299–304. doi:10.1097/AJP.0b013e318164d2cc PMID:18427228

Hoffman, H. G., Richards, T. L., Bills, A. R., Van Oostrom, T., Magula, J., Seibel, E. J., & Sharar, S. R. (2006). Using fMRI to study the neural correlates of virtual reality analgesia. *CNS Spectrums*, *11*(01), 45–51. doi:10.1017/S1092852900024202 PMID:16400255

Hoffman, H. G., Seibel, E. J., Richards, T. L., Furness, T. A., Patterson, D. R., & Sharar, S. R. (2006). Virtual Reality Helmet Display Quality Influences the Magnitude of Virtual Reality Analgesia. *The Journal of Pain*, *7*(11), 843–850. doi:10.1016/j.jpain.2006.04.006 PMID:17074626

Hunfeld, J. a, Perquin, C. W., Duivenvoorden, H. J., Hazebroek-Kampschreur, a a, Passchier, J., van Suijlekom-Smit, L. W., & van der Wouden, J. C. (2001). Chronic pain and its impact on quality of life in adolescents and their families. *Journal of Pediatric Psychology*. doi:10.1093/jpepsy/26.3.145

Ilgen, M. A., Kleinberg, F., Ignacio, R. V., Bohnert, A. S. B., Valenstein, M., & McCarthy, J. F. … Katz, I. R. (2013). Noncancer Pain Conditions and Risk of Suicide. *JAMA Psychiatry*. doi:10.1001/jamapsychiatry.2013.908

Jäncke, L., Cheetham, M., & Baumgartner, T. (2009). Virtual reality and the role of the prefrontal cortex in adults and children. *Frontiers in Neuroscience*, *3*(1). doi:10.3389/neuro.01.006.2009 PMID:19753097

Jeon, B., Cho, S., & Lee, J.-H. (2014). Application of Virtual Body Swapping to Patients with Complex Regional Pain Syndrome: A Pilot Study. *Cyberpsychology, Behavior, and Social Networking*, *17*(6), 366–370. doi:10.1089/cyber.2014.0046 PMID:24892199

Jones, T., Moore, T., & Choo, J. (2016). The impact of virtual reality on chronic pain. *PLoS One*, *11*(12), e0167523. doi:10.1371/journal.pone.0167523 PMID:27997539

Kashikar-Zuck, S., Goldschneider, K. R., Powers, S. W., Vaught, M. H., & Hershey, A. D. (2001). Depression and functional disability in chronic pediatric pain. *The Clinical Journal of Pain*, *17*(4), 341–349. doi:10.1097/00002508-200112000-00009 PMID:11783815

Katz, J., Rosenbloom, B. N., & Fashler, S. (2015). Chronic pain, psychopathology, and DSM-5 somatic symptom disorder. *Canadian Journal of Psychiatry*, *60*(4), 160–167. doi:10.1177/070674371506000402 PMID:26174215

Keefe, F. J., Lefebvre, J. C., Egert, J. R., Affleck, G., Sullivan, M. J., & Caldwell, D. S. (2000). The relationship of gender to pain, pain behavior, and disability in osteoarthritis patients: The role of catastrophizing. *Pain*, *87*(3), 325–334. doi:10.1016/S0304-3959(00)00296-7 PMID:10963912

King, S., Chambers, C. T., Huguet, A., MacNevin, R. C., McGrath, P. J., Parker, L., & MacDonald, A. J. (2011). The epidemiology of chronic pain in children and adolescents revisited: A systematic review. *Pain*, *152*(12), 2729–2738. doi:10.1016/j.pain.2011.07.016 PMID:22078064

Kokinsky, E., Enska, K., Nilsson, S., & Finnstro, B. (2009). The use of Virtual Reality for needle-related procedural pain and distress in children and adolescents in a paediatric oncology unit. *European Journal of Oncology Nursing, 13*, 102–109. doi:10.1016/j.ejon.2009.01.003

Mahrer, N. E., & Gold, J. I. (2009). The use of virtual reality for pain control: A review. *Current Pain and Headache Reports*, *13*(2), 100–109. doi:10.100711916-009-0019-8 PMID:19272275

Malloy, K. M., & Milling, L. S. (2010). The effectiveness of virtual reality distraction for pain reduction: A systematic review. *Clinical Psychology Review*, *30*(8), 1011–1018. doi:10.1016/j.cpr.2010.07.001 PMID:20691523

Melzack, R. (1999). From the gate to the neuromatrix. *Pain*, *82*, S121–S126. doi:10.1016/S0304-3959(99)00145-1 PMID:10491980

Melzack, R. (2001). Pain and the neuromatrix in the brain. *Journal of Dental Education*. PMID:11780656

Melzack, R., & Wall, P. D. (1965). Pain mechanisms: A new theory. *Science*, *150*(3699), 971–978. doi:10.1126cience.150.3699.971 PMID:5320816

Moayedi, M., & Davis, K. D. (2013). Theories of pain: From specificity to gate control. *Journal of Neurophysiology*, *109*(1), 5–12. doi:10.1152/jn.00457.2012 PMID:23034364

Moseley, G. L., Gallace, A., & Spence, C. (2012). Bodily illusions in health and disease: Physiological and clinical perspectives and the concept of a cortical "body matrix.". *Neuroscience and Biobehavioral Reviews*, *36*(1), 34–46. doi:10.1016/j.neubiorev.2011.03.013 PMID:21477616

Neugebauer, V., Li, W., Bird, G. C., & Han, J. S. (2004). The amygdala and persistent pain. *The Neuroscientist*, *10*(3), 221–234. doi:10.1177/1073858403261077 PMID:15155061

Oneal, B. J., Patterson, D. R., Soltani, M., Teeley, A., & Jensen, M. P. (2008). Virtual reality hypnosis in the treatment of chronic neuropathic pain: A case report. *The International Journal of Clinical and Experimental Hypnosis*, *56*(4), 451–462. doi:10.1080/00207140802255534 PMID:18726807

Palermo, T. M., Eccleston, C., Lewandowski, A. S., Williams, A. C. de C., & Morley, S. (2010). Randomized controlled trials of psychological therapies for management of chronic pain in children and adolescents: An updated meta-analytic review. *Pain*. doi:10.1016/j.pain.2009.10.004 PMID:19910118

Perquin, C. W., Hazebroek-Kampschreur, A. A. J. M., Hunfeld, J. A. M., Bohnen, A. M., Van Suijlekom-Smit, L. W. A., Passchier, J., & Van Der Wouden, J. C. (2000). Pain in children and adolescents: A common experience. *Pain*, *87*(1), 51–58. doi:10.1016/S0304-3959(00)00269-4 PMID:10863045

Ramachandran, V. S. (1993). Behavioral and magnetoencephalographic correlates of plasticity in the adult human brain. *Proceedings of the National Academy of Sciences*. 10.1073/pnas.90.22.10413

Ramachandran, V. S., & Altschuler, E. L. (2009). The use of visual feedback, in particular mirror visual feedback, in restoring brain function. *Brain*, *132*(7), 1693–1710. doi:10.1093/brain/awp135 PMID:19506071

Ramachandran, V. S., & Rogers-Ramachandran, D. (2000). Phantom Limbs and Neural Plasticity. *Archives of Neurology*, *57*(3), 317. doi:10.1001/archneur.57.3.317 PMID:10714655

Ramachandran, V. S., Rogers-Ramachandran, D., & Cobb, S. (1995). Touching the phantom limb. *Nature*, *377*(6549), 489–490. doi:10.1038/377489a0 PMID:7566144

Ramachandran, V. S., Stewart, M., & Rogers-Ramachandran, D. C. (1992). Perceptual correlates of massive cortical reorganization. *Neuroreport*, *3*(7), 583–586. doi:10.1097/00001756-199207000-00009 PMID:1421112

Reid, G. J., Lang, B. A., & McGrath, P. J. (1997). Primary juvenile fibromyalgia: Psychological adjustment, family functioning, coping, and functional disability. *Arthritis and Rheumatism*, *40*(4), 752–760. doi:10.1002/art.1780400423 PMID:9125260

Rhee, H. (2000). Prevalence and predictors of headaches in US adolescents. *Headache*, *40*(7), 528–538. doi:10.1046/j.1526-4610.2000.00084.x PMID:10940091

Roth-Isigkeit, A. (2005). Pain Among Children and Adolescents: Restrictions in Daily Living and Triggering Factors. *Pediatrics*, *115*(2), e152–e162. doi:10.1542/peds.2004-0682 PMID:15687423

Shahrbanian, S., Ma, X., Aghaei, N., Korner-bitensky, N., & Simmonds, M. J. (2012). Use of virtual reality (immersive vs. non immersive) for pain management in children and adults: A systematic review of evidence from randomized controlled trials. *European Journal of Experimental Biology*.

Sharar, S. R., Carrougher, G. J., Nakamura, D., Hoffman, H. G., Blough, D. K., & Patterson, D. R. (2007). Factors Influencing the Efficacy of Virtual Reality Distraction Analgesia During Postburn Physical Therapy: Preliminary Results from 3 Ongoing Studies. *Archives of Physical Medicine and Rehabilitation*, *88*(12), S43–S49. doi:10.1016/j.apmr.2007.09.004 PMID:18036981

Sillanpää, M., & Anttila, P. (1996). Increasing prevalence of headache in 7-year-old schoolchildren. *Headache*, *36*(8), 466–470. doi:10.1046/j.1526-4610.1996.3608466.x PMID:8824000

Slater, M., Spanlang, B., Sanchez-Vives, M. V., & Blanke, O. (2010). First person experience of body transfer in virtual reality. *PLoS One*, *5*(5), e10564. doi:10.1371/journal.pone.0010564 PMID:20485681

Soler, M. D., Kumru, H., Pelayo, R., Vidal, J., Tormos, J. M., Fregni, F., ... Pascual-Leone, A. (2010). Effectiveness of transcranial direct current stimulation and visual illusion on neuropathic pain in spinal cord injury. *Brain*, *133*(9), 2565–2577. doi:10.1093/brain/awq184 PMID:20685806

Songer, D. (2005). Psychotherapeutic Approaches in the Treatment of Pain. *Psychiatry*. PMID:21152145

Stanford, E. A., Chambers, C. T., Biesanz, J. C., & Chen, E. (2008). The frequency, trajectories and predictors of adolescent recurrent pain: A population-based approach. *Pain*, *138*(1), 11–21. doi:10.1016/j.pain.2007.10.032 PMID:18093737

Tsakiris, M., & Haggard, P. (2005). The rubber hand illusion revisited: Visuotactile integration and self-attribution. *Journal of Experimental Psychology. Human Perception and Performance*, *31*(1), 80–91. doi:10.1037/0096-1523.31.1.80 PMID:15709864

Turk, D. C., & Okifuji, A. (2002). Psychological factors in chronic pain: Evolution and revolution. *Journal of Consulting and Clinical Psychology*, *70*(3), 678–690. doi:10.1037/0022-006X.70.3.678 PMID:12090376

Turk, D. C., Swanson, K. S., & Tunks, E. R. (2008). Psychological approaches in the treatment of chronic pain patients - When pills, scalpels, and needles are not enough. *Canadian Journal of Psychiatry*, *53*(4), 213–223. doi:10.1177/070674370805300402 PMID:18478824

Valet, M., Sprenger, T., Boecker, H., Willoch, F., Rummeny, E., & Conrad, B., … Tolle, T. R. (2004). Distraction modulates connectivity of the cingulo-frontal cortex and the midbrain during pain - An fMRI analysis. *Pain*. doi:10.1016/j.pain.2004.02.033

Vogt, B. A., Sikes, R. W., & Vogt, L. J. (1993). Anterior Cingulate Cortex and the Medial Pain System. In Neurobiology of Cingulate Cortex and Limbic Thalamus: A Comprehensive Handbook. Academic Press. doi:10.1007/978-1-4899-6704-6_11

Von Korff, M., Crane, P., Lane, M., Miglioretti, D. L., Simon, G., & Saunders, K. … Kessler, R. (2005). Chronic spinal pain and physical-mental comorbidity in the United States: Results from the national comorbidity survey replication. *Pain*. doi:10.1016/j.pain.2004.11.010

Walker, L. S., & Greene, J. W. (1991). The functional disability inventory: Measuring a neglected dimension of child health status. *Journal of Pediatric Psychology*, *16*(1), 39–58. doi:10.1093/jpepsy/16.1.39 PMID:1826329

Walker, L. S., Guite, J. W., Duke, M., Barnard, J. A., & Greene, J. W. (1998). Recurrent abdominal pain: A potential precursor of irritable bowel syndrome in adolescents and young adults. *The Journal of Pediatrics*, *132*(6), 1010–1015. doi:10.1016/S0022-3476(98)70400-7 PMID:9627595

Wiederhold, B. K., Gao, K., Sulea, C., & Wiederhold, M. D. (2014). Virtual Reality as a Distraction Technique in Chronic Pain Patients. *Cyberpsychology, Behavior, and Social Networking*, *17*(6), 346–352. doi:10.1089/cyber.2014.0207 PMID:24892196

Williams, A., Eccleston, C., & Morley, S. (2012). Psychological therapies for the management of chronic pain (excluding headache) in adults. *Cochrane Database of Systematic Reviews*. doi:10.1002/14651858.CD007407.pub3 PMID:23152245

Won, A., Bailey, J., Bailenson, J., Tataru, C., Yoon, I., & Golianu, B. (2017). Immersive Virtual Reality for Pediatric Pain. *Children*, *4*(7), 52. doi:10.3390/children4070052 PMID:28644422

Won, A. S., Bailey, J., Bailenson, J., Tataru, C., Yoon, I. A., & Golianu, B. (2017). Immersive Virtual Reality for Pediatric Pain. *Children*, *4*(52), 1–15. doi:10.3390/children4070052 PMID:28644422

Won, A. S., Tataru, C. A., Cojocaru, C. M., Krane, E. J., Bailenson, J. N., Niswonger, S. G. B., & Golianu, B. (2015). Two Virtual Reality Pilot Studies for the Treatment of Pediatric CRPS. *Pain Medicine*, *16*(8), 1644–1647. doi:10.1111/pme.12755 PMID:25930099

Yang, T. T., Gallen, C., Schwartz, B., Bloom, F. E., Ramachandran, V. S., & Cobb, S. (1994). Sensory maps in the human brain. *Nature*, *368*(6472), 592–593. doi:10.1038/368592b0 PMID:8145842

## ADDITIONAL READING

Bohil, C. J., Alicea, B., & Biocca, F. A. (2011). Virtual reality in neuroscience research and therapy. *Nature Reviews. Neuroscience*, *12*(12), 752–762. doi:10.1038/nrn3122 PMID:22048061

Gold, J. I., Belmont, K. A., & Thomas, D. A. (2007). The Neurobiology of Virtual Reality Pain Attenuation. *Cyberpsychology & Behavior*, *10*(4), 536–544. doi:10.1089/cpb.2007.9993 PMID:17711362

Gujjar, K. R., van Wijk, A., Sharma, R., & de Jongh, A. (2017). Virtual Reality Exposure Therapy for the Treatment of Dental Phobia: A Controlled Feasibility Study. *Behavioural and Cognitive Psychotherapy*. doi:10.1017/S1352465817000534 PMID:28903790

Li, L., Yu, F., Shi, D., Shi, J., Tian, Z., & Yang, J. … Jiang, Q. (2017). Application of virtual reality technology in clinical medicine. *American Journal of Translational Research*. doi:10.3969/j.issn.1673-8225.2011.30.036

Pozeg, P., Palluel, E., Ronchi, R., Solcà, M., Al-Khodairy, A. W., & Jordan, X. … Blanke, O. (2017). Virtual reality improves embodiment and neuropathic pain caused by spinal cord injury. *Neurology*. doi:10.1212/WNL.0000000000004585

Raghav, K., Van Wijk, A. J., Abdullah, F., Islam, M. N., Bernatchez, M., & De Jongh, A. (2016). Efficacy of virtual reality exposure therapy for treatment of dental phobia: A randomized control trial. *BMC Oral Health*, *16*(1), 25. doi:10.118612903-016-0186-z PMID:26920573

Ramachandran, V. S., & Altschuler, E. L. (2009). The use of visual feedback, in particular mirror visual feedback, in restoring brain function. *Brain*, *132*(7), 1693–1710. doi:10.1093/brain/awp135 PMID:19506071

Sharar, S. R., Alamdari, A., Hoffer, C., Hoffman, H. G., Jensen, M. P., & Patterson, D. R. (2016). Circumplex Model of Affect: A Measure of Pleasure and Arousal During Virtual Reality Distraction Analgesia. *Games for Health Journal*, *5*(3), 197–202. doi:10.1089/g4h.2015.0046 PMID:27171578

## KEY TERMS AND DEFINITIONS

**Biopsychosocial:** A model or approach that recognizes biologic, psychologic, and social effects.

**Chronic Pain:** Persistent pain, typically lasting three or more months.

**Cortical Reorganization:** A change in the original mapping pattern of the brain so that stimuli activate different parts of the cortex.

**Immersive Virtual Reality:** A type of virtual reality where the user is fully immersed in the virtual environment, most often achieved using a head-mounted display.

**Neuroplasticity:** The ability of the brain to adapt to the environment.

**Perception:** The conscious result of the brain's interpretation of sensory information.

**Sensation:** The physiologic detection of a stimuli through peripheral receptors.

# Chapter 14
# E-Learning and Augmented Reality (AR) for Chronic Wound Assessment:
## Promoting Learning and Quality of Care

**Nelson Ribeiro Jorge**
*Universidade Aberta, Portugal*

**Lina Morgado**
*Universidade Aberta, Portugal*

**Pedro J. S. Gaspar**
*Instituto Politécnico de Leiria, Portugal*

## ABSTRACT

*This investigation aimed to verify if augmented reality (AR) increases students' motivation and enhances the development of clinical decision-making skills in wound diagnosis and treatment. A quasi-experimental study was carried out with a sample of 54 nursing students. A comparative analysis of the progress of the control and experimental group was made using the data extracted from the simulator and a questionnaire. First, both groups used e-FER, a virtual simulator that simulates the diagnosis and treatment of virtual clinical cases. In the second moment, the control group continued using only e-FER, while the experimental group used e-FER combined with an AR application to observe the chronic wounds. The results showed that AR enhanced student performance, particularly in wound diagnostic parameters, with highly statistically significant differences (p<0,001), and registering high levels of motivation and simulator usability, even with the introduction of an additional device in the activity.*

DOI: 10.4018/978-1-5225-7168-1.ch014

## INTRODUCTION

Emerging technologies for teaching and learning have enabled the creation of environments, scenarios and virtual patients, simulating clinical practices with the purpose to promote the development of skills and knowledge in healthcare education (Lewis, Davies, Jenkins, & Tait, 2005; Hogan, Sabri & Kapralos, 2007). These simulations are considered educational techniques that bring interactivity and immersion into the teaching and learning process, allowing the recreation of clinical experiences without the risk of causing harm to patients (Maran & Glavin, 2003). The possibility learners have to practice an unlimited number of times a procedure or technique until correct realization, before applying it in real-world scenarios, is also considered a valuable advantage (Rey, Visconti, Balaguer, & Martínez, 2006).

Virtual and Augmented Reality technologies, when used in education, allow the creation of digitally enhanced learning environments. These emerging technologies are expected to have a big impact in education in the coming years, as highlighted by the Horizon reports for Higher Education in 2010, 2011 and 2016 (Johnson, Levine, Smith, & Stone,2010; Johnson et al., 2011, 2016). In fact, a positive impact of Virtual Reality (VR) and Augmented Reality (AR) can already be seen in healthcare education, where several studies have indicated the positive effect of VR and AR in developing decision making skills and practical procedures using virtual simulators, with a higher impact on participants with no experience (Zhu, Hadadgar, Masiello, & Zaryet, 2014).

However, using VR in healthcare education can be a debatable approach since it immerses learners in a synthetic environment, enabling them to see the real-world. Acting in a different environment from which learners will act in real life scenarios is another relevant concern. According to Ellaway (2010, p.791):

*(…) in medicine and medical education aspects of virtual reality have found their way into the mainstream through the use of 3D animations, digital imaging tools that can make 3D models (…) and more interactively through the use of synthetic worlds such as Second Life and haptic simulators for technical procedures such as laparoscopic surgery.*

*A key limitation however for virtual reality in medical education is that it requires participants to step away from the environment in which the practice for which they are preparing takes place. Virtual reality is therefore essentially divergent from real world practice and the embodied experiences within it.*

In AR environments, digital objects are added to the real-world, enhancing it and not replacing it. AR is a technology that allows the integration of virtual objects into the physical real-world. It supplements the real world with virtual objects in a way that they seem to coexist in the same space (Zhou, Duh & Billinghurst, 2008). The combination of real with virtual, real time interactivity and three dimensional (3D) virtual content are the three commonly accepted characteristics of AR systems indicated by Azuma (1997). In this way, AR plays an important role in education, as the 2011 Horizon report states (Johnson et al., 2011, p.22):

*Augmented reality has strong potential to provide both powerful contextual, in situ learning experiences and serendipitous exploration and discovery of the connected nature of information in the real world.*

This chapter describes part of a doctoral study where the effect of AR in nursing student's decision making skills was investigated, by comparing the usage of a virtual simulator in wound care diagnosis and treatment, with and without the support of an AR application to visualize the wounds.

There are associations between chronic wounds and mental health status (Hopman et al., 2009). Chronic wounds represent a significant burden to patients (Phillips et al., 2016), including costs associated with anxiety, depression and feelings related to social isolation (Jones, Barr, Robinson & Carlisle, 2006; Herber, Schepp & Rieger, 2007). Chronic wounds can heavily impair the patients' quality of life by causing severe pain, social isolation, restricted mobility, sleeping problems and many other negative effects on the patients' daily life (Herber et al., 2007; Gorecki, Nixon, Lamping, Alavi & Brown, 2014).

We believe that by improving care for chronic wounds through emerging technologies for teaching and learning, we are promoting the mental health of patients and their significant relatives.

A literature review was conducted to identify, select and analyse the effectiveness of AR in medical education. *Web of Science*™ was used to retrieve all studies published until 29 July 2015, according to the following query: *augmented reality OR mixed reality AND medical OR healthcare AND training OR education*. In total, 43 studies out of 163 were selected to review, after excluding papers that focused only on VR, telemedicine, technical equipment, veterinary or exclusively related to medical practices and not educational.

This literature review has shown that AR is used in several disciplines of medical education, with a higher incidence of studies related to the training of laparoscopic surgery (Botden, Buzink, Schijven, & Jakimowicz, 2008; Feifer, Delisle, & Anidjar, 2008; Oostema, Abdel, & Gould, 2008; LeBlanc et al., 2010, Brinkman et al., 2012; Nugent et al., 2013; Vera et al., 2014), surgical puncture (Vikal et al., 2010; Yeo et al., 2011; Ungi et al., 2012; Moult et al., 2013; Nugent et al., 2013; Sutherland, Hashtrudi-Zaad, Sellens, Abolmaesumi, & Mousavi, 2013) and neurosurgery (Luciano et al., 2011; Alaraj et al., 2013; Mitha, Almekhlafi, Janjua, Albuquerque, & McDougall, 2013; Abhari et al., 2015). In general, AR has shown to be an effective tool to develop clinical skills when compared with other methods, with a greater impact on unexperienced learners, and its transfer to real world scenarios. AR in medical education is seen as a safe simulation method to practice unlimitedly clinical procedures, without the risk of harming real patients.

The objectives of this chapter are to explore the possibilities and limitations of AR in education, in particular in the medical field, to describe the materials, methods, results and conclusions of the research conducted.

## BACKGROUND

### Chronic Wounds and Mental Health

A chronic wound is a wound that does not heal in an orderly set of stages and in a predictable amount of time. Having a chronic wound is a medical condition that can affect mental health status in patients and caregivers.

Several studies confirm this relationship between chronic wounds and mental health status and recent research has started to identify mood disorders associated with chronic wounds, which have been shown to contribute to delayed healing, poor patient well-being and a reduced quality of life.

Upton and Hender (2012) carried out a study about the cost of mood disorders in patients with chronic wounds and found that there is considerable evidence that wounds can lead to negative emotional states, such as anxiety and depression and the cost implications of mood disorders in chronic wound patients can be considerable. In this study, the authors point that successfully managing pain and using a holistic approach to patient care could have incalculable benefits for the patient and considerable economic benefits to health care providers and society.

Upton, Solowiej and Woo (2014) studied the perspective of health professionals on the prevalence of mood disorders in patients with acute and chronic wounds. The results showed a strong awareness of the prevalence of mood disorders in patients with wounds, among health professionals around the world. Additionally, these authors stress that mood disorders have shown to have a negative impact on the financial costs of service providers and also in general society regarding treatment and sickness absence.

Upton, Upton and Alexander (2015) conducted a study about the complexity of caring and the detrimental health and well-being effects of caregivers of people with chronic wounds. These authors showed that the relationship between caregiving, health and well-being is complex and many research indicates detrimental physical and psychological outcomes of caregivers of patients with wounds. However, until now there has been insufficient attention paid to the health and well-being outcomes of carers of people living with chronic wounds in the research literature, therefore it's vital to understand how to maximise health and well-being outcomes of carers of patients with chronic wounds.

Corrêa, de Brito, de Carvalho Resende, Duarte, Santos, Salomé and Ferreira (2016) studied the impact of surgical wound dehiscence on health-related quality of life and mental health. Results showed that these wounds had a negative impact on the quality of life and on mental health.

More recently, Renner and Erfurt-Berge (2017) investigated the relationship between depression and quality of life in patients with chronic wounds and found that at least 30% of those patients suffer from depressive symptoms or anxiety. Moreover, Ahn, Del Core, Wukich, Liu, Lalli, VanPelt and Raspovic (2018) found that the mental health and the quality of life in patients with diabetic foot complications were lower than in patients without these complications.

Improving the physical health care of people with diagnosed mental illness, including appropriate wound care treatment for mental health service users, is an area of care that needs more attention (Hemingway, Atkin & Stephenson, 2013). According to these authors, a strategic plan for tissue viability in mental health settings and appropriate training for health professionals is needed.

## AR Learning Environments

According to the literature, *AR learning environments can enable (1) learning content in 3D perspectives, (2) ubiquitous, collaborative and situated learning, (3) learners' senses of presence, immediacy, and immersion, (4) visualizing the invisible, and (5) bridging formal and informal learning* (Wu, Lee, Chang, & Liang, 2013, p.43). These points will be addressed below, including some examples.

### 1. Learning Content in 3D Perspectives

Using 3D content is part of Azuma's (1997) definition of AR, as mentioned earlier in this chapter. According to Arvanitis et al. (2007), virtual 3D objects can increase the visual perception of a certain AR environment. Students can explore the 3D objects in different perspectives in order to strengthen understanding (Chen et al., 2011).

AR has the potential to motivate students by allowing them to manipulate virtual objects from various perspectives (Kerawalla, Luckin, Seljeflot, & Woolard, 2006). In the study of Kaufmann, Steinbugl, Dunser, and Gluck (2005), a geometric and dynamic 3D system (Construct 3D) was used to facilitate learning mathematics and geometry. According to these authors, Construct 3D not only promoted a collaborative learning context for students, but also promoted the understanding of spatial relationships by enabling the manipulation and measurement of virtual 3D objects.

The importance of studying Anatomy in medicine made a group of researchers develop an AR application to create an interactive learning system, allowing students to better understand and memorize the 3D anatomical structure (Chien et al., 2010). Another example of AR is the LearnAR tool that allows visualization and interaction with 3D content in the area of science, mathematics, and languages.

As presented in the introduction of the chapter, this research is based on the use of 3D digital content that represent chronic wounds, to be observed by students using AR. Although interaction with the 3D content is minimal, since the system only allows to observe the wound, this is a critical task in order to perform a correct diagnosis and subsequent treatment of the clinical case to be solved.

## 2. Ubiquitous, Collaborative and Situated Learning

Mobile devices with wireless and GPS technology can enable collaborative, ubiquitous and situated learning, enhanced by the use of games, computer simulations, models and virtual objects in real environments (Broll et al., 2008; Dunleavy, Dede, & Mitchell, 2009). Their characteristics may also include portability, social interaction, context sensitivity, connectivity and individuality (Klopfer, 2008; Squire & Jan, 2007; Squire & Klopfer, 2007).

The AR-mobile games Environmental Detectives (Squire & Klopfer, 2007; Klopfer, 2008) and Mad City Mystery (Squire & Jan, 2007) are examples that promote learning outside the classroom, where students carry out investigations in order to make more informed decisions.

Providing different investigation paths can help promote individuality (Klopfer, 2008).

Birchfield and Megowan-Romanowicz (2009) report that the social interactivity can be enhanced when students collaborate using networked mobile devices, as well as in face-to-face interactions.

AR has the ability to involve students in real world investigations through virtual objects like texts, videos and images, additional elements added to their surroundings (Dede, 2009).

According to Johnson et al. (2010), geolocating certain places with overlapped information is one of the most common uses of AR.

Regarding situated learning in the context of medical education, Feng et al. (2013, p.181) refer that:

*Situated e-learning is an effective method to improve novice learners' performance. The effect of the situated e-learning on the improvement of cognitive ability is limited when compared to traditional learning. Situated e-learning may be a useful adjunct to traditional learning for medical and nursing students, but does not appear to have any benefit over traditional learning methods for practicing clinicians.*

According to these authors, situated learning in the context of e-Learning is more effective with inexperienced students, when compared to experienced professionals, an idea that is coherent with the information revealed in the literature review.

## 3. Learners' Senses of Presence, Immediacy and Immersion

Bronack (2011), in an article about the role of immersive media in online education, points out that emerging technologies such as AR, virtual worlds, simulations and serious games can convey a sense of presence, immediacy and immersion, so far unavailable to educators, both in face-to-face and distance education.

- *Sense of presence*, since AR can provide a mediated space for students that can lead to the recognition of the learning community (Squire & Jan, 2007).
- *Immediacy*, since AR can include real-time feedback and provide verbal and non-verbal information to students (Kotranza, Lind, Pugh, & Lok, 2009).
- *Immersion*, as it provides students with *the subjective impression that one is participating in a comprehensive, realistic experience* (Dede, 2009, p.66). According to this author, immersion can promote a situated learning environment where students deal with problems and issues of the real world.

A recent study with mobile-AR revealed the sense of presence, immediacy and immersion when promoting students' learning about a scientific and social issue, namely the use of nuclear energy and the impact of radioactive contamination, in the context of the nuclear power plant accidents of Fukushima Daiichi, after the earthquake in Japan (Chang, Wu & Hsu, 2013). Students used tablets to simulate collecting radiation data at their campus, in a place located 12 km away from the nuclear power plant and on the day after the explosion. This study revealed a significant correlation in students' perceptions regarding nuclear energy, showing that the AR can influence their affective domain in real-world issues.

Medical simulation is another example where immediacy and immersion are useful to recreate learning experiences that are as close to reality as possible. In medical education we can find AR educational applications for the practice, planning and guidance of surgical procedures (Shuhaiber, 2004; Reitinger, Bornik, Beichel, & Schmalstieget, 2006; De Paolis et al., 2008; Hansen, Wieferich, Ritter, Rieder, & Peitgen, 2009).

## 4. Visualizing the Invisible

Using AR to overlap virtual objects or information in real environments can enable the visualization of unseen concepts or events (Arvanitis et al., 2007; Dunleavy et al., 2009). Increasing reality creates new views that have the potential to promote the understanding of abstract and invisible concepts or phenomena.

The integration of digital educational content in the real world using AR enables to create immersive learning experiences that in some cases are difficult to recreate in the real world. AR systems can support learning about abstract concepts or unobservable phenomena, as for example convection currents, electromagnetic fields, atomic models, molecular structures, various types of forces, among others.

Klopfer and Squire (2008) have shown that AR enables students to experience scientific phenomena that are difficult to recreate in the real world. Liu, Cheok, Mei-Ling, and Theng (2007) have also created several educational applications with AR for this purpose, enabling students to view the solar system as if it was in their classroom, and the photosynthesis process. In the area of chemistry AR enables students to visualize 3D molecular models (Fjeld & Voegtli, 2002; Chen, 2006). Other example in the field of chemistry is an application that uses AR to explore the atomic orbitals of hydrogen (Trindade et al., 2004).

### 5. Bridging Formal and Informal Learning

Other purpose identified in research is the potential of AR to bridge formal and informal learning contexts. The CONNECT project combined AR with other technologies to develop a virtual Science Park that contained a museum and a school (Sotiriou & Bogner, 2008). A first evaluation of this project indicated that the environment positively influenced students' motivation and learning of science.

## Limitations of Educational Augmented Reality Systems

Several authors have identified a number of problems in the use of AR in education, both at a technological and at a pedagogical level.

From a technological point of view, the use of traditional HMD (Head Mounted Display) equipment can be considered a problem, since the weight and design of these devices may cause discomfort and impair depth perception, despite the developments in their construction (Kerawalla et al., 2006).

Although AR systems with geolocation may offer more contextualized environments, they present limitations regarding portability and flexibility, as they require a specific location for their implementation (Klopfer & Sheldon, 2010).

At a pedagogical level, there may be a natural resistance to change in the teaching practices, more active, learner-centred and contextualized with AR, as opposed to the traditional, teacher-centred information transfer method (Kerawalla et al., 2006; Mitchell, 2011; Squire & Jan, 2007).

However, the obstacles to the integration of new teaching methodologies or emerging technologies are common in education, and not specific to AR. Thus, it is important to determine how, when and where AR should be integrated in the educational processes, in order to potentiate significant learning and maximize the benefits to students.

The planning of educational activities with AR, namely how the information should be distributed between the two worlds and the different devices, is another challenge identified by Klopfer and Squire (2008). The inflexibility of some AR systems, very difficult or even impossible to modify, prevent teachers from adapting the contents to the defined learning goals and to students' needs. The use of authoring tools may help to overcome this limitation (Bergig, Hagbi, El-Sana, & Billinghurst, 2009), allowing teachers and students to edit and create AR activities and applications (Klopfer & Squire, 2008).

When it comes to learning, however, students may experience cognitive overload because of the sheer amount of information they encounter, the simultaneous use of several devices and the complexity of the tasks to perform (Wu et al., 2013).

The intertwining of physical reality and virtual reality may also cause some confusion in learners, although this can be seen as a positive thing due to the authenticity of the process.

As Dunleavy et al. (2009) point out, losing sense of the real physical environment might not be productive for learners and present a threat to their safety.

Although AR involves the use of technologies, not always easy to access and use, the focus should be on the way these technologies can support and facilitate significant learning. This is how AR should be perceived, i.e. as a concept, and not merely as a technology.

Nevertheless, system usability is a very important aspect to take into account, and something the authors also investigated in this study.

## AR in Medical Education

In general, the articles that discuss AR in medical education refer to its potential, limitations, and examples. As described, the pedagogical potential of AR in education is evident, although several authors state that more research is needed to prove its effectiveness. It is therefore critical to understand its impact in order to prevent risk for patients and improve the quality of care.

Monkman and Kushniruk (2015) report that AR will be increasingly present in medicine in general. However, they caution against the need to investigate its benefits over traditional methods, and that AR applications should be carefully tested in order to avoid introducing new errors into clinical practice, thereby compromising patient safety.

Kamphuis et al. (2014, p.300) believe that AR has the "potential to offer a highly realistic situated learning experience supportive of complex medical learning and transfer". According to this author (*ibid*) AR presents organizational and particular advantages, namely:

- The physical training environment with AR can be similar to the professional working environment;
- A variety of possible tasks to perform;
- Real-time feedback;
- The fact that a trainer isn't needed all the time;
- The fact that AR provides a just-in-time and just-in-place learning experience.

Zhu et al. (2014) carried out an integrative review of the literature on AR in health education by analyzing 25 articles in detail, in order to identify the potential and limitations in this field. Although most of the AR applications analyzed by the authors were still in the prototype phase, the results suggest several educational potentialities, allowing the learner to:

- Understand spatial relationships and concepts;
- Acquire skills and knowledge;
- Strengthen their cognitive and psychomotor skills;
- Decrease their learning curve;
- Extend their learning retention;
- Increase their interest and attractiveness to the topics through simulated authentic experiences.

Regarding the forms in which AR is used, the study emphasizes:

- Learning through feedback or guidance system;
- Immersion in a scenario;
- Participatory reality;
- Innovative interface;
- Application with relevant information;
- Evaluation and remote training;
- Simulated practice.

As a limitation, in addition to the fact that most of the studies focus on prototypes, that is, in applications under development and tests that lead to optimization, there was a gap from the educational point of view, since the theoretical pedagogical models that support the activities developed in the studies were not explicit. Finally, another limitation refers to the adopted learning strategies – traditional *observation-practice* approach – and the fact that they do not integrate clinical competences that assure patient safety.

## MATERIALS AND METHODS

### Equipment

A web based learning simulator (e-FER) that holds several virtual cases of patients with chronic wounds was developed by Monguet et al. (2009) to improve wound care training. The clinical cases were developed by healthcare specialists and include a detailed description with pictorial (real picture of wounds) and non-pictorial information. The e-FER simulator allows users to simulate decision-making when treating wounds, providing immediate feedback to the answers submitted (Figure 1). The main goal is to promote the healing of the patient's wound by selecting the best diagnosis and treatment solution, in this order.

The effectiveness of e-FER was demonstrated by Costa (2010), showing that students developed their skills in all assessment parameters – infection, type of wound, type of tissue, wound cleaning, wound-dressing material and complementary procedure – except for the wound depth. The e-FER simulator saves all participants data in a file that can easily be extracted for further analysis of performance.

The AR component was created using user-friendly technology, both for the production of the 3D objects and its implementation in an AR mobile application. For this study 6 clinical cases were created and added to e-FER.

*Figure 1. View of a clinical case in the e-FER web based simulator that shows feedback given after answer submission*

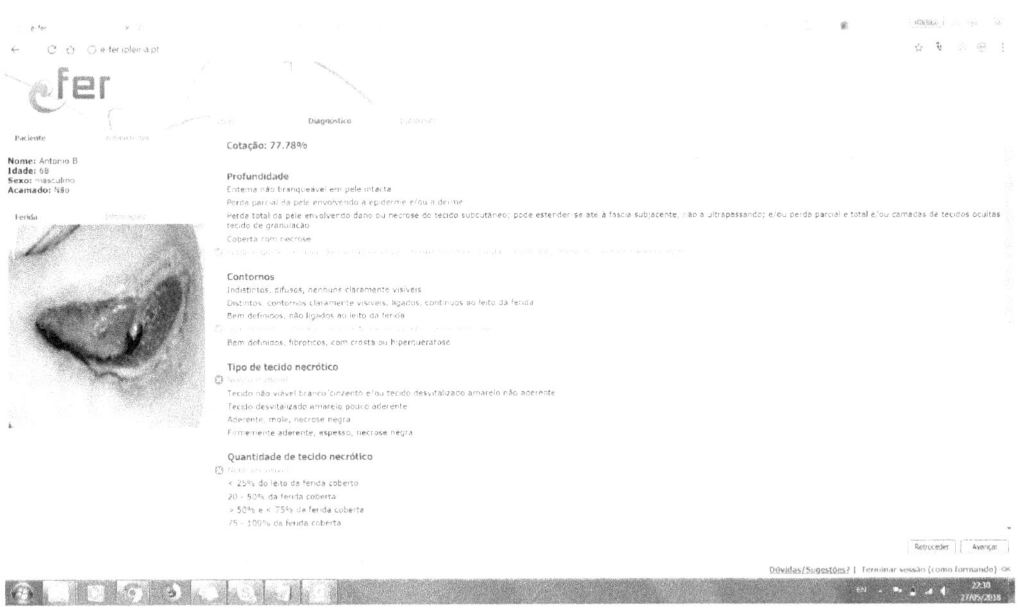

The objects for these new cases were produced using Autodesk® 123D® Catch, a software that generates 3D objects based on several pictures taken from different angles, as shown in figure 2.

After producing the objects the files were uploaded to ViewAR, a software that uses printed markers to show the 3D objects in AR, when detected by an iPad with the application installed.

## Sample

In total, 54 participants completed the 4 week training period on wound care using the e-FER simulator. All participants were Nursing students in their first year of study with no previous clinical wound care experience. Informed consent was given by all participants, who voluntarily participated in this study.

## Procedure

A quasi experimental study with pre and post test was conducted with 54 participants that started the activity by solving clinical cases on e-FER during 2 weeks. After this period participants were split into control group (n=24) and experimental group (n=30) for the second part of the activity. The control group kept solving clinical cases as they were used to in the e-FER simulator. The experimental group also solved the clinical cases using e-FER, but observed and analysed the wounds with AR (figure 3).

Since the e-FER simulator is web based, participants could solve the clinical cases at their own time and pace. However, due to technical reasons, a room with 4 laptops and 2 iPads was arranged in order to facilitate participants from the experimental group to carry out the activity. After 4 weeks the data with the participants performance was extracted from e-FER. All data from the 4 week period of training was extracted only in the end, since it could easily be split into pre test and post test data by dates. In this way, the data from the pre test corresponded to the first 2 weeks, whereas the data from the post

*Figure 2. Creating a 3D wound with Autodesk® 123D® Catch*

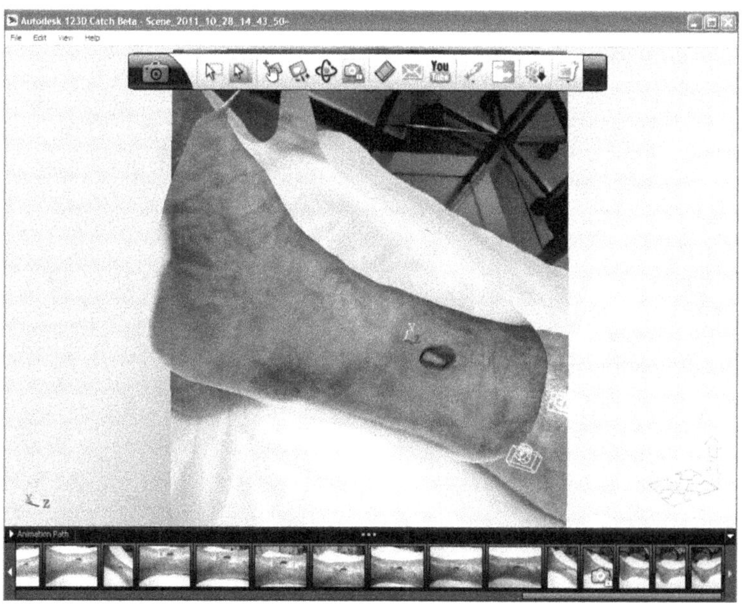

*Figure 3. Students from the experimental group solving clinical cases with e-FER while using AR to observe the chronic wounds*

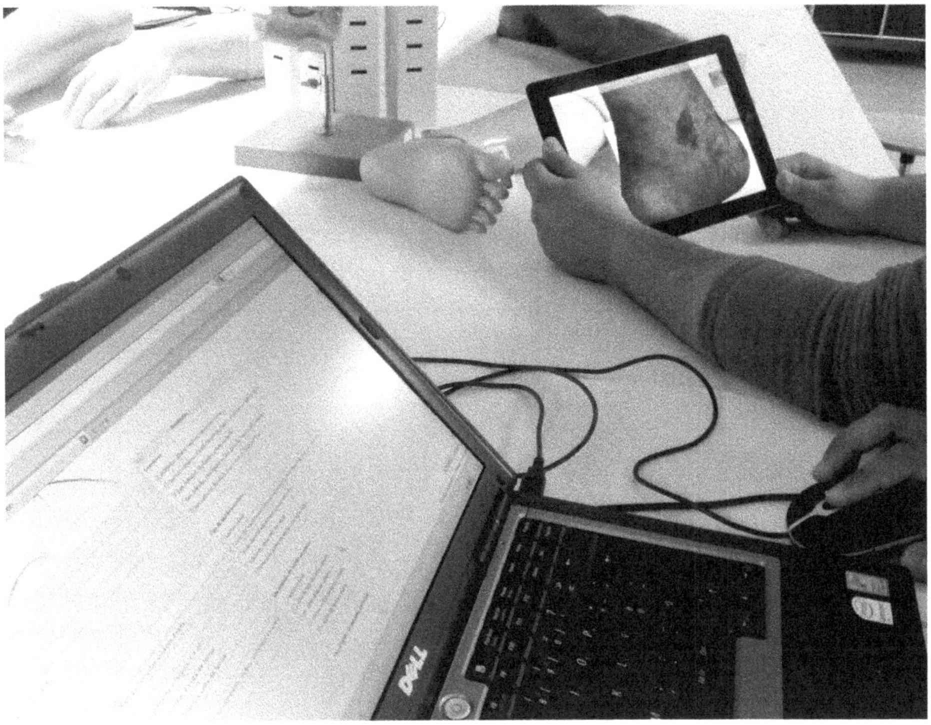

test corresponded to the last 2 weeks. Regarding student's motivation and the usability of the system, a validated survey was conducted after each moment of the investigation, each corresponding to a 2 week period, as explained previously.

## Data Analysis

All data was collected from the motivation and usability survey and extracted from the e-FER simulator, processed and analysed anonymously using Statistical Package for the Social Sciences 20.0 for Windows (SPSS Inc., Chicago, IL). The Mann–Whitney U test and Wilcoxon signed-rank test were used to compare and analyse the differences in performance, motivation and usability, between and within groups respectively. A p value $< 0.05$ was considered statistically significant.

## Results and Discussion

The results after statistical treatment of the data extracted from e-FER are based on the correct number of answers per clinical case given by students. The Mann-Whitney U test was used to compare groups. As shown in table 1, no statistically significant differences were found between the two groups in the pre test, which validates the homogeneity of the groups before manipulating the independent variable, when both groups were using the traditional e-FER without AR.

*Table 1. Parameters of both groups (n = 54) in the diagnosis and comparison (Mann-Whitney U test) in the pre test*

| Parameters | Control (n=24) | | Experimental (n=30) | | Mann-Whitney U Test |
|---|---|---|---|---|---|
| | M | SD | M | SD | p Value |
| Depth | 2,47 | 1,49 | 2,37 | 1,14 | 0,924 |
| Edges | 2,08 | 1,07 | 2,01 | 0,87 | 0,828 |
| Type of necrotic tissue | 2,20 | 1,14 | 2,15 | 0,98 | 1,000 |
| Amount of necrotic tissue | 2,24 | 1,11 | 2,09 | 1,04 | 0,531 |
| Color of surrounding tissue | 2,04 | 0,89 | 1,89 | 0,73 | 0,554 |
| Granulation tissue | 2,15 | 1,05 | 2,08 | 0,83 | 0,979 |
| Epithelial tissue | 2,41 | 1,09 | 2,32 | 0,92 | 0,958 |
| Wound type | 2,79 | 1,65 | 2,64 | 1,42 | 0,754 |
| Infection | 2,86 | 1,66 | 2,74 | 1,47 | 0,774 |
| Diagnosis (total) | 21,23 | 10,87 | 20,28 | 9,14 | 0,889 |

In the second moment, when the experimental group used e-FER with AR, statistically significant differences were revealed in all parameters, except for the Type of necrotic tissue, as shown in table 2. The means (M) obtained by the experimental group raised significantly in the second moment, while the control group had a similar performance.

In the treatment phase no statistically significant differences were revealed in all parameters, after applying the same statistical tests to the extracted data. In fact, it's in the diagnosis phase that observing the wound is critical for a correct decision. In the treatment step, observation takes a secondary role, since it depends on the correct diagnosis previously realized.

*Table 2. Parameters of both groups (n = 54) in the diagnosis and comparison (Mann-Whitney U test) in the post test*

| Parameters | Control (n=24) | | Experimental (n=30) | | Mann-Whitney U Test |
|---|---|---|---|---|---|
| | M | SD | M | SD | p Value |
| Depth | 2,03 | 0,99 | 4,28 | 2,18 | 0,000 |
| Edges | 1,86 | 0,79 | 3,72 | 1,56 | 0,000 |
| Type of necrotic tissue | 1,92 | 0,93 | 2,29 | 1,10 | 0,182 |
| Amount of necrotic tissue | 1,85 | 0,89 | 2,85 | 0,80 | 0,000 |
| Color of surrounding tissue | 1,83 | 0,91 | 3,52 | 1,31 | 0,000 |
| Granulation tissue | 1,78 | 0,96 | 2,48 | 0,97 | 0,002 |
| Epithelial tissue | 2,27 | 1,35 | 4,14 | 1,20 | 0,000 |
| Wound type | 2,38 | 1,47 | 4,69 | 1,58 | 0,000 |
| Infection | 2,43 | 1,51 | 5,13 | 1,91 | 0,000 |
| Diagnosis (total) | 18,35 | 8,92 | 33,10 | 11,05 | 0,000 |

In this way, observing the wound with AR proved to have a positive effect in the overall diagnosis phase on the experimental group, with highly statistically significant differences ($p<0.001$).

Regarding students' motivation and usability of the system, no statistically significant differences were found between groups and moments. Both motivation and usability variables kept at high levels when comparing the experimental and control group in the different moments of the investigation.

## FUTURE RESEARCH DIRECTIONS

From a usability point of view, it would be interesting to develop a single system, accessible via mobile device, that would show in the same screen the 3D wound, additional information to support the clinical decision-making and the diagnosis and treatment questionnaires.

The use of AR glasses would also be a path to develop and explore, since it would create a more similar experience to what students will encounter in their future professional practice, since it would free both hands instead of having to hold a mobile device.

Additionally, adding a haptic feedback system would enable to practice the treatment stage by performing proper wound care, including wound cleaning and applying wound dressing. This would offer a more comprehensive learning simulator system that includes decision-making and practical procedures, closer to real-life practice.

Developing these ideas and understanding their effect on learning, motivation and usability are therefore future research possibilities to consider.

## CONCLUSION

In this study an AR component was added to an online clinical decision-making simulator, with new clinical cases, creating an augmented learning environment where students could observe 3D chronic wounds in a more realistic and natural way, simulating real practice.

The goal of this investigation (a quasi experimental study with pre and post test was conducted with 54 participants that started the activity by solving clinical cases without AR during 2 weeks) was to verify if AR enhances the development of clinical decision-making skills in wound diagnosis and treatment. The results showed that AR enhanced students' performance in wound diagnostic parameters, with highly statistically significant differences ($p<0.001$) in the Mann-Whitney U test.

Factors such as motivation and usability, also object of this study, maintained high levels without interfering with the results. The high motivation of the participants is a positive result as well as the usability of the system since an additional device was used for AR, a condition that could have interfered with this last factor.

As for many studies of AR in medical education that were found in the literature review, we're aware that the size and convenience of the sample limits the generalization of these results. However, we believe that this study may represent another step in creating augmented learning environments, closer to what students will encounter in real-world scenarios, and that the intelligent use of technologies like AR is making possible.

## REFERENCES

Abhari, K., Baxter, J. S. H., Chen, E. C. S., Khan, A. R., Peters, T. M., de Ribaupierre, S., & Eagleson, R. (2015). Training for Planning Tumour Resection: Augmented Reality and Human Factors. *IEEE Transactions on Biomedical Engineering*, *62*(6), 1466–1477. doi:10.1109/TBME.2014.2385874 PMID:25546854

Ahn, J., Del Core, M. A., Wukich, D. K., Liu, G. T., Lalli, T., VanPelt, M. D., & Raspovic, K. M. (2018). Scoring Mental Health Quality of Life With the SF-36 in Patients With and Without Diabetes Foot Complications. *The International Journal of Lower Extremity Wounds*, *17*(1), 30–35. doi:10.1177/1534734618762226 PMID:29546783

Alaraj, A., Charbel, F. T., Birk, D., Tobin, M., Luciano, C., Banerjee, P. P., ... Roitberg, B. (2013). Role of cranial and spinal virtual and augmented reality simulation using immersive touch modules in neurosurgical training. *Neurosurgery*, *72*(1), 115–123. doi:10.1227/NEU.0b013e3182753093 PMID:23254799

Arvanitis, T. N., Petrou, A., Knight, J. F., Savas, S., Sotiriou, S., Gargalakos, M., & Gialouri, E. (2007). Human factors and qualitative pedagogical evaluation of a mobile augmented reality system for science education used by learners with physical disabilities. *Personal and Ubiquitous Computing*, *13*(3), 243–250. doi:10.100700779-007-0187-7

Azuma, R. (1997). A Survey of Augmented Reality. *Presence (Cambridge, Mass.)*, *6*(4), 355–385. doi:10.1162/pres.1997.6.4.355

Bergig, O., Hagbi, N., El-Sana, J., & Billinghurst, M. (2009). In-place 3D sketching for authoring and augmenting mechanical systems. In *Mixed and Augmented Reality, 2009. ISMAR 2009. 8th IEEE International Symposium on* (pp. 87-94). IEEE. doi: 10.1109/ISMAR.2009.5336490

Birchfield, D., & Megowan-Romanowicz, C. (2009). Earth science learning in SMALLab: A design experiment for mixed reality. *International Journal of Computer-Supported Collaborative Learning*, *4*(4), 403–421. doi:10.100711412-009-9074-8

Botden, S. M. B. I., Buzink, S. N., Schijven, M. P., & Jakimowicz, J. J. (2008). ProMIS Augmented Reality Training of Laparoscopic Procedures Face Validity. *Simulation in Healthcare*, *3*(2), 97–102. doi:10.1097/SIH.0b013e3181659e91 PMID:19088648

Brinkman, W. M., Havermans, S. Y., Buzink, S. N., Botden, S. M. B. I., Jakimowicz, J. J., & Schoot, B. C. (2012). Single versus multimodality training basic laparoscopic skills. *Surgical Endoscopy and Other Interventional Techniques, 26*(8), 2172-2178. doi:10.100700464-012-2184-9

Broll, W., Lindt, I., Herbst, I., Ohlenburg, J., Braun, A. K., & Wetzel, R. (2008). Toward next-gen mobile AR games. *Computer Graphics and Applications, IEEE, 28*(4), 40–48. doi:10.1109/MCG.2008.85

Bronack, S. C. (2011). The role of immersive media in online education. *Journal of Continuing Higher Education*, *59*(2), 113–117. doi:10.1080/07377363.2011.583186

Chang, H. Y., Wu, H. K., & Hsu, Y. S. (2013). Integrating a mobile augmented reality activity to contextualize student learning of a socioscientific issue. *British Journal of Educational Technology*, *44*(3), E95–E99. doi:10.1111/j.1467-8535.2012.01379.x

Chen, Y.-C. (2006). A study of comparing the use of augmented reality and physical models in chemistry education. In *Proceedings of the 2006 ACM international conference on Virtual reality continuum and its applications* (pp. 369-372). Hong Kong, China: ACM. 10.1145/1128923.1128990

Chen, Y.-C., Chi, H.-L., Hung, W.-H., & Kang, S.-C. (2011). Use of tangible and augmented reality models in engineering graphics courses. *Journal of Professional Issues in Engineering Education and Practice*, *137*(4), 267–276. doi:10.1061/(ASCE)EI.1943-5541.0000078

Chien, C. H., Chen, C. H., & Jeng, T. S. (2010, March). An Interactive Augmented Reality System for Learning Anatomy Structure. *Proceedings of the International MultiConference of Engineers and Computer Scientists*, *1*, 17–19.

Corrêa, N. F. M., de Brito, M. J. A., de Carvalho Resende, M. M., Duarte, M. F. P., Santos, F. S., Salomé, G. M., & Ferreira, L. M. (2016). Impact of surgical wound dehiscence on health-related quality of life and mental health. *Journal of Wound Care*, *25*(10), 561–570. doi:10.12968/jowc.2016.25.10.561 PMID:27681586

Costa, J. (2010). *Efetividade de um Web Based Learning para o desenvolvimento de competências no âmbito das feridas crónicas* (Unpublished Doctoral dissertation). Polytechnic University of Catalonia, Barcelona, Spain.

De Paolis, L. T., Pulimeno, M., & Aloisio, G. (2008). An augmented reality application for minimally invasive surgery. In *IFMBE Proceedings 14th Nordic-Baltic Conference on Biomedical Engineering and Medical Physics* (pp. 489-492). Springer. 10.1007/978-3-540-69367-3_131

Dede, C. (2009). Immersive interfaces for engagement and learning. *Science*, *323*(5910), 66–69. doi:10.1126cience.1167311 PMID:19119219

Dunleavy, M., Dede, C., & Mitchell, R. (2009). Affordances and limitations of immersive participatory augmented reality simulations for teaching and learning. *Journal of Science Education and Technology*, *18*(1), 7–22. doi:10.100710956-008-9119-1

Ellaway, R. (2010). eMedical Teacher. *Medical Teacher*, *32*(9), 791–793. doi:10.3109/0142159X.2010.513223 PMID:20795817

Feifer, A., Delisle, J., & Anidjar, M. (2008). Hybrid augmented reality simulator: Preliminary construct validation of laparoscopic smoothness in a urology residency program. *The Journal of Urology*, *180*(4), 1455–1459. doi:10.1016/j.juro.2008.06.042 PMID:18710760

Feng, J. Y., Chang, Y. T., Chang, H. Y., Erdley, W. S., Lin, C. H., & Chang, Y. J. (2013). Systematic review of effectiveness of situated e-learning on medical and nursing education. *Worldviews on Evidence-Based Nursing*, *10*(3), 174–183. doi:10.1111/wvn.12005 PMID:23510119

Fjeld, M., & Voegtli, B. M. (2002). *Augmented chemistry: An interactive educational workbench.* International symposium on mixed and augmented reality (ISMAR), Darmstadt, Germany. doi:10.1109/ISMAR.2002.1115100

Fjeld, M., & Voegtli, B. M. (2002, September). Augmented chemistry: An interactive educational workbench. In *Proceedings of the 1st international Symposium on Mixed and Augmented Reality* (p. 259). IEEE Computer Society. 10.1109/ISMAR.2002.1115100

Gorecki, C., Nixon, J., Lamping, D. L., Alavi, Y., & Brown, J. M. (2014). Patient-reported outcome measures for chronic wounds with particular reference to pressure ulcer research: A systematic review. *International Journal of Nursing Studies*, *51*(1), 157–165. doi:10.1016/j.ijnurstu.2013.03.004 PMID:23522938

Hansen, C., Wieferich, J., Ritter, F., Rieder, C., & Peitgen, H.-O. (2009). Illustrative visualization of 3D planning models for augmented reality in liver surgery. *International Journal of Computer Assisted Radiology and Surgery*, *5*(2), 133–141. doi:10.100711548-009-0365-3 PMID:20033519

Hemingway, S., Atkin, L., & Stephenson, J. (2013). Assessing and managing wounds in mental health settings. *Wounds UK*, *9*(3), 34–40.

Herber, O. R., Schepp, W., & Rieger, M. A. (2007). A systematic review on the impact of leg ulceration on patients' quality of life. *Health and Quality of Life Outcomes*, *5*(1), 44. doi:10.1186/1477-7525-5-44 PMID:17651490

Hogan, M., Sabri, H., & Kapralos, B. (2007). Interactive community simulation environment for community health nursing. In *Proceedings of the 2007 conference on Future Play* (pp. 237-240). ACM. 10.1145/1328202.1328248

Hopman, W. M., Harrison, M. B., Coo, H., Friedberg, E., Buchanan, M., & VanDenKerkhof, E. G. (2009). Associations between chronic disease, age and physical and mental health status. *Chronic Diseases in Canada*, *29*(3), 108–116. PMID:19527569

Johnson, L., Adams Becker, S., Cummins, M., Estrada, V., Freeman, A., & Hall, C. (2016). *NMC Horizon Report: 2016 Higher Education Edition.* Austin, TX: The New Media Consortium.

Johnson, L., Levine, A., Smith, R., & Stone, S. (2010). *The 2010 Horizon Report.* Austin, TX: The New Media Consortium.

Johnson, L., Smith, R., Willis, H., Levine, A., & Haywood, K. (2011). *The 2011 Horizon Report.* Austin, TX: The New Media Consortium.

Jones, J., Barr, W., Robinson, J. & Carlisle, C. (2006). Depression in patients with chronic venous ulceration. *British Journal of Nursing, 15*(Sup2), S17-S23.

Kamphuis, C., Barsom, E., Schijven, M., & Christoph, N. (2014). Augmented reality in medical education? *Perspectives on Medical Education*, *3*(4), 300–311. doi:10.100740037-013-0107-7 PMID:24464832

Kaufmann, H., Steinbugl, K., Dunser, A., & Gluck, J. (2005). General training of spatial abilities by geometry education in augmented reality. *Cyberpsychology & Behavior*, *8*(4), 330.

Kerawalla, L., Luckin, R., Seljeflot, S., & Woolard, A. (2006). "Making it real": Exploring the potential of augmented reality for teaching primary school science. *Virtual Reality (Waltham Cross)*, *10*(3-4), 163–174. doi:10.100710055-006-0036-4

Klopfer, E. (2008). *Augmented learning: Research and design of mobile educational games*. Cambridge, MA: MIT Press. doi:10.7551/mitpress/9780262113151.001.0001

Klopfer, E., & Sheldon, J. (2010). Augmenting your own reality: Student authoring of science-based augmented reality games. *New Directions for Youth Development*, *2010*(128), 85–94. doi:10.1002/yd.378 PMID:21240956

Klopfer, E., & Squire, K. (2008). Environmental detectives: The development of an augmented reality platform for environmental simulations. *Educational Technology Research and Development*, *56*(2), 203–228. doi:10.100711423-007-9037-6

Kotranza, A., Lind, D. S., Pugh, C. M., & Lok, B. (2009). Real-time in-situ visual feedback of task performance in mixed environments for learning joint psychomotorcognitive tasks In *Mixed and Augmented Reality, 2009. ISMAR 2009. 8th IEEE International Symposium on* (pp. 125-134). IEEE. doi: 10.1109/ISMAR.2009.5336485

Leblanc, F., Delaney, C. P., Ellis, C. N., Neary, P. C., Champagne, B. J., & Senagore, A. J. (2010). Hand-Assisted Versus Straight Laparoscopic Sigmoid Colectomy on a Training Simulator: What is the Difference? A Stepwise Comparison of Hand-Assisted Versus Straight Laparoscopic Sigmoid Colectomy Performance on an Augmented Reality Simulator. *World Journal of Surgery*, *34*(12), 2909–2914. doi:10.100700268-010-0765-0 PMID:20740283

Lewis, M. J., Davies, R., Jenkins, D., & Tait, M. I. (2005). A review of evaluative studies of computer-based learning in nursing education. *Nurse Education Today*, *25*(8), 586–597. doi:10.1016/j.nedt.2005.09.006 PMID:16289489

Liu, W., Cheok, A. D., Mei-Ling, C. L., & Theng, Y. L. (2007, September). Mixed reality classroom: learning from entertainment. In *Proceedings of the 2nd international conference on Digital interactive media in entertainment and arts* (pp. 65-72). ACM.

Luciano, C. J., Banerjee, P. P., Bellotte, B., Oh, G. M., Lemole, M. Jr, Charbel, F. T., & Roitberg, B. (2011). Learning Retention of Thoracic Pedicle Screw Placement Using a High-Resolution Augmented Reality Simulator With Haptic Feedback. *Neurosurgery*, *69*, 14–19. doi:10.1227/NEU.0b013e31821954ed PMID:21471846

Maran, N. J., & Glavin, R. J. (2003). Low- to high-fidelity simulation – a continuum of medical education? *Medical Education*, *37*(1), 22–28. doi:10.1046/j.1365-2923.37.s1.9.x PMID:14641635

Mitha, A. P., Almekhlafi, M. A., Janjua, M. J. J., Albuquerque, F. C., & McDougall, C. G. (2013). Simulation and augmented reality in endovascular neurosurgery: Lessons from aviation. *Neurosurgery*, *72*(1), 107–114. doi:10.1227/NEU.0b013e31827981fd PMID:23254798

Monguet, J. M., Costa, J., Gaspar, P., & Costa, R. (2009). Web Based Learning Environment for medical education: E-fer, a practical tool for diagnosis and treatment of chronic wounds. In M. Manuela Cunha, A. Tavares, & R. Simões (Eds.), *Handbook of Research on Developments in e-Health and Telemedicine: Technological and Social Perspectives* (pp. 728–755). Hershey, PA: IGI Global.

Monkman, H., & Kushniruk, A. W. (2015). A see through future: Augmented reality and health information systems. *Studies in Health Technology and Informatics*, *208*, 281–285. PMID:25676988

Moult, E., Ungi, T., Welch, M., Lu, J., McGraw, R. C., & Fichtinger, G. (2013). Ultrasound-guided facet joint injection training using Perk Tutor. *International Journal of Computer Assisted Radiology and Surgery*, *8*(5), 831–836. doi:10.100711548-012-0811-5 PMID:23329279

Nugent, E., Shirilla, N., Hafeez, A., O'Riordain, D. S., Traynor, O., Harrison, A. M., & Neary, P. (2013). Development and evaluation of a simulator-based laparoscopic training program for surgical novices. *Surgical Endoscopy and other Interventional Techniques*, *27*(1), 214-221. doi:10.100700464-012-2423-0

Oostema, J. A., Abdel, M. P., & Gould, J. C. (2008). Time-efficient laparoscopic skills assessment using an augmented-reality simulator. *Surgical Endoscopy and other Interventional Techniques*, *22*(12), 2621-2624. doi:10.100700464-008-9844-9

Phillips, C. J., Humphreys, I., Fletcher, J., Harding, K., Chamberlain, G., & Macey, S. (2016). Estimating the costs associated with the management of patients with chronic wounds using linked routine data. *International Wound Journal*, *13*(6), 1193–1197. doi:10.1111/iwj.12443 PMID:25818405

Reitinger, B., Bornik, A., Beichel, R., & Schmalstieg, D. (2006). Liver surgery planning using virtual reality. *IEEE Computer Graphics and Applications*, *26*(6), 36–47. doi:10.1109/MCG.2006.131 PMID:17120912

Renner, R., & Erfurt-Berge, C. (2017). Depression and quality of life in patients with chronic wounds: Ways to measure their influence and their effect on daily life. *Chronic Wound Care Management and Research*, *4*, 143–151. doi:10.2147/CWCMR.S124917

Rey, G., Visconti, A., Balaguer, E., & Martínez, J. (2006). Uso de simuladores en ginecología y obstetricia: Experiencia en la enseñanza de pregrado. *Educação Médica*, *9*(4b), 229–233.

Shuhaiber, J. H. (2004). Augmented reality in surgery. *Archives of Surgery*, *139*(2), 170–174. doi:10.1001/archsurg.139.2.170 PMID:14769575

Sotiriou, S., & Bogner, F. X. (2008). Visualizing the invisible: Augmented reality as an innovative science education scheme. *Advanced Science Letters*, *1*(1), 114–122. doi:10.1166/asl.2008.012

Squire, K., & Jan, M. (2007). Mad city mystery: Developing scientific argumentation skills with a place-based augmented reality game on handheld computers. *Journal of Science Education and Technology*, *16*(1), 5–29. doi:10.100710956-006-9037-z

Squire, K., & Klopfer, E. (2007). Augmented reality simulations on handheld computers. *Journal of the Learning Sciences*, *16*(3), 371–413. doi:10.1080/10508400701413435

Sutherland, C., Hashtrudi-Zaad, K., Sellens, R., Abolmaesumi, P., & Mousavi, P. (2013). An Augmented Reality Haptic Training Simulator for Spinal Needle Procedures. *IEEE Transactions on Biomedical Engineering*, *60*(11), 3009–3018. doi:10.1109/TBME.2012.2236091 PMID:23269747

Trindade, J., Kirner, C., & Fiolhais, C. (2004). Orbitário: Exploração de Orbitais Hidrogenoides com Realidade Aumentada. In J. Pérez, J. Pulido, M. Rodríguez, B. Manjón, J. Rodríguez (Eds.), Avances en Informática Educativa, artículos selecionados del VI Simpósio Internacional de Informática Educativa. Academic Press.

Ungi, T., Sargent, D., Moult, E., Lasso, A., Pinter, C., McGraw, R. C., & Fichtinger, G. (2012). Perk Tutor: An Open-Source Training Platform for Ultrasound-Guided Needle Insertions. *IEEE Transactions on Biomedical Engineering*, *59*(12), 3475–3481. doi:10.1109/TBME.2012.2219307 PMID:23008243

Upton, D., & Hender, C. (2012). The cost of mood disorders in patients with chronic wounds. *Wounds UK*, *8*(1), 107–109.

Upton, D., Solowiej, K., & Woo, K. Y. (2014). A multinational health professional perspective of the prevalence of mood disorders in patients with acute and chronic wounds. *International Wound Journal*, *11*(6), 627–635. doi:10.1111/iwj.12018 PMID:23289905

Upton, D., Upton, P., & Alexander, R. (2015). The complexity of caring (Part 1): Detrimental health and well-being outcomes for caregivers of people with chronic wounds. *Wound Practice & Research: Journal of the Australian Wound Management Association*, *23*(3), 104.

Vera, A. M., Russo, M., Mohsin, A., & Tsuda, S. (2014). Augmented reality telementoring (ART) platform: a randomized controlled trial to assess the efficacy of a new surgical education technology. *Surgical Endoscopy and other Interventional Techniques*, *28*(12), 3467-3472. doi:10.100700464-014-3625-4

Vikal, S., U-Thainual, P., Carrino, J. A., Iordachita, I., Fischer, G. S., & Fichtinger, G. (2010). Perk Station-Percutaneous surgery training and performance measurement platform. *Computerized Medical Imaging and Graphics*, *34*(1), 19–32. doi:10.1016/j.compmedimag.2009.05.001 PMID:19539446

Wu, H.-K., Lee, S. W.-Y., Chang, H.-Y., & Liang, J.-C. (2013). Current status, opportunities and challenges of augmented reality in education. *Computers & Education*, *62*, 41–49. doi:10.1016/j.compedu.2012.10.024

Yeo, C. T., Ungi, T., U-Thainual, P., Lasso, A., McGraw, R. C., & Fichtinger, G. (2011). The Effect of Augmented Reality Training on Percutaneous Needle Placement in Spinal Facet Joint Injections. *IEEE Transactions on Biomedical Engineering*, *58*(7), 2031–2037. doi:10.1109/TBME.2011.2132131 PMID:21435970

Zhou, F., Duh, H. B.-L., & Billinghurst, M. (2008). Trends in augmented reality tracking, interaction and display: A review of ten years of ISMAR. In *Proceedings of the 7th IEEE/ACM International Symposium on Mixed and Augmented Reality* (pp.193-202). IEEE Computer Society.

Zhu, E., Hadadgar, A., Masiello, I., & Zary, N. (2014). Augmented reality in healthcare education: An integrative review. *PeerJ*, *2*, e469. doi:10.7717/peerj.469 PMID:25071992

## ADDITIONAL READING


Gupta, N., & Rohil, M. K. (2017, February). Exploring possible applications of augmented reality in education. In *Signal Processing and Integrated Networks (SPIN), 2017 4th International Conference on* (pp. 437-441). IEEE 10.1109/SPIN.2017.8049989

Jorge, N. (2016). *Realidade aumentada num simulador virtual de tomada de decisão clínica.* (Unpublished doctoral dissertation). Universidade Aberta, Lisboa. Retrieved May 3, 2017, from http://hdl.handle.net/10400.2/6676

Kuehn, B. M. (2018). Virtual and Augmented Reality Put a Twist on Medical Education. *Journal of the American Medical Association*, *319*(8), 756–758. doi:10.1001/jama.2017.20800 PMID:29417140

Marescaux, J., Rubino, F., Arenas, M., Mutter, D., & Soler, L. (2004). Augmented reality–assisted laparoscopic adrenalectomy. *Journal of the American Medical Association*, *292*(18), 2211–2215. doi:10.1001/jama.292.18.2214-c PMID:15536106

Meng, M., Fallavollita, P., Blum, T., Eck, U., Sandor, C., Weidert, S., . . . Navab, N. (2013, October). Kinect for interactive AR anatomy learning. In *Mixed and Augmented Reality (ISMAR), 2013 IEEE International Symposium* on (pp. 277-278). IEEE. 10.1109/ISMAR.2013.6671803

Moro, C., Štromberga, Z., Raikos, A., & Stirling, A. (2017). The effectiveness of virtual and augmented reality in health sciences and medical anatomy. *Anatomical Sciences Education*, *10*(6), 549–559. doi:10.1002/ase.1696 PMID:28419750

Portalés, C., Gimeno, J., Vera, L., & Fernández, M. (2015). Towards a guidance system to aid in the dosimetry calculation of intraoperative electron radiation therapy. *Journal of Imaging*, *1*(1), 180–192. doi:10.3390/jimaging1010180

Ruiz, J. G., Mintzer, M. J., & Leipzig, R. M. (2006). The impact of e-learning in medical education. *Academic Medicine*, *81*(3), 207–212. doi:10.1097/00001888-200603000-00002 PMID:16501260

Sen, A., Chuen, C. L., & Hta, A. C. Z. (2018). Toward Smart Learning Environments: Affordances and Design Architecture of Augmented Reality (AR) Applications in Medical Education. In *Proceedings of First International Conference on Smart System, Innovations and Computing* (pp. 843-861). Springer, Singapore. 10.1007/978-981-10-5828-8_80

Sen, A., Chuen, C. L., Liew, S. H., & Hta, A. C. Z. (2017, July). Augmented Reality as a Tool for Authentic Learning of Clinical Skills in Early Years of Medical Training. In *IFIP World Conference on Computers in Education* (pp. 231-242). Springer, Cham. 10.1007/978-3-319-74310-3_25

van Oosterom, M. N., van der Poel, H. G., Navab, N., van de Velde, C. J., & van Leeuwen, F. W. (2018). Computer-assisted surgery: Virtual-and augmented-reality displays for navigation during urological interventions. *Current Opinion in Urology*, *28*(2), 205–213. PMID:29278582

Wilhelm, D., Vogel, T., Ostler, D., Marahrens, N., Kohn, N., Koller, S., Friess, H. & Kranzfelder, M. (2018). Enhanced Visualization: From Intraoperative Tissue Differentiation to Augmented Reality. *Visceral Medicine*, 34.

## KEY TERMS AND DEFINITIONS

**Augmented Reality:** A technology that allows the live integration of digital content into the physical real world, in order to enrich the users' environment and experience.

**Clinical Decision Making:** A type of informal decision-making that combines clinical expertise, patient concerns, and evidence gathered from scientific literature to arrive at a diagnosis and treatment recommendations.

**Digital Learning:** A method that uses digital content, activities, tools, and technologies to facilitate learning.

**Medical Education:** The provision of instruction and information in the sciences basic to medicine and in clinical practice, ideally in such a manner as to inculcate in the student the desire to continue the process, spontaneously, throughout life.

**Situated Learning:** A theory that argues that learning occurs naturally when students are immersed in contextual, cultural, and authentic real-life activities.

**Virtual Reality:** A technology that creates a simulated environment to replace the existing real world.

**Web-Based Learning Simulator (e-FER):** Software developed for training, certification, modeling, and demonstrating problems in the management of healthcare, namely in diagnosis and treatment of chronic wounds.

# Chapter 15
# Look of Life:
## The Wonder Therapy

**Vittoria Sichi**
*ANT Foundation, Italy*

**Giacomo Ercolani**
*ANT Foundation, Italy*

**Luca Franchini**
*ANT Foundation, Italy*

**Luca Golfari**
*ANT Foundation, Italy*

**Silvia Varani**
*ANT Foundation, Italy*

**Daniela Rizzoli**
*ANT Foundation, Italy*

**Raffaella Pannuti**
*ANT Foundation, Italy*

**Daniele Roganti**
*ANT Foundation, Italy*

## ABSTRACT

*The use of virtual reality (VR) shows promising results in improving the emotional wellbeing of cancer patients, reducing anxiety, depression, and pain symptoms. No data exist concerning the use of VR in cancer patients assisted at home. The ANT Foundation decided to conduct a pilot study to test the use of VR in cancer patients assisted at home. Fifty-eight ANT patients were randomized and assigned to a control group that didn't use VR devices and to an experimental group that used them. The primary objective of the pilot study was to determine whether VR device could be a viable instrument in homecare patients. Furthermore, the aim of the study was to discover if VR could have beneficial effects on patients' quality of life as well as discover which kind of videos were more effective. The innovative aspect of this study was to test the use of VR directly at home of patients, proposing a use of VR that is compatible with the needs and the daily rhythms of families, and investigating its effectiveness through appropriate validated psychometric questionnaires and semi-structured interviews.*

DOI: 10.4018/978-1-5225-7168-1.ch015

## INTRODUCTION

The experience of a cancer diagnosis and progression of the disease in its different phases can lead to psychological distress, relationship problems, cognitive limitations and numerous physical symptoms of a strong emotional impact. Besides compromising the physical health of the patient, cancer often causes psychological discomfort characterized by anxious and depressive symptoms that may be clinically significant in some cases. These factors can seriously affect the quality of life of the person and his family environment, hampering the adherence to treatment, the efficacy of therapies and deteriorating the clinical prognosis. Cancer greatly interferes with all aspects of daily life of the person affected, from family and personal relationships to business and financial areas. Numerous studies confirm that a high number of cancer patients experience severe levels of psychological distress such as depression and anxiety, with a percentage people affected respectively of 20% and 10% (Pitman et al., 2018). Contrary to expectations, percentages of people suffering of depression and anxiety in end-of-life phase do not differ significantly from those of patients in non-palliative care settings (Mitchell et al., 2011). In addition to the emotional distress related to the anguish of confronting death, advanced stages of the disease very often imply a progressive loss of functional autonomy. This puts the patient in a state of deprivation and forced isolation from a relational and social aspect that was hitherto part of their life. This state of psychological distress naturally adds to the burden of the physical symptoms caused by the disease and/or invasive therapies, above pain. The reduction of the opportunities in which it is possible to experience positive emotions and meaningful social interactions often corresponds to an intensification of the concerns and the obsessive thoughts, which in turn increase stress and connect to further negative emotional experiences. This vicious circle, in absence of rapid and effective intervention, risks to worsen patients' quality of life. Beyond pharmacological approach, complementary psychological techniques aiming to deflect patient's attention from unpleasant symptoms have been employed (e.g. muscular progressive relaxation, mindfulness, guided imagery). By moving attention towards neutral or positive emotions and sensations, these techniques may help patients to manage distress and pain.

## BACKGROUND

Alongside traditional interventions, in recent years several studies have tested the effectiveness of the use of immersive audiovisual technologies, which are able to emotionally involve the person, capture his attention and directing it to new stimuli (Nichols & Patel 2002; Spagnolli et al., 2003; Spagnolli & Gamberini, 2005; Scozzari & Gamberini, 2011; Gamberini & Spagnolli, 2015). Moreover, such a technology offers the significant advantage of being used in low mobility conditions and without specific and complicated training. In recent years, Virtual Reality (VR) has been employed with great success to manage anxiety in different anxiety disorders – through the Virtual Reality Exposure Therapy – chronic pain and acute pain in patients undergoing routine and invasive medical interventions (Li et al., 2011; Morina et al., 2015). Indeed, use of VR has shown promising results in reducing emotional and physical discomfort among cancer patients. A common disturbing experience relating to cancer is definitely pain: chronic cancer pain often involves persistent pain – which may last all day – and breakthrough pain–a brief flare-up of severe pain occurring even while patient is regularly taking pain medication. Cancer-related pain affects about 70% of patients and recent data suggest that it may be inadequately controlled in up to 50% of patients (Neufeld et al. 2017). VR has gained recognition as means of attenuating pain in several medical procedure, such as burn care procedures (Morris et al., 2009; Malloy & Milling, 2010). Scientific rationale behind the employment of this technology refers to Melzack and Wall's Gate Control Theory (1968) and to the observation of McCaul and Malot (1984) about role of attention and effect of distraction on the perception of painful stimuli. From a neurobiological point of view VR likely act differently from other known pain interventions. In particular, VR may affect the pain modulation system of body by acting directly and not on pain perception and signaling through senses, attention, memory and emotions: indeed, both attention and emotions are able to affect significantly pain perception via the descending pain-control system (Gold et al. 2007). Authors who have investigated feasibility and effectiveness of VR in cancer patients have applied this tool to pediatric settings certainly because of its playful character. In addition, several studies have investigated feasibility and effectiveness of VR as a tool for supporting and monitoring treatments in cancer adult patients by influencing their psychological and physiological functions (Chirico et al., 2016). As early as the late 1990's, Oyama (1997) already explored potential of VR for cancer patients in palliative care: the author argued that VR could enhance possibilities of communication both by creating a medical cyberspace to provide mental care and by allowing patients and relatives to communicate and support each other – reducing as a result loneliness and despair. Even though attention of research is currently concentrating on symptoms management, it is possible that these applications could be future directions of investigations on integration of technology in health system. Although this research field is steadily increasing – also because of the ongoing technological innovation –there is a lack of robust data concerning the use of VR in cancer patients assisted at home. It will be interesting testing the use of VR in this particular setting for two main reasons: first of all, nowadays VR is accessible almost to everyone, due to its partial low-cost; secondly, there is a growing interest in home care in term of cost and benefits for patients and his relatives. Therefore, the ANT Italian Foundation in collaboration with the Human Inspired Technology Research Centre (HIT) of University of Padova and with the cultural association MenoMale, decided to conduct a pilot exploratory study to test the feasibility of VR in cancer patients assisted at home.

## ANT ITALIA FOUNDATION

ANT is one of the leading organization, working in Italy in the field of palliative home care and pain management. ANT provides free social-health assistance at home to cancer sufferers and, depending on the resources available in the local area, runs free of charge cancer prevention initiatives. ANT's philosophy can be summed up by the term *Eubiosia* (from ancient Greek 'good life'), meaning overall quality to guarantee a dignified life right up until one's last breath. Since 1985, ANT has assisted more than 110.000 sufferers, completely free of charge, in 20home oncology clinics (ODO-ANT) in 9 Italian regions. There are currently 4.000patients receiving care throughout Italy every day. ANT offers specialized care provided by 433 healthcare professionals, including physicians, nurses, psychologists, nutritionists, physiotherapists, social-health workers, pharmacists who are able to provide patients with round the clock care, 365 days of the year.

## AIM

The primary objective of the pilot study was to determine whether VR device could be a viable instrument in home care patients. Furthermore, the aim of the study was to discover if VR could have beneficial effects on patient's quality of life as well as discover which kind of videos were more effective. The innovative aspect of this study was to test the use of VR directly at home of patients, proposing a use of VR that is compatible with the needs and the daily rhythms of families, and investigating its effectiveness through appropriate validated psychometric questionnaires and semi-structured interviews.

## VIRTUAL REALITY HEAD-MOUNTED DISPLAY

The VR device employed in the study is the Samsung Gear VR headset, a portable VR viewer developed from Samsung Electronics in collaboration with Oculus. The device is used in combination with Samsung Galaxy S6 Edge Plus, which performs the function of VR display. The Gear VR contains a sensor capable of perceiving the movement and rotation of the head and able to modulate the image according to the movement of the subject, giving the illusion of being immersed in a three-dimensional scenario. In this way Oculus reproduces 3D environments of everyday life giving you the feeling of actually being immersed in a virtual environment. There are twenty infrared sensors positioned on the viewer, which, when combined with a camera placed in front of the user, are able to detect any shifts in movement in 3 directions, thus allowing the users to be able to move in a 3D environment. The model also integrates the control box in the head-mounted display, a small box containing the control board that acts as a link between the screen and the device. It has a 7-inch LCD screen with a colour depth of 24 bits per pixel and is 3D stereoscopic enabled. The field of vision is of more than 90 degrees horizontally (110 degrees diagonal), which is more than double when compared to other competing devices. The resolution is 1280x800 (16:10 aspect ratio), i.e. 640 × 800 per eye (4: 5 aspect ratio).The viewer can be calibrated to compensate for visual disturbances such as myopia, thanks to a wheel on the front of the viewer that adjusts the focal distance of the lenses. The Gear VR used by the authors was released in November 2015 and it is one of the first devices for virtual reality to be used by a significant number of users.

## SAFETY PRECAUTIONS

The scientific literature has reported the possibility of some episodes of nausea during the exposure to VR, especially with the first types of devices, with particular contents and in predisposed subjects. However, in the case of the specific technology used by the authors (Samsung Gear VR), adverse effects have been reported only in very few cases, as demonstrated by the study of Mosadeghi et al. (2016), in which there was a single subject who experience nausea and therefore interrupted the vision. Video used in *The Look Of Life* have been selected because they contain the least possible amount of stimuli that can hinder motion sickness or emotional distress. At the same time, videos should provide audiovisual experiences considered pleasant and comfortable by the vast majority of users, according to reviews on the appropriate Samsung Gear VR market.All the videos have been specifically selected for content and duration by the scientific committee of the ANT Research Department in collaboration with the interdepartmental research center 'Human Inspired Technologies research center-HIT' of the University of Padova, headed by Professor Luciano Gamberini.

## SANITARY AND HYGIENIC PRECAUTIONS

Regarding the hygiene measures, authors followed the guidelines of the Health and Social Agency of Emilia-Romagna (Mongardi et al., 2011), concerning the disinfection of medical devices and equipment. Prior to each use by the subjects the viewer was disinfected with special disposable wipes (Clorox Disinfectant Wipes - Clorox Germicidal Wipes) and the lenses were cleaned with specific cloths based on alcohol. As an additional measure of safety, the viewer has not been placed directly in contact with the head and face of the subjects, but special disposable sterilized cloths have been used in order to minimize any direct contact with the device.

## SAMPLE

The study involved 58 ANT patients in the metropolitan area of Bologna. Exclusion criteria were: age> 18; presence of brain cancer or brain metastases; epilepsy; had a heart attack in the last year; suffering from a severe psychopathology (e.g. bipolar disorder, schizophrenia); inability to speak and read the Italian language. After the recruitment phase, the participants were randomized and assigned to a control group which didn't use VR device and to an intervention group that used it. Overall, the sample was composed by 32 females and 26 males and the average age was 50 years (between 25 and 60 years old) and most of participants were married or cohabited with partners (67%). As for occupation, 43% of sample worked at the time of the study whereas 39% were retired or in sick leave. Average Karnofsky Performance Status (KPS) score – a measure of functional impairment which allows physicians to assess how a patient's disease is progressing– was 72 ($\sigma = 15$). Average KPS did not differ significantly between control and intervention groups – respectively 72 and 73. Intervention group was composed by 14 females and 15 males and 76% of them were involved with someone and cohabited with their spouses or partners whereas 17% lived alone. As for level of education, half the group had high school diploma and 20% had a university degree or a postgraduate degree. Almost all of participants within intervention group were familiar with PC and smartphone, however none of them has reported to use virtual reality devices usually.

## PROCEDURE

ANT psychologists, adequately trained, met each patient in the experimental group four times in a week and during each meeting patients had the opportunity to see an immersive video. Videos shown to patients were selected on the basis of two focus groups conducted in October 2016 with groups of cancer patients followed by ANT. During the first and last meetings, intervention group also completed (before watching the first video and after watching the last video) a personal data card and two questionnaires: the Hospital Anxiety and Depression Scale (HADS) and the Brief Pain Inventory (BPI). During second and third meeting, before and after watching the videos, Edmonton Symptom Assessment Scale (ESAS), a visual-analogue scale for the assessment of symptoms in patients receiving palliative care, has been administered. The evaluated symptoms concerned pain, fatigue, nausea, depression, anxiety, drowsiness, loss of appetite, discomfort and difficulty in breathing. On the fourth day the patients of the experimental group were asked some questions about the frequency with which they would use the VR if they had the device at home. Patients were requested to describe the VR experience just ended: the purpose of the recorded audio interview was to investigate the opinions of the respondents about the effects experienced with VR and preferences for a hypothetical video specifically created for them. Answers to the questions were audio recorded and then categorized. As for patients in the control group, they only met the psychologist twice in a week for filling in the personal registry form and answering the same questionnaire of the experimental group, except for ESAS, which they did not complete. The quantitative data,related to the questionnaires compiled by the two groups, were statistically analyzed using the SPSS software. The authors conducted a qualitative analysis of the frequencies for the answers of the interviews. In particular, the answers were grouped into four thematic or macro-category areas (VR effects, attitude towards VR, preference for interactive videos, comfort) and each of them contained a different number of categories. This chapter will treat exclusively the qualitative results of the study.

## MEASURES

*Acute and chronic pain.* Acute and chronic pain were assessed using four items taken from the Italian version of Brief Pain Inventory - Short Form (Bonezzi et al., 2002), an easy-to-use pain assessment questionnaire which quantify the intensity of pain. It is characterized by a series of questions (descriptors) concerning the intensity of pain. Besides the intensity of current pain, levels of pain investigated are the maximum, minimum and average during the 24 hours before the test.

*Anxiety and depression.* Mood status, in particular anxiety and depression, was assessed through the Hospital Anxiety and Depression Scale - HADS (Zigmond & Snaith, 1983). This is a very simple scale consisting of 14 items which explore both anxiety and depression symptoms, keeping the two scores divided. The main characteristic of the scale is that it excludes the somatic symptomatology from the evaluation. The scale instead focuses, especially for depression, on the reduction of hedonic capacity, considering it among the most sensitive indicators in the diagnosis of this disorder.

*Other symptoms.* Other various symptoms were assessed through the ESAS (Edmonton Symptom Assessment Scale), which represents a scale composed by nine visual analog scales (VAS) that investigate specific symptoms such as pain, general activity, nausea, depression, anxiety, drowsiness, appetite, general well-being and shortness of breath.The patient attributes a severity score on a 100 mm line for each of these symptoms.

## RESULTS

From the qualitative analysis of the interviews, it appears that most of patients in the experimental group(73%) said they would like to have the instrument at home and that they would use it for a total daily duration ranging from 10 to 60 minutes. The experience of VR, has been defined as "pleasant" (term reported by 16 patients) and "innovative" (reported by 6).

*It was definitely a very good experience! After each use I'd go to speak, extremely enthusiastic, with my mother and sister and I told them "you know, I saw that thing and I tried to take it with my hands... wow!". Yes, it was a very impactful experience (Maria 25 years old)*

*It is something new (VR)... [..] Well it is something funny and innovative to do (Matteo 59 years old)*

Relaxation (reported by 10) and distraction (reported by 8) were the most commonly reported effects, followed by reassurance, amusement and amazement (reported by 4).

*mh... actually it helps to detach your mind from what you are doing and it casts you in something different... so it calms you down*

If a video could be created specifically for them all the patients said they would like to see natural scenarios. In addition, eleven patients (36%) said they preferred interactive videos while ten (33%) wanted to see videos in which they were more aloof as simple observers. All patients, even those who have openly declared themselves unfamiliar with technology, have found the viewer comfortable and easy to use. On the basis of the interviews and focus groups, ANT produced a video of the concert of the Oscar-winning composer Nicola Piovani, a video shot inside the Sigurtà garden park and one at Arte Sella, a contemporary art exhibition inserted in a natural context.These immersive videos were made through the use of complex equipment consisting of 14 cameras recording two spherical videos, one for the left hemisphere and one for the right hemisphere, able to faithfully reproduce the environment where the experience took place.

## CONCLUSION

The objective of this pilot study was to evaluate the home use of an innovative technology which has shown to have the potential to alleviate and improve some particular clinical and psychological conditions linked to disabling cancer diseases (Chirico et al., 2016).The VR device has also been appreciated by older patients and this suggests that its use could be extended to subjects with advanced age. More unambiguous and specific conclusions about effects of VR on psychological and physical state of patients can be drawn after that quantitative data will be analyzed. Of course, preliminary data are encouraging. Indeed, employment of VR among patients assisted by ANT seems to have brought positive effects in terms of physical sensations and emotions. Relaxation is definitely the most reported physical effect although short-lived and mild unpleasant physical sensations have been found in rare cases (e.g. mild lightheadedness during the use of device). However, it is reassuring to note that an extremely involving and potentially effective technology such as VR does not cause particular side effects in patients living a condition of frailty and sufferance. The study carried out by ANT Foundation is showing the great potential of VR with respect to the management of particular mood states such as anxiety, boredom and discomfort due to cancer disease and related therapies. Moreover, most of interviews conducted suggest that some experiences can generate positive emotions such as happiness and wonder, which have the potential to balance the empty often caused by being compelled at home and limited in daily activities and relationships.

## REFERENCES

Bonezzi, C., Nava, A., Barbieri, M., Demartini, L., Miotti, D., & Paulin, D. (2002). Validazione della versione italiana del Brief Pain Inventory nei pazienti con dolore cronico. *Minerva Anestesiologica*, *68*(7-8), 607–611. PMID:12244292

Chirico, A., Lucidi, F., De Laurentiis, M., Milanese, C., Napoli, A., & Giordano, A. (2016). Virtual Reality in health system: Beyond entertainment. A mini-review on the efficacy of VR during cancer treatment. *Journal of Cellular Physiology*, *231*(2), 275–287. doi:10.1002/jcp.25117 PMID:26238976

Gamberini, L., & Spagnolli, A. (2015). An Action-Based Approach to Presence: Foundations and Methods. In M. Lombard, F. Biocca, J. Freeman, W. IJsselsteijn, & R. Schaevitz (Eds.), *Immersed in Media: Telepresence Theory, Measurement & Technology* (pp. 101–114). Cham: Springer. doi:10.1007/978-3-319-10190-3_6

Gold, J. I., Belmont, K. A., & Thomas, D. A. (2007). The neurobiology of virtual reality pain attenuation. *Cyberpsychology & Behavior*, *10*(4), 536–544. doi:10.1089/cpb.2007.9993 PMID:17711362

Li, A., Montaño, Z., Chen, V. J., & Gold, J. L. (2011). Virtual reality and pain management: Current trends and future directions. *Pain Management*, *1*(2), 147–157. doi:10.2217/pmt.10.15 PMID:21779307

Malloy, K. M., & Milling, L. S. (2010). The effectiveness of virtual reality distraction for pain reduction: A systematic review. *Clinical Psychology Review*, *30*(8), 1011–1018. doi:10.1016/j.cpr.2010.07.001 PMID:20691523

McCaul, K. D., & Malott, J. M. (1984). Distraction and coping with pain. *Psychological Bulletin*, *95*(3), 516–533. doi:10.1037/0033-2909.95.3.516 PMID:6399756

Melzack, R., & Wall, P. D. (1965). Pain mechanisms: A new theory. *Science*, *150*(3699), 971–979. doi:10.1126cience.150.3699.971 PMID:5320816

Mitchell, A. J., Chan, M., Bhatti, H., Halton, M., Grassi, L., Johansen, C., & Meader, N. (2011). Prevalence of depression, anxiety, and adjustment disorder in oncological, haematological, and palliative-care settings: A meta-analysis of 94 interview-based studies. *The Lancet Oncology*, *12*(2), 160–174. doi:10.1016/S1470-2045(11)70002-X PMID:21251875

Morina, N., Ijntema, H., Meyerbröker, K., & Emmelkamp, P. M. (2015). Can virtual reality exposure therapy gains be generalized to real-life? A meta-analysis of studies applying behavioral assessments. *Behaviour Research and Therapy*, *74*, 18–24. doi:10.1016/j.brat.2015.08.010 PMID:26355646

Morris, L. D., Louw, Q. A., & Grimmer-Somers, K. (2009). The effectiveness of virtual reality on reducing pain and anxiety in burn injury patients: A systematic review. *The Clinical Journal of Pain*, *25*(9), 815–826. doi:10.1097/AJP.0b013e3181aaa909 PMID:19851164

Neufeld, N. J., Elnahal, S. M., & Alvarez, R. H. (2017). Cancer pain: A review of epidemiology, clinical quality and value impact. *Future Oncology (London, England)*, *13*(9), 833–841. doi:10.2217/fon-2016-0423 PMID:27875910

Nichols, S., & Patel, H. (2002). Health and safety implications of virtual reality: A review of empirical evidence. *Applied Ergonomics*, *33*(3), 251–271. doi:10.1016/S0003-6870(02)00020-0 PMID:12164509

Oyama, H. (1998). Virtual reality for the palliative care of cancer. *Studies in Health Technology and Informatics*, *58*, 140–150. PMID:10350914

Scozzari, S., & Gamberini, L. (2011). Virtual Reality as a Tool for Cognitive Behavioral Therapy: A Review. In S. Brahnam & L. C. Jain (Eds.), *Advanced Computational Intelligence Paradigms in Healthcare 6. Virtual Reality in Psychotherapy, Rehabilitation, and Assessment. Studies in Computational Intelligence* (Vol. 337). Berlin: Springer. doi:10.1007/978-3-642-17824-5_5

Spagnolli, A., & Gamberini, L. (2005). A Place for presence. Understanding the human involvement in mediated interactive environments. *PsychNology Journal*, *3*(1), 6–15. PMID:16190023

Spagnolli, A., Gamberini, L., Cottone, P., & Mantovani, G. (2003). Ergonomics of virtual environments for clinical use. *Studies in Health Technology and Informatics*, *99*, 217–230. PMID:15295153

Zigmond, A. S., & Snaith, R. P. (1983). The hospital anxiety and depression scale. *Acta Psychiatrica Scandinavica*, *67*(6), 361–370. doi:10.1111/j.1600-0447.1983.tb09716.x PMID:6880820

## KEY TERMS AND DEFINITIONS

**Breakthrough Cancer Pain (BTcP):** Transient exacerbation of pain occurring in a patient with otherwise stable, persistent pain. Breakthrough pain is relatively common among cancer patients, particularly those with moderate to severe background pain, and is one of the most difficult pain syndromes to treat.

**End-of-Life Care:** Care given to people who are near the end of life and have stopped treatment to cure or control their disease. End-of-life care includes physical, emotional, social, and spiritual support for patients and their families.

**Home Oncological Clinic:** ANT oncological home care service.

**Mindfulness:** The psychological process of bringing one's attention to the internal and external experiences occurring in the present moment, which can be developed through the practice of meditation and other training.

**Palliative Care (PC):** Palliative care is an approach that improves the quality of life of patients and their families facing the problem associated with life-threatening illness, through the prevention and relief of suffering by identification, assessment and treatment of pain and other problems, physical, psychosocial, and spiritual.

**Psychological Distress (Distress):** Is a general term used to describe unpleasant feelings or emotions that impact your level of functioning. Sadness, anxiety, distraction, and symptoms of mental illness are manifestations of psychological distress.

**Virtual Reality (VR):** The possibility to immerse in a completely virtual world using a device to visualize computer graphics or computer sound.

# Compilation of References


Abell, F., Happe, F., & Frith, U. (2000). Do triangles play tricks? Attribution of mental states to animated shapes in normal and abnormal development. *Cognitive Development*, *15*(1), 1–16. doi:10.1016/S0885-2014(00)00014-9

Abhari, K., Baxter, J. S. H., Chen, E. C. S., Khan, A. R., Peters, T. M., de Ribaupierre, S., & Eagleson, R. (2015). Training for Planning Tumour Resection: Augmented Reality and Human Factors. *IEEE Transactions on Biomedical Engineering*, *62*(6), 1466–1477. doi:10.1109/TBME.2014.2385874 PMID:25546854

Abichou, K., La Corte, V., & Piolino, P. (2017). Does virtual reality have a future for the study of episodic memory in aging? *Gériatrie et Psychologie Neuropsychiatrie du Vieillissement*, *15*(1), 65–74. doi:10.1684/pnv.2016.0648 PMID:28266343

Adjorlu, A., Høeg, E. R., Mangano, L., & Serafin, S. (2017, October). Daily Living Skills Training in Virtual Reality to Help Children with Autism Spectrum Disorder in a Real Shopping Scenario. In *Mixed and Augmented Reality (ISMAR-Adjunct), 2017 IEEE International Symposium on* (pp. 294-302). IEEE. 10.1109/ISMAR-Adjunct.2017.93

Adjorlu, A., Hussain, A., Mødekjær, C., & Warming Austad, N. (2018). Head-Mounted Display-Based Virtual Reality Social Story as a Tool to Teach Social Skills to Children Diagnosed with Autism Spectrum Disorder. In *K-12 Embodied Learning through Virtual & Augmented Reality (KELVAR), 2018 IEEE Virtual Reality Workshop on* (pp. 1-4). IEEE.

Adjorlu, A. (2018). Virtual Reality Therapy. In *Encyclopedia of Computer Graphics and Games (ecgg)*. Springer. doi:10.1007/978-3-319-08234-9_244-1

Ahn, J., Del Core, M. A., Wukich, D. K., Liu, G. T., Lalli, T., VanPelt, M. D., & Raspovic, K. M. (2018). Scoring Mental Health Quality of Life With the SF-36 in Patients With and Without Diabetes Foot Complications. *The International Journal of Lower Extremity Wounds*, *17*(1), 30–35. doi:10.1177/1534734618762226 PMID:29546783

Ahn, S. J., Bostick, J., Ogle, E., Nowak, K. L., McGillicuddy, K. T., & Bailenson, J. N. (2016). Experiencing nature: Embodying animals in immersive virtual environments increases inclusion of nature in self and involvement with nature. *Journal of Computer-Mediated Communication*, *21*(6), 399–419. doi:10.1111/jcc4.12173

Aiello, P., D'Elia, F., Di Tore, S., & Sibilio, M. (2012). A constructivist approach to virtual reality for experiential learning. *E-Learning and Digital Media*, *9*(3), 317–324. doi:10.2304/elea.2012.9.3.317

Akil, H., Mayer, D. J., & Liebeskind, J. C. (1976). Antagonism of stimulation-produced analgesia by naloxone, a narcotic antagonist. *Science*, *191*(4230), 961–962. doi:10.1126cience.1251210 PMID:1251210

Alamri, A., Jongeun, C., & El Saddik, A. (2010). AR-REHAB: An Augmented Reality Framework for Poststroke-Patient Rehabilitation. *IEEE Transactions on* Instrumentation and Measurement, *59*(10), 2554–2563. doi:10.1109/tim.2010.2057750

Alaraj, A., Charbel, F. T., Birk, D., Tobin, M., Luciano, C., Banerjee, P. P., ... Roitberg, B. (2013). Role of cranial and spinal virtual and augmented reality simulation using immersive touch modules in neurosurgical training. *Neurosurgery*, *72*(1), 115–123. doi:10.1227/NEU.0b013e3182753093 PMID:23254799

Albiol-Pérez, S., Gil-Gómez, J. A., Muñoz-Tomás, M. T., Gil-Gómez, H., Vial-Escolano, R., & Lozano-Quilis, J.-A. (2017). The effect of balance training on postural control in patients with Parkinson's disease using a virtual rehabilitation system. *Methods of Information in Medicine*, *56*(2), 138–144. doi:10.3414/ME16-02-0004 PMID:28244545

Alhamid, M. F., Eid, M., & El Saddik, A. (2012, May 18-19). A multi-modal intelligent system for biofeedback interactions. *Paper presented at the 2012 IEEE International Symposium on Medical Measurements and Applications Proceedings (MeMeA).*

Al-Heeti, A. (2018). *VR could be your next painkiller.* Retrieved from https://www.cnet.com/news/virtual-reality-at-hospitals-could-be-your-next-painkiller/

Altschuler, E. L., Wisdom, S. B., Stone, L., Foster, C., Galasko, D., Llewellyn, D. M. E., & Ramachandran, V. S. (1999). Rehabilitation of hemiparesis after stroke with a mirror. *Lancet*, *353*(9169), 2035–2036. doi:10.1016/S0140-6736(99)00920-4 PMID:10376620

Ambron, E., Miller, A., Kuchenbecker, K. J., Buxbaum, L. J., & Coslett, H. (2018). Immersive low-cost Virtual reality Treatment for Phantom limb Pain: Evidence from Two cases. *Frontiers in Neurology*, *9*, 67. doi:10.3389/fneur.2018.00067 PMID:29515513

American Academy of Pediatrics (AAP). (n.d.). Retrieved from https://www.aap.org/

American Psychiatric Association. (2013). *Diagnostic and Statistical Manual of Mental Disorders* (5th ed.). Washington, DC.

American Psychiatric Association. (2013). *Diagnostic and statistical manual of mental disorders (DSM-5®).* American Psychiatric Pub.

American Psychiatric Association. (2013). *Diagnostic and statistical manual of mental disorders: DSM-5*. Washington, DC: American Psychiatric Publishing.

American Psychological Association (APA). (n.d.). Retrieved from http://www.apa.org/

Amsterdam, B. (1972). Mirror self-image reactions before age two. *Developmental Psychobiology*, *5*(4), 297–305. doi:10.1002/dev.420050403 PMID:4679817

Anda, R. F., Whitfield, C. L., Felitti, V. J., Chapman, D., Edwards, V. J., Dube, S. R., & Williamson, D. F. (2002). Adverse childhood experiences, alcoholic parents, and later risk of alcoholism and depression. *Psychiatric Services (Washington, D.C.)*, *53*(8), 1001–1009. doi:10.1176/appi.ps.53.8.1001 PMID:12161676

Andersen, M. (2016). A conceptual framework for understanding characteristics of self-awareness associated with autism spectrum disorder. *Scandinavian Journal of Child and Adolescent Psychiatry and Psychology*, *4*(3), 109–114. doi:10.21307jcapp-2016-017

Andrews, G., Creamer, M., Crino, R., Hunt, C., Lampe, L., & Page, A. (2003). *Trattamento dei disturbi d'ansia, Guida per il clinico e manuali per chi soffre del disturbo*. Turin, Italy: Centro Scientifico Editore.

Anketell, P., Saunders, K., Gallagher, S., Bailey, C., & Little, J. A. (2013). Visual findings in children with Autistic Spectrum Disorder. *Investigative Ophthalmology & Visual Science*, *54*(15), 569–569.

Anthes, C., García-Hernández, R. J., Wiedemann, M., & Kranzlmüller, D. (2016). State of the art of virtual reality technology. *Paper presented at the 2016 IEEE Aerospace Conference*. 10.1109/AERO.2016.7500674

Arnold-Saritepe, A. M., Phillips, K. J., Mudford, O. C., De Rozario, K. A., & Taylor, S. A. (2009). Generalization and maintenance. In *Applied behavior analysis for children with autism spectrum disorders* (pp. 207–224). Springer. doi:10.1007/978-1-4419-0088-3_12

Arvanitis, T. N., Petrou, A., Knight, J. F., Savas, S., Sotiriou, S., Gargalakos, M., & Gialouri, E. (2007). Human factors and qualitative pedagogical evaluation of a mobile augmented reality system for science education used by learners with physical disabilities. *Personal and Ubiquitous Computing*, *13*(3), 243–250. doi:10.100700779-007-0187-7

Ascott, R. (1988). Art and Education in the Telematic Culture. *Leonardo*, (1), 7-11.

Ascott, R. (2001). *When the Jaguar lies down with the Lamb: speculations on the post-biological culture.* Paper presented at CAiiA-STAR Symposium: 'Extreme parameters. New dimensions of interactivity', Barcelona, Spain. 10.7238/a.v0i1.677

Ascott, R. (2013). *Interstitial Creativity Art/Mind/Technology.* Paper presented at COST Arts & Technologies Workshop - CAT, Zagreb, Croatia.

Ascott, R. (Ed.). (1999). *Reframing Consciousness: Art, Mind and Technology*. Bristol, UK: Intellect.

Attril, A. (2012). Self-disclosure online. In Encyclopedia of Cyber Behaviour (pp. 855-872). Oxford, UK: Encyclopedia of Cyber Behaviour. doi:10.4018/978-1-4666-0315-8.ch071

Azuma, R. T. (1997). A Survey of Augmented Reality. *Presence (Cambridge, Mass.)*, *6*(4), 355–385. doi:10.1162/pres.1997.6.4.355

Bach, F., Schmitz, B., Maaß, H., Çakmak, H., & Diers, M., B-Bodmann, R. … Flor, H. (2010). Using interactive immersive VR/AR for the therapy of phantom limb pain. *Paper presented at the 13th International Conference on Humans and Computers.*

Badcock, N. A., Mousikou, P., Mahajan, Y., De Lissa, P., Thie, J., & McArthur, G. (2013). Validation of the Emotiv EPOC® EEG gaming system for measuring research quality auditory ERPs. *PeerJ*, *1*, e38. doi:10.7717/peerj.38 PMID:23638374

Baglivio, M. T., Epps, N., Swartz, K., Huq, M. S., Sheer, A., & Hardt, N. S. (2014). The prevalence of adverse childhood experiences (ACE) in the lives of juvenile offenders. *Journal of Juvenile Justice*, *3*(2), 1.

Bai, Z. (2012). Augmenting imagination for children with autism. *Paper presented at the 11th International Conference on Interaction Design and Children.*

Bai, Z., Blackwell, A. F., & Coulouris, G. (2013). Through the looking glass: Pretend play for children with autism. *Paper presented at the 2013 IEEE International Symposium on Mixed and augmented reality (ISMAR).* 10.1109/ISMAR.2013.6671763

Bailenson, J. N., Beall, A. C., Loomis, J., Blascovich, J., & Turk, M. (2004). Transformed social interaction: Decoupling representation from behavior and form in collaborative virtual environments. *Presence (Cambridge, Mass.)*, *13*(4), 428–441. doi:10.1162/1054746041944803

Bailey, J. O., & Bailenson, J. N. (2018). *Immersive Virtual Reality and the Developing Child. In Cognitive Development in Digital Contexts* (pp. 181–200). Elsevier.

Baldini, M., & Balestrini, N. (2005). *La parola nella galassia elettronica.* Milan, Italy: Armando Editore.

Bandell-Hoekstra, I. E. N. G., Abu-Saad, H. H., Passchier, J., Frederiks, C. M. A., Feron, F. J. M., & Knipschild, P. (2001). Prevalence and characteristics of headache in Dutch schoolchildren. *European Journal of Pain (London, England)*, *5*(2), 145–153. doi:10.1053/eujp.2001.0234 PMID:11465980

Bantick, S. J., Wise, R. G., Ploghaus, A., Clare, S., Smith, S. M., & Tracey, I. (2002). Imaging how attention modulates pain in humans using functional MRI. *Brain*, *125*(2), 310–319. doi:10.1093/brain/awf022 PMID:11844731

Barak, A. (2007). Emotional support and suicide prevention through the Internet: A field project report. *Computers in Human Behavior*, *23*(2), 971–984. doi:10.1016/j.chb.2005.08.001

Bashiri, A., Ghazisaeedi, M., & Shahmoradi, L. (2017). The opportunities of virtual reality in the rehabilitation of children with attention deficit hyperactivity disorder: A literature review. *Korean Journal of Pediatrics*, *60*(11), 337–343. doi:10.3345/kjp.2017.60.11.337 PMID:29234356

Bateson, G. (1972). Steps to an ecology of mind: Collected essays. In *Anthropology, Psychiatry, Evolution, and Epistemology*. University of Chicago Press.

Baudrillard, J. (1980). *Simulacres et simulation*. Paris: Galilée.

Bauman, Z. (2000). *Liquid Modernity*. Cambridge, UK: Polity Press.

Baumgartner, T. (2008). Feeling present in arousing virtual reality worlds: Prefrontal brain regions differentially orchestrate presence experience in adults and children. *Frontiers in Human Neuroscience*, *2*. doi:10.3389/neuro.09.008.2008 PMID:18958209

Beach, J., & Wendt, J. (2014). *Social Interaction Development through Immersive Virtual Environments*. International Association for Development of the Information Society.

Bellani, M., Fornasari, L., Chittaro, L., & Brambilla, P. (2011).*Virtual reality in autism: state of the art*. Retrieved from https://www.ncbi.nlm.nih.gov/pubmed/21922965

Bellani, M., Fornasari, L., Chittaro, L., & Brambilla, P. (2011). Virtual reality in autism: State of the art. *Epidemiology and Psychiatric Sciences*, *20*(3), 235–238. doi:10.1017/S2045796011000448 PMID:21922965

Benyoucef, Y., Lesport, P., & Chassagneux, A. (2017). The emergent role of virtual reality in the treatment of neuropsychiatric disease. *NCBI*. Retrieved May 10, 2018 from https://www.ncbi.nlm.nih.gov/pmc/articles/PMC5591848/

Benyoucef, Y., Lesport, P., & Chassagneux, A. (2017). *The Emergent Role of Virtual Reality in the Treatment of Neuropsychiatric Disease*. Retrieved from https://www.ncbi.nlm.nih.gov/pmc/articles/PMC5591848/

Bergig, O., Hagbi, N., El-Sana, J., & Billinghurst, M. (2009). In-place 3D sketching for authoring and augmenting mechanical systems. In *Mixed and Augmented Reality, 2009. ISMAR 2009. 8th IEEE International Symposium on* (pp. 87-94). IEEE. doi: 10.1109/ISMAR.2009.5336490

Bezerra, Í. M. P., Crocetta, T. B., Massetti, T., Silva, T. D. D., Guarnieri, R., Meira, C. M. Jr, ... Monteiro, C. B. M. (2018). Functional performance comparison between real and virtual tasks in older adults: A cross-sectional study. *Medicine*, *97*(4), e9612–e9612. doi:10.1097/MD.0000000000009612 PMID:29369177

Bhatt, S., De Leon, N., & Al-Jumaily, A. (2014). Augmented reality game therapy for children with autism spectrum disorder. *International Journal on Smart Sensing and Intelligent Systems*, *7*(2), 519–536. doi:10.21307/ijssis-2017-668

Billstedt, E., Gillberg, C., & Gillberg, C. (2005). Autism after adolescence: Population-based 13-to 22-year follow-up study of 120 individuals with autism diagnosed in childhood. *Journal of Autism and Developmental Disorders*, *35*(3), 351–360. doi:10.100710803-005-3302-5 PMID:16119476

Bimber, O., & Raskar, R. (2005). *Spatial Augmented Reality: Merging Real and Virtual Worlds*. A. K. Peters, Ltd. doi:10.1201/b10624

Birchfield, D., & Megowan-Romanowicz, C. (2009). Earth science learning in SMALLab: A design experiment for mixed reality. *International Journal of Computer-Supported Collaborative Learning*, *4*(4), 403–421. doi:10.100711412-009-9074-8

Birkfellner, W., Figl, M., Huber, K., Watzinger, F., Wanschitz, F., Hummel, J., ... Bergmann, H. (2002). A head-mounted operating binocular for augmented reality visualization in medicine--design and initial evaluation. *IEEE Transactions on Medical Imaging*, *21*(8), 991–997. doi:10.1109/TMI.2002.803099 PMID:12472271

Bisson, J., & Andrew, M. (2009). Psychological treatments of post-traumatic stress disorder (PTSD). *The Cochrane Library*. Retrieved from http://www.thecochranelibrary.com

Bitner, J. (2017). *11 Tools for VR Developers*. Retrieved from: https://www.lullabot.com/articles/11-tools-for-vr-developers

Bitsika, V., & Sharpley, C. F. (2014). Understanding, experiences, and reactions to bullying experiences in boys with an autism spectrum disorder. *Journal of Developmental and Physical Disabilities*, *26*(6), 747–761. doi:10.100710882-014-9393-1

Blake, E. H., & Winterbottom, C. (2008). Constructivism, virtual reality and tools to support design. In *Proceedings of the 7th ACM conference on Designing interactive systems*, (pp. 230-239), New York, NY: ACM.

Blum, T., Kleeberger, V., Bichlmeier, C., & Navab, N. (2012). mirracle: An augmented reality magic mirror system for anatomy education. In *Virtual Reality Conference*, Costa Mesa, CA. doi: http://doi.ieeecomputersociety.org/10.1109/VR.2012.6180909 doi:10.1109/VR.2012.6180909

Bölte, S., Golan, O., Goodwin, M. S., & Zwaigenbaum, L. (2010). What can innovative technologies do for Autism Spectrum Disorders? *Autism*, *14*(3), 155–159. doi:10.1177/1362361310365028 PMID:20603897

Bonezzi, C., Nava, A., Barbieri, M., Demartini, L., Miotti, D., & Paulin, D. (2002). Validazione della versione italiana del Brief Pain Inventory nei pazienti con dolore cronico. *Minerva Anestesiologica*, *68*(7-8), 607–611. PMID:12244292

Bonnet, L., Lotte, F., & Lecuyer, A. (2013). Two brains, one game: Design and evaluation of a multi-user BCI video game based on motor imagery. *IEEE Transactions on Computational Intelligence and AI in Games*, *5*(2), 185–198.

Booth, V., Masud, T., Connell, L., & Bath-Hextall, F. (2014). The effectiveness of virtual reality interventions in improving balance in adults with impaired balance compared with standard or no treatment: A systematic review and meta-analysis. *Clinical Rehabilitation*, *28*(5), 419–431. doi:10.1177/0269215513509389 PMID:24188913

Boot, W. R., Kramer, A. F., Simons, D. J., Fabiani, M., & Gratton, G. (2008). The effects of video game playing on attention, memory, and executive control. *Acta Psychologica*, *129*(3), 387–398. doi:10.1016/j.actpsy.2008.09.005 PMID:18929349

Bordnick, P. S., Yoon, J. H., Kaganoff, E., & Carter, B. (2013). Virtual reality cue reactivity assessment: A comparison of treatment-vs. nontreatment-seeking smokers. *Research on Social Work Practice*, *23*(4), 419–425. doi:10.1177/1049731513482377

Bork, F., Barmaki, R., Eck, U., Yu, K., Sandor, C., & Navab, N. (2017). Empirical Study of Non-Reversing Magic Mirrors for Augmented Reality Anatomy Learning. *Paper presented at the 2017 IEEE International Symposium on Mixed and Augmented Reality (ISMAR)*. 10.1109/ISMAR.2017.33

Borrego, A., Latorre, J., Alcaniz, M., & Llorens, R. (2018). Comparison of Oculus Rift and HTC Vive: Feasibility for Virtual Reality-Based Exploration, Navigation, Exergaming, and Rehabilitation. *Games for Health Journal*, *7*(3), 151–156. doi:10.1089/g4h.2017.0114 PMID:29293369

Bos, D. P. O., Reuderink, B., Van De Laar, B., Gurkok, H., Muhl, C., Poel, M., . . . Nijholt, A. (2010). Human-computer interaction for bci games: Usability and user experience. In *Cyberworlds (CW), 2010 International Conference on* (pp. 277-281). IEEE.

Botden, S. M. B. I., Buzink, S. N., Schijven, M. P., & Jakimowicz, J. J. (2008). ProMIS Augmented Reality Training of Laparoscopic Procedures Face Validity. *Simulation in Healthcare*, *3*(2), 97–102. doi:10.1097/SIH.0b013e3181659e91 PMID:19088648

Botella, C. M., Juan, M. C., Banos, R. M., Alcaniz, M., Guillen, V., & Rey, B. (2005). Mixing realities? An application of augmented reality for the treatment of cockroach phobia. *Cyberpsychology & Behavior*, *8*(2), 162–171. doi:10.1089/cpb.2005.8.162 PMID:15938656

Botella, C., Bretón-López, J., Quero, S., Baños, R., & García-Palacios, A. (2010). Treating cockroach phobia with augmented reality. *Behavior Therapy*, *41*(3), 401–413. doi:10.1016/j.beth.2009.07.002 PMID:20569788

Botella, C., Garcia-Palacios, A., Vizcaíno, Y., Herrero, R., Baños, R. M., & Belmonte, M. A. (2013). Virtual Reality in the Treatment of Fibromyalgia: A Pilot Study. *Cyberpsychology, Behavior, and Social Networking*, *16*(3), 215–223. doi:10.1089/cyber.2012.1572 PMID:23496678

Botella, C., Quero, S., Baños, R. M., Perpiña, C., García Palacios, A., & Riva, G. (2004). Virtual Reality and psychotherapy. *Studies in Health Technology and Informatics*, *99*, 37–54. PMID:15295145

Botvinick, M., & Cohen, J. (1998). Rubber hands "feel" touch that eyes see [8]. *Nature*, *391*(6669), 756. doi:10.1038/35784 PMID:9486643

Boyer, S. A. (2009). *SCADA: supervisory control and data acquisition*. International Society of Automation.

Breivik, H., Collett, B., Ventafridda, V., Cohen, R., & Gallacher, D. (2006). Survey of chronic pain in Europe: Prevalence, impact on daily life, and treatment. *European Journal of Pain (London, England)*, *10*(4), 287. doi:10.1016/j.ejpain.2005.06.009 PMID:16095934

Brignell, A., Morgan, A. T., Woolfenden, S., Klopper, F., May, T., Sarkozy, V., & Williams, K. (2018). A systematic review and meta-analysis of the prognosis of language outcomes for individuals with autism spectrum disorder. *Autism & Developmental Language Impairments*. Retrieved July 3, 2018 from http://journals.sagepub.com/doi/10.1177/2396941518767610

Brinkman, W. M., Havermans, S. Y., Buzink, S. N., Botden, S. M. B. I., Jakimowicz, J. J., & Schoot, B. C. (2012). Single versus multimodality training basic laparoscopic skills. *Surgical Endoscopy and Other Interventional Techniques, 26*(8), 2172-2178. doi:10.100700464-012-2184-9

Broll, W., Lindt, I., Herbst, I., Ohlenburg, J., Braun, A. K., & Wetzel, R. (2008). Toward next-gen mobile AR games. *Computer Graphics and Applications, IEEE*, *28*(4), 40–48. doi:10.1109/MCG.2008.85

Bronack, S. C. (2011). The role of immersive media in online education. *Journal of Continuing Higher Education*, *59*(2), 113–117. doi:10.1080/07377363.2011.583186

Brunner, I., Skouen, J. S., Hofstad, H., Aßmus, J., Becker, F., Sanders, A. M., ... Verheyden, G. (2017). Virtual reality training for upper extremity in subacute stroke (VIRTUES): A multicenter RCT. *Neurology*, *89*(24), 2413–2421. doi:10.1212/WNL.0000000000004744 PMID:29142090

Buckley, A. W., & Holmes, G. L. (2016). Epilepsy and autism. *Cold Spring Harbor Perspectives in Medicine*, *6*(4), a022749. doi:10.1101/cshperspect.a022749 PMID:26989064

Buescher, A. V., Cidav, Z., Knapp, M., & Mandell, D. S. (2014). Costs of autism spectrum disorders in the United Kingdom and the United States. *JAMA Pediatrics*, *168*(8), 721–728. doi:10.1001/jamapediatrics.2014.210 PMID:24911948

Butler, A. C., Chapman, J. E., Forman, E. M., & Beck, A. T. (2006). The empirical status of cognitive-behavioral therapy: A review of meta-analyses. *Clinical Psychology Review*, *26*(1), 17–31. doi:10.1016/j.cpr.2005.07.003 PMID:16199119

Calderoni, A. (2013). *Psicologia digitale*. Rome, Italy: Ecomind.

Cameirão, M. S., Bermúdez, S., & Verschure, P. F. M. J. (2008). Virtual reality based upper extremity rehabilitation following stroke: A review. *Journal of Cyber Therapy and Rehabilitation*, *1*(1), 63–74.

Campo, J. V., Di Lorenzo, C., Chiappetta, L., Bridge, J., Colborn, D. K., & Gartner, J. C. Jr. … Brent, D. (2001). Adult Outcomes of Pediatric Recurrent Abdominal Pain: Do They Just Grow Out of It? *Pediatrics*. doi:10.1542/peds.108.1.e1

Canevacci, M. (2012). Digital Auratic Reproducibility: Ubiquitous Ethnographies and Communicational Metropolis. In *An Ethnography of Global Landscapes and Corridors*. Retrieved July 8, 2018, from http://www.intechopen.com/books/an-ethnography-of-global-landscapes-and- corridors/digital-auratic-reproducibility

Cantelmi, T. (2013). *Tecnoliquidità. La psicologia ai tempi di internet: La mente tecno-liquida*. Milan, Italy: San Paolo.

Cantelmi, T., & Grifo, L. (2003). *La mente virtuale*. Milan, Italy: San Paolo.

Capucci, P. L. (1993). *Realtà del Virtuale. Rappresentazioni tecnologiche, comunicazione, arte*. Bologna: CLUEB.

Cardinale, J. (2018). *Does Virtual Reality Balance Training Utilizing the Wii Balance Board Improve Balance in Community Dwelling Older Adults: A Meta-Analysis* [Doctoral dissertation]. California State University, Fresno, CA.

Caronia, A. (1996). *Il corpo virtuale. Dal corpo robotizzato al corpo disseminato nelle reti*. Padova: FrancoMuzzio Editore.

Carrino, F., Rizzotti, D., Gheorghe, C., Kabasu Bakajika, P., Francescotti-Paquier, F., & Mugellini, E. (2014). Augmented Reality Treatment for Phantom Limb Pain. In R. Shumaker & S. Lackey (Eds.), *Virtual, Augmented and Mixed Reality. Applications of Virtual and Augmented Reality* (pp. 248–257). Springer International Publishing. doi:10.1007/978-3-319-07464-1_23

Carson, E. (2015). *6 cool uses for augmented reality in healthcare*. Retrieved from https://www.techrepublic.com/article/6-cool-uses-for-augmented-reality-in-healthcare/

Casas Yrurzum, S. (2014). *Mejoras en la generación de claves gravito-inerciales en simuladores de vehículos no aéreos [PhD thesis]*. Universitat de València.

Casas, X., Herrera, G., Coma, I., & Fernández, M. (2012). A kinect-based augmented reality system for individuals with autism spectrum disorders. In *Proceedings of the International Conference on Computer Graphics Theory and Applications and International Conference on Information Visualization Theory and Applications* (vol. 1, pp. 440-446). GRAPP.

Casas, X., Herrera, G., Coma, I., & Fernández, M. (2012). A Kinect-based augmented reality system for individuals with autism spectrum disorders. *Paper presented at the Computer Graphics Theory and Applications*, Rome, Italy.

Casas, S., Coma, I., Portalés, C., & Fernández, M. (2016). Towards a simulation-based tuning of motion cueing algorithms. *Simulation Modelling Practice and Theory*, *67*, 137–154. doi:10.1016/j.simpat.2016.06.002

Casas, X., Herrera, G., Coma, I., & Fernández, M. (2012). *A Kinect-based Augmented Reality System for Individuals with Autism Spectrum Disorders* (pp. 440–446). GRAPP/IVAPP.

Catren, N. R. (2017). *Virtual reality may be a help to autistic children in the classroom*. Retrieved March 5, 2018 from http://www.independent.co.uk/news/science/virtual-reality-may-be-a-help-to-autistic-children-in-the-classroom-a7676391.html

Catren, N. R. (2017). *Virtual reality may be a help to autistic children in the classroom*. Retrieved March 5, 2018, from http://www.independent.co.uk/news/science/virtual-reality-may-be-a-help-to-autistic-children-in-the-classroom-a7676391.html

Cederlund, M., Hagberg, B., Billstedt, E., Gillberg, I. C., & Gillberg, C. (2008). Asperger syndrome and autism: A comparative longitudinal follow-up study more than 5 years after original diagnosis. *Journal of Autism and Developmental Disorders*, *38*(1), 72–85. doi:10.100710803-007-0364-6 PMID:17340200

Centers for Disease Control and Prevention. (n.d.). Adverse Childhood Experiences (ACE's). Retrieved from https://www.cdc.gov/violenceprevention/acestudy/index.html

Centre for Youth Wellness. (n.d.). Children can thrive: Report. Retrieved July 18, 2018 from https://centerforyouthwellness.org/wp-content/themes/cyw/build/img/building-a-movement/children-can-thrive.pdf

Chan, B. L., Witt, R., Charrow, A. P., Magee, A., Howard, R., Pasquina, P. F., ... Tsao, J. W. (2007). Mirror Therapy for Phantom Limb Pain. *The New England Journal of Medicine*, *357*(21), 2206–2207. doi:10.1056/NEJMc071927 PMID:18032777

Chandra, G., & Tang, S. (2017). *Virtual Reality:Components*. Retrieved from http://web.tecnico.ulisboa.pt/ist188480/cmul/devices.html

Chang, H. Y., Wu, H. K., & Hsu, Y. S. (2013). Integrating a mobile augmented reality activity to contextualize student learning of a socioscientific issue. *British Journal of Educational Technology*, *44*(3), E95–E99. doi:10.1111/j.1467-8535.2012.01379.x

Chang, L. C., Wang, C. Y., & Yu, P. (2014). Virtual reality improves sleep quality amongst older adults with disabilities. *International Journal of Geriatric Psychiatry*, *29*(12), 1312–1313. doi:10.1002/gps.4172 PMID:25394270

Charles, A. (2013). The evolution of a migraine attack–a review of recent evidence. *Headache*, *53*(2), 413–419. doi:10.1111/head.12026 PMID:23278169

Charlop-Christy, M. H., & Daneshvar, S. (2003). Using video modeling to teach perspective taking to children with autism. *Journal of Positive Behavior Interventions*, *5*(1), 12–21. doi:10.1177/10983007030050010101

Chau, B., Phelan, I., Dunn, J., Yeo, E., & Hata, J. H. S. (2016). *Complex Regional Pain Syndrome: A Case Report*. Academic Press.

Chen, Z., Hood, R. W., Jr., Yang, L., & Watson, P. J. (2011). Mystical experience among Tibetan Buddhists: The common core thesis revisited. *Journal for the Scientific Study of Religion*, *50*(2), 328-338.

Chen, C.-H., Lee, I.-J., & Lin, L.-Y. (2015). Augmented reality-based self-facial modeling to promote the emotional expression and social skills of adolescents with autism spectrum disorders. *Research in Developmental Disabilities*, *36*, 396–403. doi:10.1016/j.ridd.2014.10.015 PMID:25462499

Cheng, Y., Huang, C. L., & Yang, C. S. (2015). Using a 3D immersive virtual environment system to enhance social understanding and social skills for children with autism spectrum disorders. *Focus on Autism and Other Developmental Disabilities*, *30*(4), 222–236. doi:10.1177/1088357615583473

Chen, S. S. A., & Bernard-Opitz, V. (1993). Comparison of personal and computer-assisted instruction for children with autism. *Mental Retardation*, *31*(6), 368. PMID:8152382

Chen, Y.-C. (2006). A study of comparing the use of augmented reality and physical models in chemistry education. In *Proceedings of the 2006 ACM international conference on Virtual reality continuum and its applications* (pp. 369-372). Hong Kong, China: ACM. 10.1145/1128923.1128990

Chen, Y.-C., Chi, H.-L., Hung, W.-H., & Kang, S.-C. (2011). Use of tangible and augmented reality models in engineering graphics courses. *Journal of Professional Issues in Engineering Education and Practice*, *137*(4), 267–276. doi:10.1061/(ASCE)EI.1943-5541.0000078

Chi, B., Chau, B., Phelan, I., Ta, P., & Hata, J. H. S. (2017). *Successful Complex Regional Pain Syndrome Treatment with Immersive Virtual Reality: Case Report*. Academic Press.

Chiang, I. T., Chen, M. L., Chang, P. S., & Lee, J. Y. (2011). Effects of a video game-based intervention on balance learning for institution-dwelling elderly in veterans home. In *The 2011 International Educational Technology Conference Proceedings Book* (Vol. 1, pp. 393-398).

Chiarovano, E., Wang, W., Reynolds, P., & MacDougall, H. G. (2018). Imbalance: Objective measures versus subjective self-report in clinical practice. *Gait & Posture*, *59*, 217–221. doi:10.1016/j.gaitpost.2017.10.019 PMID:29080510

Chicchi Giglioli, I. A., Pallavicini, F., Pedroli, E., Serino, S., & Riva, G. (2015). Augmented reality: A brand new challenge for the assessment and treatment of psychological disorders. *Computational and Mathematical Methods in Medicine*. PMID:26339283

Chien, C. H., Chen, C. H., & Jeng, T. S. (2010, March). An Interactive Augmented Reality System for Learning Anatomy Structure. *Proceedings of the International MultiConference of Engineers and Computer Scientists*, *1*, 17–19.

Chimes, G. P., Bernstein, C. D., Cortazzo, M. H., & Huber, L. M. (2009). Poster presentation. *PM & R*, *1*(9 Suppl.), S220. doi:10.1016/j.pmrj.2009.08.290

Chirico, A., Lucidi, F., De Laurentiis, M., Milanese, C., Napoli, A., & Giordano, A. (2016). Virtual Reality in Health System: Beyond Entertainment. A Mini-Review on the Efficacy of VR During Cancer Treatment. *Journal of Cellular Physiology*, *231*(2), 275–287. doi:10.1002/jcp.25117 PMID:26238976

Choinière, M., Dion, D., Peng, P., Banner, R., Barton, P. M., Boulanger, A., … Ware, M. (2010). The Canadian STOP-PAIN project - Part 1: Who are the patients on the waitlists of multidisciplinary pain treatment facilities? *Canadian Journal of Anaesthesia = Journal Canadien d'anesthésie*. doi:10.100712630-010-9305-5

Christensen, D. L., Baio, J., Braun, K. V. N., Bilder, D., Charles, J., Constantino, J. N., ... Yeargin-Allsopp, M. (2016). Prevalence and characteristics of autism spectrum disorder among children aged 8 years — autism and developmental disabilities monitoring network, 11 sites, United States, 2012. *MMWR. Surveillance Summaries*, *65*(3), 1–23. doi:10.15585/mmwr.ss6503a1 PMID:27031587

Chukoskie, L., Westerfield, M., & Townsend, J. (2017). A novel approach to training attention and gaze in ASD: A feasibility and efficacy pilot study. *Developmental Neurobiology*, *78*(5), 546–554. doi:10.1002/dneu.22563 PMID:29218791

Cipolletta, G. (2014). *Passages metrocorporei. Per un'estetica della transizione*. Macerata: eum.

Coates, G. (1992). *Program from Invisible Site—a virtual sho*. San Francisco, CA: Performance Works.

Cobb, S., Nichols, S. C., Ramsey, A., & Wilson, J. (1999). Virtual reality induced symptoms and effects (VRISE). *Presence (Cambridge, Mass.)*, *8*(2), 169–186. doi:10.1162/105474699566152

Coffey, A. L., Leamy, D. J., & Ward, T. E. (2014). A novel BCI-controlled pneumatic glove system for home-based neurorehabilitation. In *Engineering in Medicine and Biology Society (EMBC), 2014 36th Annual International Conference of the IEEE* (pp. 3622-3625). IEEE. 10.1109/EMBC.2014.6944407

Colby, K. M. (1968). Computer-aided language development in nonspeaking children. *Archives of General Psychiatry*, *19*(6), 641–651. doi:10.1001/archpsyc.1968.01740120001001 PMID:4177129

*Collins English dictionary*. (2014). Glasgow, UK: HarperCollins Publishers.

Colomer, C., Noe, E., & Rodríguez, R. L. (2016). Mirror therapy in chronic stroke survivors with severely impaired upper limb function: a randomized controlled trial. *Paper presented at the European journal of physical and rehabilitation medicine.*

Common Sense Report Highlights Potential Impact of Virtual Reality on Children's Development, (2018). Common Sense Media. Retrieved from https://www.commonsensemedia.org/about-us/news/press-releases/common-sense-report-highlights-potential-impact-of-virtual-reality-on

Connelly, L., Jia, Y., Toro, M. L., Stoykov, M. E., Kenyon, R. V., & Kamper, D. G. (2010). A pneumatic glove and immersive virtual reality environment for hand rehabilitative training after stroke. *IEEE Transactions on Neural Systems and Rehabilitation Engineering*, *18*(5), 551–559. doi:10.1109/TNSRE.2010.2047588 PMID:20378482

Connors, M. H., & Coltheart, M. (2011). On the behaviour of senile dementia patients vis-à-vis the mirror: Ajuriaguerra, Strejilevitch and Tissot (1963). *Neuropsychologia*, *49*(7), 1679–1692. doi:10.1016/j.neuropsychologia.2011.02.041 PMID:21356221

Correa, A. G. D., Ficheman, I. K., do Nascimento, M., & De Deus Lopes, R. (2009, 15-17 July 2009). Computer assisted music therapy: a case study of an augmented reality musical system for children with cerebral palsy rehabilitation. *Paper presented at the Ninth IEEE International Conference on Advanced Learning Technologies ICALT 2009.*

Corrêa, N. F. M., de Brito, M. J. A., de Carvalho Resende, M. M., Duarte, M. F. P., Santos, F. S., Salomé, G. M., & Ferreira, L. M. (2016). Impact of surgical wound dehiscence on health-related quality of life and mental health. *Journal of Wound Care*, *25*(10), 561–570. doi:10.12968/jowc.2016.25.10.561 PMID:27681586

Costa, J. (2010). *Efetividade de um Web Based Learning para o desenvolvimento de competências no âmbito das feridas crónicas* (Unpublished Doctoral dissertation). Polytechnic University of Catalonia, Barcelona, Spain.

Costantini, M., & Haggard, P. (2007). The rubber hand illusion: Sensitivity and reference frame for body ownership. *Consciousness and Cognition*, *16*(2), 229–240. doi:10.1016/j.concog.2007.01.001 PMID:17317221

Covanis, A. (2005). Photosensitivity in idiopathic generalized epilepsies. *Epilepsia*, *46*(s9), 67–72. doi:10.1111/j.1528-1167.2005.00315.x PMID:16302877

Cox, D. J., Brown, T., Ross, V., Moncrief, M., Schmitt, R., Gaffney, G., & Reeve, R. (2017). Can youth with autism spectrum disorder use virtual reality driving simulation training to evaluate and improve driving performance? An exploratory study. *Journal of Autism and Developmental Disorders*, *47*(8), 2544–2555. doi:10.100710803-017-3164-7 PMID:28540452

Cox, D. J., Davis, M., Singh, H., Barbour, B., Nidiffer, F. D., Trudel, T., ... Moncrief, R. (2010). Driving rehabilitation for military personnel recovering from traumatic brain injury using virtual reality driving simulation: A feasibility study. *Military Medicine*, *175*(6), 411–416. doi:10.7205/MILMED-D-09-00081 PMID:20572473

Crane, L., Goddard, L., & Pring, L. (2009). Specific and general autobiographical knowledge in adults with autism spectrum disorders: The role of personal goals. *Memory (Hove, England)*, *17*(5), 557–576. doi:10.1080/09658210902960211 PMID:19499459

Cruz-Neira, C., Leigh, J., Papka, M., Barnes, C., Cohen, S. M., Das, S., . . . Siegel, L. (1993). Scientists in wonderland: A report on visualization applications in the CAVE virtual reality environment. *Paper presented at the IEEE 1993 Symposium on Research Frontiers in Virtual Reality.* 10.1109/VRAIS.1993.378262

Csikszentmihalyi, M. (1997). *Finding flow: The psychology of engagement with everyday life*. Basic Books.

Cuomo-Granston, A., & Drummond, P. D. (2010). Migraine and motion sickness: What is the link? *Progress in Neurobiology*, *91*(4), 300–312. doi:10.1016/j.pneurobio.2010.04.001 PMID:20416353

Cushman, L., Stein, K., & Duffy, C. (2008). Detecting navigational deficits in cognitive aging and Alzheimer disease using virtual reality. *Neurology*, *71*(12), 888–895. doi:10.1212/01.wnl.0000326262.67613.fe PMID:18794491

Dahlquist, L. M., McKenna, K. D., Jones, K. K., Dillinger, L., Weiss, K. E., & Ackerman, C. S. (2007). Active and Passive Distraction Using a Head-Mounted Display Helmet: Effects on Cold Pressor Pain in Children. *Health Psychology*, *26*(6), 794–801. doi:10.1037/0278-6133.26.6.794 PMID:18020853

Dahlquist, L. M., Weiss, K. E., Law, E. F., Sil, S., Herbert, L. J., & Horn, S. B. … Ackerman, C. S. (2010). Effects of videogame distraction and a virtual reality type head-mounted display helmet on cold pressor pain in young elementary school-aged children. *Journal of Pediatric Psychology*. doi:10.1093/jpepsy/jsp082

Darnall, B. D. (2009). Self-Delivered Home-Based Mirror Therapy for Lower Limb Phantom Pain. *American Journal of Physical Medicine & Rehabilitation*, *88*(1), 78–81. doi:10.1097/PHM.0b013e318191105b PMID:19096290

Darvasi, P. (2016). Five ethical considerations for using virtual reality with children and adolescents. *KQED*. Retrieved July 3, 2018 from https://www.kqed.org/mindshift/46103/five-ethical-considerations-for-using-virtual-reality-with-children-and-adolescents

Darvasi, P. (2016). *Five ethical considerations for using virtual reality with children and adolescents*. Retrieved July 3, 2018 from https://www.kqed.org/mindshift/46103/five-ethical-considerations-for-using-virtual-reality-with-children-and-adolescents

Daw, N. W. (1997). Critical periods and strabismus: What questions remain? *Optometry and Vision Science*, *74*(9), 690–694. doi:10.1097/00006324-199709000-00002 PMID:9380366

Day, K., Carreon, D., & Stump, C. (2000). The therapeutic design of environments for people with dementia: A review of the empirical research. *The Gerontologist*, *40*(4), 397–416. doi:10.1093/geront/40.4.397 PMID:10961029

De Paolis, L. T., Pulimeno, M., & Aloisio, G. (2008). An augmented reality application for minimally invasive surgery. In *IFMBE Proceedings 14th Nordic-Baltic Conference on Biomedical Engineering and Medical Physics* (pp. 489-492). Springer. 10.1007/978-3-540-69367-3_131

Deconinck, F. J., Smorenburg, A. R., Benham, A., Ledebt, A., Feltham, M. G., & Savelsbergh, G. J. (2015). Reflections on mirror therapy: A systematic review of the effect of mirror visual feedback on the brain. *Neurorehabilitation and Neural Repair*, *29*(4), 349–361. doi:10.1177/1545968314546134 PMID:25160567

Dede, C. (2009). Immersive interfaces for engagement and learning. *Science, 323*(5910), 66-69.

Dede, C. (2009). Immersive interfaces for engagement and learning. *Science*, *323*(5910), 66–69. doi:10.1126cience.1167311 PMID:19119219

Deleuze, G. (1968). *Spinoza et le problème de l'expression*. Paris: Les Editions de Minuit.

Deleuze, G., & Guattarì, F. (1983). *Anti-Oedipus*. Minneapolis, MN: University of Minnesota.

Deleuze, G., & Parnet, C. (2002). *Dialogues II*. New York: Columbia University Press.

Deluze, G., & Guattarì, F. (1987). *A Thousand Plateaus*. Minneapolis, MN: University of Minnesota.

Demyttenaere, K., Bruffaerts, R., Lee, S., Posada-Villa, J. A., Kovess, V., & Angermeyer, M. … Von Korff, M. (2007). Mental disorders among persons with chronic back or neck pain: Results from the World Mental Health Surveys. *Pain*. doi:10.1016/j.pain.2007.01.022

Desmond, D. M., O'neill, K., De Paor, A., McDarby, G., & MacLachlan, M. (2006). Augmenting the reality of phantom limbs: Three case studies using an augmented mirror box procedure. *JPO: Journal of Prosthetics and Orthotics*, *18*(3), 74–79.

Desmond, D. M., O'Neill, K., Paor, A. D., McDarby, G., & MacLachlan, M. (2006). Augmenting the Reality of Phantom Limbs: Three Case Studies Using an Augmented Mirror Box Procedure. *Journal of Prosthetics and Orthotics*, *18*(3), 74–79. doi:10.1097/00008526-200607000-00005

Deutsch, J. E., & Westcott McCoy, S. (2017). Virtual reality and serious games in neurorehabilitation of children and adults: Prevention, plasticity, and participation. *Pediatric Physical Therapy: The Official Publication of The Section on Pediatrics of the American Physical Therapy Association*, *29*(Suppl. 3), S23–S36. doi:10.1097/PEP.0000000000000387 PMID:28654475

di Pellegrino, G., Fadiga, L., Fogassi, L., Gallese, V., & Rizzolatti, G. (1992). Understanding motor events: A neurophysiological study. *Experimental Brain Research*, *91*(1), 176–180. doi:10.1007/BF00230027 PMID:1301372

Díaz, D., Boj, C., & Portalés, C. (2016). HybridPLAY: A New Technology to Foster Outdoors Physical Activity, Verbal Communication and Teamwork. *Sensors (Basel)*, *16*(4), 586. doi:10.339016040586 PMID:27120601

Didehbani, N., Allen, T., Kandalaft, M., Krawczyk, D., & Chapman, S. (2016). Virtual Reality Social Cognition Training for children with high functioning autism. *Computers in Human Behavior*, *62*, 703–711. doi:10.1016/j.chb.2016.04.033

Difende, J., & Hoffman, H. G. (2002). Virtual reality exposure therapy for World Trade Center Posttraumatic Stress Disorder: A case report. *Cyberpsychology & Behavior: The Impact of the Internet. Multimedia and Virtual Reality on Behavior and Society*, *5*(6), 529–535.

Diodato, R. (2018). Virtual. In *International Lexicon of Aesthetics. Spring 2018 Edition.* Retrieved July 8, 2018, from https://lexicon.mimesisjournals.com/archive/2018/spring/Virtual.pdf

Diodato, R. (2012). *Aesthetics of the Virtual*. New York: Suny Press.

Djaouti, D., Alvarez, J., Jessel, J. P., Methel, G., & Molinier, P. (2007). Towards a classification of video games. In *Artificial and Ambient Intelligence convention*. Artificial Societies for Ambient Intelligence.

Dohle, C., Pullen, J., Nakaten, A., Kust, J., Rietz, C., & Karbe, H. (2009). Mirror therapy promotes recovery from severe hemiparesis: A randomized controlled trial. *Neurorehabilitation and Neural Repair*, *23*(3), 209–217. doi:10.1177/1545968308324786 PMID:19074686

Doi, K. (2007). Computer-Aided Diagnosis in Medical Imaging: Historical Review, Current Status and Future Potential. *Computerized Medical Imaging and Graphics*, *31*(4-5), 198–211. doi:10.1016/j.compmedimag.2007.02.002

Dommes, A., & Cavallo, V. (2012). Can simulator-based training improve street-crossing safety for elderly pedestrians? *Transportation Research Part F: Psychology and Behaviour*, *15*(2), 206–218. doi:10.1016/j.trf.2011.12.004

Dommès, A., Le Lay, T., Vienne, F., Dang, N. T., Beaudoin, A. P., & Do, M. C. (2015). Towards an explanation of age-related difficulties in crossing a two-way street. *Accident; Analysis and Prevention*, *85*, 229–238. doi:10.1016/j.aap.2015.09.022 PMID:26476193

Duff, C. K., & Flattery, J. J. (2014). Developing mirror self awareness in students with autism spectrum disorder. *Journal of Autism and Developmental Disorders*, *44*(5), 1027–1038. doi:10.100710803-013-1954-0 PMID:24077784

Dunaway, M. O. (2000). Assessing the potential of online psychotherapy. *The Psychiatric Times*, (17): 10.

Dunleavy, M., & Dede, C. (2014). *Augmented reality teaching and learning. In Handbook of research on educational communications and technology* (pp. 735–745). Springer. doi:10.1007/978-1-4614-3185-5_59

Dunleavy, M., Dede, C., & Mitchell, R. (2009). Affordances and limitations of immersive participatory augmented reality simulations for teaching and learning. *Journal of Science Education and Technology*, *18*(1), 7–22. doi:10.100710956-008-9119-1

Dunn, J., Yeo, E., Moghaddampour, P., Chau, B., & Humbert, S. (2017). Virtual and augmented reality in the treatment of phantom limb pain: A literature review. *NeuroRehabilitation*, *40*(4), 595–601. doi:10.3233/NRE-171447 PMID:28211829

Duric, N. S., Assmus, J., Gundersen, D., & Elgen, I. B. (2012). Neurofeedback for the treatment of children and adolescents with ADHD: A randomized and controlled clinical trial using parental reports. *BMC Psychiatry*, *12*(1), 107. doi:10.1186/1471-244X-12-107 PMID:22877086

Eggenberger, P., Theill, N., Holenstein, S., Schumacher, V., & de Bruin, E. D. (2015). Multicomponent physical exercise with simultaneous cognitive training to enhance dual-task walking of older adults: A secondary analysis of a 6-month randomized controlled trial with 1-year follow-up. *Clinical Interventions in Aging*, *10*, 1711–1732. doi:10.2147/CIA.S91997 PMID:26604719

Ehde, D. M., Dillworth, T. M., & Turner, J. A. (2014). Cognitive-Behavioral Therapy for Individuals With Chronic Pain. *The American Psychologist*, *69*(2), 153–166. doi:10.1037/a0035747 PMID:24547801

Ehrlich, J., & Munger, J. (2012). Utilizing head mounted displays as a learning tool for children with autism. In Proceedings of 4th European Immersive Education Summit, Vienna, Austria.

Ehrsson, H. H., Spence, C., & Passingham, R. E. (2004). That's my hand! Activity in premotor cortex reflects feeling of ownership of a limb. *Science*, *305*(5685), 875–877. doi:10.1126cience.1097011 PMID:15232072

Ellaway, R. (2010). eMedical Teacher. *Medical Teacher*, *32*(9), 791–793. doi:10.3109/0142159X.2010.513223 PMID:20795817

Elsley, C. (2018). *About - Dementia Training from Forget Me Not - Dementia Training | Forget Me Not Dementia Training*. Retrieved July 10, 2018 from http://www.forgetmenotdementia.co.uk/about/

Ely, E., Chen-Lim, M. L., Carpenter, K. M. II, Wallhauser, E., & Friedlaender, E. (2016). Pain assessment of children with autism spectrum disorders. *Journal of Developmental and Behavioral Pediatrics*, *37*(1), 53–61. doi:10.1097/DBP.0000000000000240 PMID:26703326

Erzegovesi, S., & Gorini, A. (2003). *Bella come sei. Vincere la Bulimia*. Milan, Italy: San Paolo.

Escobedo, L., Tentori, M., Quintana, E., Favela, J., & Garcia-Rosas, D. (2014). Using augmented reality to help children with autism stay focused. *IEEE Pervasive Computing*, *13*(1), 38–46. doi:10.1109/MPRV.2014.19

Escribano, L. R., Herrera, G., Jordan, R., & Gimeno, J. (2010). Pictogram-Room: uso de la realidad aumentada para el aprendizaje visual de personas con Autismo. *Paper presented at the Investigaciones sobre autismo en español: problemas y perspectivas.*

Esguerra, S., Ben, J., & Johnson, K. (2017). Improving Balance through Virtual Reality and Physical Therapy Integration. *International Journal of Clinical Medicine*, *8*(5). doi:10.4236/ijcm.2017.85030

Fabri, M., & Moore, D. J. (2005). The use of emotionally expressive avatars in Collaborative Virtual Environments. In *Proceedings of Symposium on Empathic Interaction with Synthetic Characters, held at Artificial Intelligence and Social Behaviour Convention 2005*. University of Hertfordshire.

Fabri, M., Elzouki, S., & Moore, D. (2007). Emotionally expressive avatars for chatting, learning and therapeutic intervention. *Proceedings of the 12th International Conference on Human-Computer Interaction (HCI International), 4552*(3), 275–285.

Fair, A. (2015). *3D Scanning - OnCorVid.* Oncor Digital. Retrieved July 10, 2018 from https://oncorvideo.co.uk/3d-scanning/

Fang, X., Brown, D. S., Florence, C. S., & Mercy, J. A. (2012). The economic burden of child maltreatment in the United States and implications for prevention. *Child Abuse & Neglect, 36*(2), 156–165. doi:10.1016/j.chiabu.2011.10.006 PMID:22300910

Feifer, A., Delisle, J., & Anidjar, M. (2008). Hybrid augmented reality simulator: Preliminary construct validation of laparoscopic smoothness in a urology residency program. *The Journal of Urology, 180*(4), 1455–1459. doi:10.1016/j.juro.2008.06.042 PMID:18710760

Feintuch, U., Tuchner, M., Lorber-Haddad, A., Meiner, Z., & Shiri, S. (2009, June 29-July 2). VirHab - A virtual reality system for treatment of chronic pain and disability. *Paper presented at the Virtual Rehabilitation International Conference.*

Felitti, V. J., & Anda, R. F. (2010). The relationship of adverse childhood experiences to adult medical disease, psychiatric disorders, and sexual behavior: Implications for healthcare. In The impact of early life trauma on health and disease: The hidden epidemic (pp. 77-87).

Feltham, M. G., Ledebt, A., Deconinck, F. J. A., & Savelsbergh, G. J. P. (2010). Mirror visual feedback induces lower neuromuscular activity in children with spastic hemiparetic cerebral palsy. *Research in Developmental Disabilities, 31*(6), 1525–1535. doi:10.1016/j.ridd.2010.06.004 PMID:20591615

Feng, J. Y., Chang, Y. T., Chang, H. Y., Erdley, W. S., Lin, C. H., & Chang, Y. J. (2013). Systematic review of effectiveness of situated e-learning on medical and nursing education. *Worldviews on Evidence-Based Nursing, 10*(3), 174–183. doi:10.1111/wvn.12005 PMID:23510119

Fernandez Montenegro, J. M., & Argyriou, V. (2017). Cognitive evaluation for the diagnosis of Alzheimer's disease based on Turing Test and Virtual Environments. *Physiology & Behavior, 173*, 42–51. doi:10.1016/j.physbeh.2017.01.034 PMID:28137425

Ferrari, M., & Matthews, W. S. (1983). Self-recognition deficits in autism: Syndrome-specific or general developmental delay? *Journal of Autism and Developmental Disorders, 13*(3), 317–324. doi:10.1007/BF01531569 PMID:6196346

Ferrie, C. D., De Marco, P., Grünewald, R. A., Giannakodimos, S., & Panayiotopoulos, C. P. (1994). Video game induced seizures. *Journal of Neurology, Neurosurgery, and Psychiatry, 57*(8), 925–931. doi:10.1136/jnnp.57.8.925 PMID:8057115

Ferri, P. (2011). *Nativi digitali.* Milan, Italy: Pearson.

Finansministeriet. (2017). *Udgiftslofter og statens finanser.* Center for udgiftspolitik og modernisering.

Finkelstein, S., Nickel, A., Lipps, Z., Barnes, T., Wartell, Z., & Suma, E. (2011). Astrojumper: Motivating exercise with an immersive virtual reality exergame. *Presence (Cambridge, Mass.), 20*(1), 78–92. doi:10.1162/pres_a_00036

Fisher, C., & Fried, A. (2003). Internet-mediated psychological services and the American Psychological Association ethics code. *Psychoterapy: Theory, Research, Practise. Training (New York, N.Y.)*, (40): 103–111.

Fisher, E., Heathcote, L., & Palermo, T. M. de C., Williams, A. C., Lau, J., & Eccleston, C. (2014). Systematic Review and Meta-Analysis of Psychological Therapies for Children With Chronic Pain. *Journal of Pediatric Psychology.* doi:10.1093/jpepsy/jsu008

Fjeld, M., & Voegtli, B. M. (2002). *Augmented chemistry: An interactive educational workbench.* International symposium on mixed and augmented reality (ISMAR), Darmstadt, Germany. doi:10.1109/ISMAR.2002.1115100

Flickr. (2008). *OneAvatar @ Milano in Digitale*. Retrieved from https://www.flickr.com/photos/xdxd_vs_xdxd/3033590996/in/photostream/

Flickr. (2010). *Torley*. Retrieved from https://www.flickr.com/photos/torley/5054603928

Flusser, V. (1996). *Kommunikologie*. Frankfurt am Main, Germany: Fisher Taschenbuch Verlag.

Flusser, V. (1997). *Medienkultur*. Frankfurt am Main, Germany: Fischer Taschenbuch Verlag.

Flusser, V. (2000). *Towards a Philosophy of Photography*. London: Reaktion Books.

Flynn, D., Schaik, P., Blackman, T., Femcott, C., Hobbs, B., & Calderon, C. (2003). Developing a virtual reality–based methodology for people with dementia: A feasibility study. *Cyberpsychology & Behavior*, *6*(6), 591–611. doi:10.1089/109493103322725379 PMID:14756925

Foege, W. H. (1998). Adverse childhood experiences. A public health perspective. *American Journal of Preventive Medicine*, *14*(4), 354–355. PMID:9635083

Foell, J., Bekrater-Bodmann, R., Diers, M., & Flor, H. (2014). *Mirror therapy for phantom limb pain: Brain changes and the role of body representation*. European Journal of Pain. doi:10.1002/j.1532-2149.2013.00433.x

Forbes. (2018). *The Difference Between Virtual Reality, Augmented Reality And Mixed Reality.* Retrieved from https://www.forbes.com/sites/quora/2018/02/02/the-difference-between-virtual-reality-augmented-reality-and-mixed-reality/#7f235f002d07

Fordyce, W. E., & Company, M. C. V. (1977). Behavioral methods for chronic pain and illness. *Pain*, *3*(3), 291–292. doi:10.1016/0304-3959(77)90029-X

Forgeron, P. A., King, S., Stinson, J. N., McGrath, P. J., MacDonald, A. J., & Chambers, C. T. (2010). Social functioning and peer relationships in children and adolescents with chronic pain: A systematic review. *Pain Research & Management*, *15*(1), 27–41. doi:10.1155/2010/820407 PMID:20195556

Fotopoulou, A., Jenkinson, P. M., Tsakiris, M., Haggard, P., Rudd, A., & Kopelman, M. D. (2011). Mirror-view reverses somatoparaphrenia: Dissociation between first- and third-person perspectives on body ownership. *Neuropsychologia*, *49*(14), 3946–3955. doi:10.1016/j.neuropsychologia.2011.10.011 PMID:22023911

Freeman, D., & Freeman, J. (2017). *Why virtual reality could be a mental health gamechanger.* Retrieved from: https://www.theguardian.com/science/blog/2017/mar/22/all.AnesthAnalg

Freeman, D., & Freeman, J. (2017). Why virtual reality could be a mental health gamechanger. *The Guardian*. Retrieved July 10, 2018 from https://www.theguardian.com/science/blog/2017/mar/22/all.AnesthAnalg

Freina, L., & Ott, M. (2015). A literature review on immersive virtual reality in education: state of the art and perspectives. In *The International Scientific Conference eLearning and Software for Education* (vol. 1, pp. 133-141). Bucharest: eLSE.

Friedrich, E. V., Sivanathan, A., Lim, T., Suttie, N., Louchart, S., Pillen, S., & Pineda, J. A. (2015). An effective neurofeedback intervention to improve social interactions in children with autism spectrum disorder. *Journal of Autism and Developmental Disorders*, *45*(12), 4084–4100. doi:10.100710803-015-2523-5 PMID:26210513

Frossard, P., & Khasanova, R. (2017). Graph-based classification of omnidirectional images. *Proceedings of the 2017 IEEE International Conference on Computer Vision Workshop*, 860-869.

Fuchs, H., Livingston, M., Raskar, R., Colucci, D. n., Keller, K., State, A., . . . Meyer, A. (1998). Augmented reality visualization for laparoscopic surgery. In W. Wells, A. Colchester & S. Delp (Eds.), Medical Image Computing and Computer-Assisted Interventation — MICCAI'98 (pp. 934-943). Springer. doi:10.1007/BFb0056282

Gaitatzes, A., Christopoulos, D., & Roussou, M. (2001). Reviving the past: cultural heritage meets virtual reality. *Paper presented at the 2001 conference on Virtual reality, archeology, and cultural heritage.* 10.1145/584993.585011

Galatis, P., Gavalas, D., Kasapakis, V., Pantziou, G., & Zaroliagis, C. (2016). Mobile augmented reality guides in cultural heritage. *Paper presented at the 8th EAI International Conference on Mobile Computing, Applications and Services.* 10.4108/eai.30-11-2016.2266954

Gallagher, S., & Cole, J. (1995). Body image and body schema in a deafferented subject. *Journal of Mind and Behavior.*

Gamberini, L., & Spagnolli, A. (2015). An Action-Based Approach to Presence: Foundations and Methods. In M. Lombard, F. Biocca, J. Freeman, W. IJsselsteijn, & R. Schaevitz (Eds.), *Immersed in Media: Telepresence Theory, Measurement & Technology* (pp. 101–114). Cham: Springer. doi:10.1007/978-3-319-10190-3_6

Gamito, P., Oliveira, J., Coelho, C., Morais, D., Lopes, P., Pacheco, J., ... Barata, F. A. (2015). Cognitive training on stroke patients via virtual reality-based serious games. *Disability and Rehabilitation*, *39*(4), 385–388. doi:10.3109/09638288.2014.934925 PMID:25739412

García-Betances, R., Waldmeyer, M., Fico, G., & Cabrera-Umpiérrez, M. (2015). A succinct overview of virtual reality technology use in Alzheimer's disease. *Frontiers in Aging Neuroscience*, 7.

Garrett, B., Taverner, T., & McDade, P. (2017). Virtual Reality as an Adjunct Home Therapy in Chronic Pain Management: An Exploratory Study. *JMIR Medical Informatics*, *5*(2), e11. doi:10.2196/medinform.7271 PMID:28495661

Garzotto, F., Gelsomini, M., Clasadonte, F., Montesano, D., & Occhiuto, D. (2016). Wearable Immersive Storytelling for Disabled Children. In *Proceedings of the International Working Conference on Advanced Visual Interfaces - AVI '16* (pp. 196–203). New York, NY: ACM Press.

Gatchel, R. J., Peng, Y. B., Peters, M. L., Fuchs, P. N., & Turk, D. C. (2007). The Biopsychosocial Approach to Chronic Pain: Scientific Advances and Future Directions. *Psychological Bulletin*, *133*(4), 581–624. doi:10.1037/0033-2909.133.4.581 PMID:17592957

Gavish, N., Gutiérrez, T., Webel, S., Rodríguez, J., Peveri, M., Bockholt, U., & Tecchia, F. (2015). Evaluating virtual reality and augmented reality training for industrial maintenance and assembly tasks. *Interactive Learning Environments*, *23*(6), 778–798. doi:10.1080/10494820.2013.815221

Gee, J. P. (2005). Learning by design: Good video games as learning machines. *E-Learning and Digital Media*, *2*(1), 5–16. doi:10.2304/elea.2005.2.1.5

Gelsomini, M., Garzotto, F., Montesano, D., & Occhiuto, D. (2016, August). Wildcard: A wearable virtual reality storytelling tool for children with intellectual developmental disability. In *2016 IEEE 38th Annual International Conference of the Engineering in Medicine and Biology Society (EMBC)* (pp. 5188-5191). IEEE. 10.1109/EMBC.2016.7591896

Gernsbacher, M. A., Morson, E. M., & Grace, E. J. (2016). Language and speech in autism. *Annual Review of Linguistics*, *2*(1), 413–425. doi:10.1146/annurev-linguistics-030514-124824 PMID:28127576

Gershon, J., Zimand, E., Pickering, M., Rothbaum, B. O., & Hodges, L. (2004). A pilot and feasibility study of virtual reality as a distraction for children with cancer. *Journal of the American Academy of Child and Adolescent Psychiatry*, *43*(10), 1243–1249. doi:10.1097/01.chi.0000135621.23145.05 PMID:15381891

Gil, J. (1998). *Metemorphoses of the Body*. Minneapolis, MN: Minnesota University Press.

Gimeno, J., Morillo, P., Casas, S., & Fernández, M. (2011). An augmented reality (AR) CAD system at construction sites. In *Augmented Reality-Some Emerging Application Areas*. InTech.

Gimeno, J., Fernández, M., Morillo, P., Coma, I., & Pérez, M. (2007). A reconfigurable immersive workbench and wall-system for designing and training in 3D environments. *Virtual Reality*, 458–467.

Gimeno, J., Portalés, C., Coma, I., Fernández, M., & Martínez, B. (2017). Combining Traditional and Indirect Augmented Reality for Indoor Crowded Environments. A Case Study on the Casa Batlló Museum. *Computers & Graphics*, *69*, 92–103. doi:10.1016/j.cag.2017.09.001

Giner Martínez, F., & Portalés Ricart, C. (2005, October 3-7). The Augmented User: A Wearable Augmented Reality Interface. *Paper presented at the International Conference on Virtual Systems and Multimedia (VSMM'05)*, Ghent, Belgium.

Glaser, D. (2002). Emotional abuse and neglect (psychological maltreatment): A conceptual framework. *Child Abuse & Neglect*, *26*(6-7), 697–714. doi:10.1016/S0145-2134(02)00342-3 PMID:12201163

Gold, J.I., Kim, S., Kant, J.A., Joseph, H.M., & Rizzo, A. (2006). Effectiveness of Virtual Reality for Pediatric Pain Distraction during IV Placement. *CyberPsychology & Behavior, 9*(2), 207-212.

Gold, J. I., Belmont, K. A., & Thomas, D. A. (2007). The Neurobiology of Virtual Reality Pain Attenuation. *Cyberpsychology & Behavior*, *10*(4), 536–544. doi:10.1089/cpb.2007.9993 PMID:17711362

Gold, J. I., Kim, S. H., Kant, A. J., Joseph, M. H., & Rizzo, A. "Skip." (2006). Effectiveness of Virtual Reality for Pediatric Pain Distraction during IV Placement. *Cyberpsychology & Behavior*. doi:10.1089/cpb.2006.9.207

Gold, J. I., & Mahrer, N. E. (2017). Is Virtual Reality Ready for Prime Time in the Medical Space? A Randomized Control Trial of Pediatric Virtual Reality for Acute Procedural Pain Management. *Journal of Pediatric Psychology*. doi:10.1093/jpepsy/jsx129 PMID:29053848

Gonzalez-Franco, M., Perez-Marcos, D., Spanlang, B., & Slater, M. (2010). The contribution of real-time mirror reflections of motor actions on virtual body ownership in an immersive virtual environment. *Paper presented at the 2010 IEEE Virtual Reality Conference (VR)*. 10.1109/VR.2010.5444805

Gorecki, C., Nixon, J., Lamping, D. L., Alavi, Y., & Brown, J. M. (2014). Patient-reported outcome measures for chronic wounds with particular reference to pressure ulcer research: A systematic review. *International Journal of Nursing Studies*, *51*(1), 157–165. doi:10.1016/j.ijnurstu.2013.03.004 PMID:23522938

Goršič, M., Cikajlo, I., Goljar, N., & Novak, D. (2017). A multisession evaluation of an adaptive competitive arm rehabilitation game. *Journal of Neuroengineering and Rehabilitation*, *14*(1), 128–128. doi:10.118612984-017-0336-9 PMID:29208017

Grace-Martin, M., & Gay, G. (2001). Web Browsing, Mobile Computing and Academic Performance. *Journal of Educational Technology & Society*, *4*, 95–107.

Gray, C. A., & Garand, J. D. (1993). Social stories: Improving responses of students with autism with accurate social information. *Focus on Autistic Behavior*, *8*(1), 1–10. doi:10.1177/108835769300800101

Greenbaum, P. (1992). The lawnmower man. Film and Video, *9*(3), 58-62.

Greenhill, L. L. (1998). Diagnosing attention-deficit/hyperactivity disorder in children. *The Journal of Clinical Psychiatry*, *59*, 31–41. PMID:9680051

Green, V. A., Pituch, K. A., Itchon, J., Choi, A., O'Reilly, M., & Sigafoos, J. (2006). Internet survey of treatments used by parents of children with autism. *Research in Developmental Disabilities*, *27*(1), 70–84. doi:10.1016/j.ridd.2004.12.002 PMID:15919178

Gregg, L., Barrowclough, C., & Haddock, G. (2007). Reasons for increased substance use in psychosis. *Clinical Psychology Review*, *27*(4), 494–510. doi:10.1016/j.cpr.2006.09.004 PMID:17240501

Grohol, J. (1993). *Best Practices in eTherapy. Definition and scope of e-therapy*. Retrieved from http://psychcentral.com/best/best3.htm

Grohol, J. (2010). From Netscape to Twitter: Fifteen Years of Mental Health Online. In A. Brunet & F. Herbert (Eds.), *Internet Use in the Aftermath of Trauma* (pp. 3–20). Amsterdam: Ios Press.

Gromala, D., Tong, X., Choo, A., Karamnejad, M., & Shaw, C. D. (2015). The Virtual Meditative Walk: Virtual Reality Therapy for Chronic Pain Management. *Paper presented at the 33rd Annual ACM Conference on Human Factors in Computing Systems*, Seoul, Republic of Korea. 10.1145/2702123.2702344

Groom, V., Bailenson, J. N., & Nass, C. (2009). The influence of racial embodiment on racial bias in immersive virtual environments. *Social Influence*, *4*(3), 231–248. doi:10.1080/15534510802643750

Gross, A. (2018). Pediatrician Nadine Burke Harris explains how childhood trauma can have lasting health impacts. *KNKX*. Retrieved July 18, 2018 from http://knkx.org/post/pediatrician-nadine-burke-harris-explains-how-childhood-trauma-can-have-lasting-health-impacts

Grynszpan, O., Weiss, P. L., Perez-Diaz, F., & Gal, E. (2014). Innovative technology-based interventions for autism spectrum disorders: A meta-analysis. *Autism*, *18*(4), 346–361. doi:10.1177/1362361313476767 PMID:24092843

Guazzaroni, G. (2017). The impact of augmented reality and virtual reality study material in the future of learning: a teamwork experience. In G. Kurubacak & H. Altinpulluk (Eds.), *Mobile Technologies and Augmented Reality in Open Education* (pp. 77–94). Hershey, PA: IGI Global. doi:10.4018/978-1-5225-2110-5.ch004

Gustafsson, L., & Papliński, A. P. (2004). Self-Organization of an Artificial Neural Network Subjected to Attention Shift Impairments and Familiarity Preference, Characteristics Studied in Autism. *Journal of Autism and Developmental Disorders*, *34*(2), 189–198. doi:10.1023/B:JADD.0000022609.31371.4d PMID:15162937

Halabi, O., El-Seoud, S. A., Alja'am, J. M., Alpona, H., Al-Hemadi, M., & Al-Hassan, D. (2017). Immersive virtual reality in improving communication skills in children with autism. *International Journal of Interactive Mobile Technologies*, *2*(11). Retrieved from http://online-journals.org/index.php/i-jim/article/view/6555/4365

Hansen, C., Wieferich, J., Ritter, F., Rieder, C., & Peitgen, H.-O. (2009). Illustrative visualization of 3D planning models for augmented reality in liver surgery. *International Journal of Computer Assisted Radiology and Surgery*, *5*(2), 133–141. doi:10.100711548-009-0365-3 PMID:20033519

Hansen, M. B. N. (2006). *Bodies in code. Interface with digital media*. New York: Routledge Taylor & Francis Group.

Hardt, J., & Rutter, M. (2004). Validity of adult retrospective reports of adverse childhood experiences: Review of the evidence. *Journal of Child Psychology and Psychiatry, and Allied Disciplines*, *45*(2), 260–273. doi:10.1111/j.1469-7610.2004.00218.x PMID:14982240

Harmsen, W. J., Bussmann, J. B., Selles, R. W., Hurkmans, H. L., & Ribbers, G. M. (2015). A mirror therapy–based action observation protocol to improve motor learning after stroke. *Neurorehabilitation and Neural Repair*, *29*(6), 509–516. doi:10.1177/1545968314558598 PMID:25416737

Hashimoto, A. (2015). *The Long Defeat Cultural Trauma, Memory and Identity in Japan*. New York, NY: Oxford University Press. doi:10.1093/acprof:oso/9780190239152.001.0001

Hassett, A. L., Aquino, J. K., & Ilgen, M. A. (2014). The risk of suicide mortality in chronic pain patients. *Current Pain and Headache Reports*, *18*(8), 436. doi:10.100711916-014-0436-1 PMID:24952608

Havik, T., Bru, E., & Ertesvåg, S. K. (2015). Assessing reasons for school non-attendance. *Scandinavian Journal of Educational Research*, *59*(3), 316–336. doi:10.1080/00313831.2014.904424

Heinz, B. R. (1981). *The origins of meditation: Perspectives beyond the scientific research* (Unpublished doctoral dissertation). Loyola University Chicago. Retrieved July 10, 2018 from https://ecommons.luc.edu/luc_diss/2065

Hemingway, S., Atkin, L., & Stephenson, J. (2013). Assessing and managing wounds in mental health settings. *Wounds UK*, *9*(3), 34–40.

Hendry, C. (2018). *Creative Aero – Craig French Hendry*. Retrieved July 10, 2018 from https://creative.aero/

Henriksen, B., Nielsen, R., Szabo, L., Evers, N., Kraus, M., & Geng, B. (2016). An affordable virtual reality system for treatment of phantom limb pain. *Paper presented at the 2016 Virtual Reality International Conference*. 10.1145/2927929.2927932

Heppelmann, B., Messlinger, K., Neiss, W. F., & Schmidt, R. F. (1990). Ultrastructural three-dimensional reconstruction of group III and group IV sensory nerve endings ("free nerve endings") in the knee joint capsule of the cat: Evidence for multiple receptive sites. *The Journal of Comparative Neurology*, *292*(1), 103–116. doi:10.1002/cne.902920107 PMID:2312785

Herber, O. R., Schepp, W., & Rieger, M. A. (2007). A systematic review on the impact of leg ulceration on patients' quality of life. *Health and Quality of Life Outcomes*, *5*(1), 44. doi:10.1186/1477-7525-5-44 PMID:17651490

Herman, D. B., Susser, E. S., Struening, E. L., & Link, B. L. (1997). Adverse childhood experiences: Are they risk factors for adult homelessness? *American Journal of Public Health*, *87*(2), 249–255. doi:10.2105/AJPH.87.2.249 PMID:9103105

Herrador Colmenero, L., Perez Marmol, J. M., Martí-García, C., Querol Zaldivar, M. Á., Tapia Haro, R. M., Castro Sánchez, A. M., & Aguilar-Ferrándiz, M. E. (2017). Effectiveness of mirror therapy, motor imagery, and virtual feedback on phantom limb pain following amputation: A systematic review. *Prosthetics and Orthotics International*. PMID:29153043

Herrera, G., Jordan, R., & Gimeno, J. (2006). Exploring the advantages of augmented reality for intervention in autism spectrum disorders. *Paper presented at the Second World Autism Congress*, Cape Town, South Africa.

Herrera, G., Alcantud, F., Jordan, R., Blanquer, A., Labajo, G., & De Pablo, C. (2008). Development of symbolic play through the use of virtual reality tools in children with autistic spectrum disorders: Two case studies. *Autism*, *12*(2), 143–157. doi:10.1177/1362361307086657 PMID:18308764

Hershey, A. D., Powers, S. W., Bentti, A. L., & DeGrauw, T. J. (2000). Effectiveness of amitriptyline in the prophylactic management of childhood headaches. *Headache*, *40*(7), 539–549. doi:10.1046/j.1526-4610.2000.00085.x PMID:10940092

Hilbert, A., Tuschen-Caffier, B., & Vögele, C. (2002). Effects of prolonged and repeated body image exposure in binge-eating disorder. *Journal of Psychosomatic Research*, *52*(3), 137–144. doi:10.1016/S0022-3999(01)00314-2 PMID:11897232

Hildebrandt, T., Loeb, K., Troupe, S., & Delinsky, S. (2012). Adjunctive mirror exposure for eating disorders: A randomized controlled pilot study. *Behaviour Research and Therapy*, *50*(12), 797–804. doi:10.1016/j.brat.2012.09.004 PMID:23089085

Hinterberger, T. (2011). The sensorium: A multimodal neurofeedback environment. *Advances in Human-Computer Interaction*, 3.

Hjelm, S. I., & Browall, C. (2000). Brainball: Using Brain Activity for Cool Competition. *Proceedings of the First Nordic Conference on Computer-Human Interaction (NordiCHI 2000).*

Hoermann, S., Ferreira Dos Santos, L., Morkisch, N., Jettkowski, K., Sillis, M., Devan, H., ... Cutfield, N. J. (2017). Computerised mirror therapy with augmented reflection technology for early stroke rehabilitation: Clinical feasibility and integration as an adjunct therapy. *Disability and Rehabilitation*, *39*(15), 1503–1514. doi:10.1080/09638288.2017.1291765 PMID:28478736

Hoffman, H.G., Patterson, D.R., & Carrougher, G.J. (2000). Use of Virtual Reality for Adjunctive Treatment of Adult Burn Pain During Physical Therapy: A Controlled Study. *The Clinical Journal of Pain, 16*(3), 244-250.

Hoffman, H. G., Chambers, G. T., Meyer, I. I. I. W. J., Arceneaux, L. L., Russell, W. J., Seibel, E. J., ... Patterson, D. R. (2011). Virtual reality as an adjunctive non-pharmacologic analgesic for acute burn pain during medical procedures. *Annals of Behavioral Medicine*, *41*(2), 183–191. doi:10.100712160-010-9248-7 PMID:21264690

Hoffman, H. G., Doctor, J. N., Patterson, D. R., Carrougher, G. J., & Furness, T. III. (2000). Virtual reality as an adjunctive pain control during burn wound care in adolescent patients. *Pain*, *85*(1), 305–309. doi:10.1016/S0304-3959(99)00275-4 PMID:10692634

Hoffman, H. G., Patterson, D. R., Seibel, E., Soltani, M., Jewett-Leahy, L., & Sharar, S. R. (2008). Virtual reality pain control during burn wound debridement in the hydrotank. *The Clinical Journal of Pain*, *24*(4), 299–304. doi:10.1097/AJP.0b013e318164d2cc PMID:18427228

Hoffman, H. G., Richards, T. L., Bills, A. R., Van Oostrom, T., Magula, J., Seibel, E. J., & Sharar, S. R. (2006). Using fMRI to study the neural correlates of virtual reality analgesia. *CNS Spectrums*, *11*(01), 45–51. doi:10.1017/S1092852900024202 PMID:16400255

Hoffman, H. G., Richards, T. L., Van, T. O., Coda, B. A., Jensen, M. P., Blough, D. K., & Sharar, S. R. (2007). The analgesic effects of opioids and immersive virtual reality distraction: Evidence from subjective and functional brain imaging assessments. *Anesthesia and Analgesia*, *105*(6), 1776–1783. doi:10.1213/01.ane.0000270205.45146.db PMID:18042882

Hoffman, H. G., Seibel, E. J., Richards, T. L., Furness, T. A., Patterson, D. R., & Sharar, S. R. (2006). Virtual Reality Helmet Display Quality Influences the Magnitude of Virtual Reality Analgesia. *The Journal of Pain*, *7*(11), 843–850. doi:10.1016/j.jpain.2006.04.006 PMID:17074626

Hogan, M., Sabri, H., & Kapralos, B. (2007). Interactive community simulation environment for community health nursing. In *Proceedings of the 2007 conference on Future Play* (pp. 237-240). ACM. 10.1145/1328202.1328248

Hopman, W. M., Harrison, M. B., Coo, H., Friedberg, E., Buchanan, M., & VanDenKerkhof, E. G. (2009). Associations between chronic disease, age and physical and mental health status. *Chronic Diseases in Canada*, *29*(3), 108–116. PMID:19527569

Howlin, P. (1997). *Autism: Preparing for Adulthood.* London: Routledge. doi:10.4324/9780203426913

Howlin, P., Moss, P., Savage, S., & Rutter, M. (2013). Social outcomes in mid-to later adulthood among individuals diagnosed with autism and average nonverbal IQ as children. *Journal of the American Academy of Child and Adolescent Psychiatry*, *52*(6), 572–581. doi:10.1016/j.jaac.2013.02.017 PMID:23702446

Hsieh, M. C., & Lee, J. J. (2018). Preliminary Study of VR and AR Applications in Medical and Healthcare Education. *Journal of Nursing and Health Studies, 3*(1).

Huang, A. X., Hughes, T. L., Sutton, L. R., Lawrence, M., Chen, X., Ji, Z., & Zeleke, W. (2017). Understanding the self in individuals with autism spectrum disorders (ASD): A review of literature. *Frontiers in Psychology*, *8*, 1422. doi:10.3389/fpsyg.2017.01422 PMID:28878717

Huang-Storms, L. (2008). *Efficacy of neurofeedback for children with histories of abuse and neglect: Pilot study and meta-analytic comparison to other treatments*. University of North Texas.

Hunfeld, J. a, Perquin, C. W., Duivenvoorden, H. J., Hazebroek-Kampschreur, a a, Passchier, J., van Suijlekom-Smit, L. W., & van der Wouden, J. C. (2001). Chronic pain and its impact on quality of life in adolescents and their families. *Journal of Pediatric Psychology*. doi:10.1093/jpepsy/26.3.145

Huster, R. J., Mokom, Z. N., Enriquez-Geppert, S., & Herrmann, C. S. (2014). Brain-computer interfaces for EEG neurofeedback: Peculiarities and solutions. *International Journal of Psychophysiology: Official Journal of the International Organization of Psychophysiology*, *91*(1), 36–45. doi:10.1016/j.ijpsycho.2013.08.011 PMID:24012908

IEEE Spectrum: Technology, Engineering, and Science News. (2017). *Silicon Valley's Latest Craze: Brain Tech*. Retrieved August, 10, 2017 from http://spectrum.ieee.org/biomedical/devices/silicon-valleys-latest-craze-brain-tech

Ienca, M., Vayena, E., & Blasimme, A. (2018). Big data and dementia: Charting the route ahead for research, ethics, and policy. *Frontiers in Medicine*, *5*, 13. doi:10.3389/fmed.2018.00013 PMID:29468161

Ikeda, J., Davitt, B. V., Ultmann, M., Maxim, R., & Cruz, O. A. (2013). Brief report: Incidence of ophthalmologic disorders in children with autism. *Journal of Autism and Developmental Disorders*, *43*(6), 1447–1451. doi:10.100710803-012-1475-2 PMID:22350452

Ilgen, M. A., Kleinberg, F., Ignacio, R. V., Bohnert, A. S. B., Valenstein, M., & McCarthy, J. F. … Katz, I. R. (2013). Noncancer Pain Conditions and Risk of Suicide. *JAMA Psychiatry*. doi:10.1001/jamapsychiatry.2013.908

Ilusio. (2016). Augmented Reality Could Revolutionize Plastic Surgery. Retrieved from http://www.illusioimaging.com/

Indovina, P., Barone, D., Gallo, L., Chirico, A., Pietro, D. G., & Antonio, G. (2018). Virtual Reality as a Distraction Intervention to Relieve Pain and Distress During Medical Procedures: A Comprehensive Literature Review. *The Clinical Journal of Pain*. Ahead of Print. Doi:10.1097/AJP.0000000000000599

Inoue, Y., Fukao, K., Araki, T., Yamamoto, S., Kubota, H., & Watanabe, Y. (1999). Photosensitive and Nonphotosensitive Electronic Screen Game-Induced Seizures. *Epilepsia*, *40*(s4), 8–16. doi:10.1111/j.1528-1157.1999.tb00900.x PMID:10487167

Ip, H. H., Wong, S. W., Chan, D. F., Byrne, J., Li, C., Yuan, V. S., & Wong, J. Y. (2016). Virtual Reality Enabled Training for Social Adaptation in Inclusive Education Settings for School-Aged Children with Autism Spectrum Disorder (ASD). *Lecture Notes in Computer Science Blended Learning: Aligning Theory with Practices,* 94-102.

Ishii, H., Kobayashi, M., & Arita, K. (1994). Iterative design of seamless collaboration media. *Communications of the ACM*, *37*(8), 83–97. doi:10.1145/179606.179687

Ito, M., Bittanti, S., & Cody, M. (2010). *Hanging out, messing around and geeking out*. Retrieved from https://mitpress.mit.edu/sites/default/files/titles/free_download/9780262013369_Hanging_Out.pdf

Jain, S. C. (1989). Standardization of international marketing strategy: Some research hypotheses. *Journal of Marketing*, *53*(1), 70–79. doi:10.2307/1251525

Jäncke, L., Cheetham, M., & Baumgartner, T. (2009). Virtual reality and the role of the prefrontal cortex in adults and children. *Frontiers in Neuroscience*, *3*(1). doi:10.3389/neuro.01.006.2009 PMID:19753097

Jansen, A., Bollen, D., Tuschen-Caffier, B., Roefs, A., Tanghe, A., & Braet, C. (2008). Mirror exposure reduces body dissatisfaction and anxiety in obese adolescents: A pilot study. *Appetite*, *51*(1), 214–217. doi:10.1016/j.appet.2008.01.011 PMID:18342397

Jansen, A., Voorwinde, V., Hoebink, Y., Rekkers, M., Martijn, C., & Mulkens, S. (2016). Mirror exposure to increase body satisfaction: Should we guide the focus of attention towards positively or negatively evaluated body parts? *Journal of Behavior Therapy and Experimental Psychiatry*, *50*, 90–96. doi:10.1016/j.jbtep.2015.06.002 PMID:26117584

Jarrold, W., Mundy, P., Gwaltney, M., Bailenson, J., Hatt, N., McIntyre, N., ... Swain, L. (2013). Social attention in a virtual public speaking task in higher functioning children with autism. *Autism Research*, *6*(5), 393–410. doi:10.1002/aur.1302 PMID:23696132

Javornik, A., Rogers, Y., Gander, D., & Moutinho, A. (2017). MagicFace: Stepping into character through an augmented reality mirror. *Paper presented at the 2017 CHI Conference on Human Factors in Computing Systems*. 10.1145/3025453.3025722

Jeng, M.-Y., Pai, F.-Y., & Yeh, T.-M. (2017). The virtual reality leisure activities experience on elderly people. *Applied Research in Quality of Life*, *12*(1), 49–65. doi:10.100711482-016-9452-0

Jeon, B., Cho, S., & Lee, J.-H. (2014). Application of Virtual Body Swapping to Patients with Complex Regional Pain Syndrome: A Pilot Study. *Cyberpsychology, Behavior, and Social Networking*, *17*(6), 366–370. doi:10.1089/cyber.2014.0046 PMID:24892199

Johnsen, K., Dickerson, R., Raij, A., Lok, B., Jackson, J., Min, S., . . . Lind, D. S. (2005, March 12-16). Experiences in using immersive virtual characters to educate medical communication skills. *Paper presented at the IEEE Proceedings Virtual Reality*.

Johnson, K. A., Kelly, S. P., Bellgrove, M. A., Barry, E., Cox, M., ... Gill, M. (2007). Response variability in attention deficit hyperactivity disorder: Evidence for neuropsychological heterogeneity. *Neuropsychologia*, *45*(4), 630–638. doi:10.1016/j.neuropsychologia.2006.03.034 PMID:17157885

Johnson, L., Adams Becker, S., Cummins, M., Estrada, V., Freeman, A., & Hall, C. (2016). *NMC Horizon Report: 2016 Higher Education Edition*. Austin, TX: The New Media Consortium.

Johnson, L., Levine, A., Smith, R., & Stone, S. (2010). *The 2010 Horizon Report*. Austin, TX: The New Media Consortium.

Johnson, L., Smith, R., Willis, H., Levine, A., & Haywood, K. (2011). *The 2011 Horizon Report*. Austin, TX: The New Media Consortium.

Jones, J., Barr, W., Robinson, J. & Carlisle, C. (2006). Depression in patients with chronic venous ulceration. *British Journal of Nursing, 15*(Sup2), S17-S23.

Jones, T., Moore, T., & Choo, J. (2016). The impact of virtual reality on chronic pain. *PLoS One*, *11*(12), e0167523. doi:10.1371/journal.pone.0167523 PMID:27997539

Josman, N., Ben-Chaim, H. M., Friedrich, S., & Weiss, P. L. (2008). Effectiveness of virtual reality for teaching street-crossing skills to children and adolescents with autism. *International Journal on Disability and Human Development*, *7*(1), 49–56. doi:10.1515/IJDHD.2008.7.1.49

Juan, M. C., Alcaniz, M., Monserrat, C., Botella, C., Banos, R. M., & Guerrero, B. (2005). Using Augmented Reality to Treat Phobias. *IEEE Computer Graphics and Applications*, *25*(6), 31–37. doi:10.1109/MCG.2005.143 PMID:16315475

Kamphuis, C., Barsom, E., Schijven, M., & Christoph, N. (2014). Augmented reality in medical education? *Perspectives on Medical Education*, *3*(4), 300–311. doi:10.100740037-013-0107-7 PMID:24464832

Kandalaft, M. R., Didehbani, N., Krawczyk, D. C., Allen, T. T., & Chapman, S. B. (2013). Virtual reality social cognition training for young adults with high-functioning autism. *Journal of Autism and Developmental Disorders*, *43*(1), 34–44. doi:10.100710803-012-1544-6 PMID:22570145

Kanner, L. (1943). Autistic disturbances of affective contact. *Nervous Child*, *2*(3), 217–250.

Kashikar-Zuck, S., Goldschneider, K. R., Powers, S. W., Vaught, M. H., & Hershey, A. D. (2001). Depression and functional disability in chronic pediatric pain. *The Clinical Journal of Pain*, *17*(4), 341–349. doi:10.1097/00002508-200112000-00009 PMID:11783815

Katz, J., Rosenbloom, B. N., & Fashler, S. (2015). Chronic pain, psychopathology, and DSM-5 somatic symptom disorder. *Canadian Journal of Psychiatry*, *60*(4), 160–167. doi:10.1177/070674371506000402 PMID:26174215

Kaufmann, H., Steinbugl, K., Dunser, A., & Gluck, J. (2005). General training of spatial abilities by geometry education in augmented reality. *Cyberpsychology & Behavior*, *8*(4), 330.

Kearney, C. A. (2001). *School refusal behavior in youth: A functional approach to assessment and treatment*. American Psychological Association. doi:10.1037/10426-000

Keefe, F. J., Lefebvre, J. C., Egert, J. R., Affleck, G., Sullivan, M. J., & Caldwell, D. S. (2000). The relationship of gender to pain, pain behavior, and disability in osteoarthritis patients: The role of catastrophizing. *Pain*, *87*(3), 325–334. doi:10.1016/S0304-3959(00)00296-7 PMID:10963912

Ke, F., & Im, T. (2013). Virtual-reality-based social interaction training for children with high-functioning autism. *The Journal of Educational Research*, *106*(6), 441–461. doi:10.1080/00220671.2013.832999

Kemeny, A., George, P., & Mérienne, F. (2017). New VR Navigation Techniques to Reduce Cybersickness. *Electronic Imaging, The Engineering Reality of Virtual Reality*, *6*, 48-53. Retrieved April 29, 2018 from http://www.ingentaconnect.com/contentone/ist/ei/2017/00002017/00000003/art00009?crawler=true&mimetype=application/pdf

Kemeny, A., George, P., & Mérienne, F. (2017). New VR Navigation Techniques to Reduce Cybersickness. *Electronic Imaging, The Engineering Reality of Virtual Reality, 6*, 48-53. Retrieved April, 29 2018, from http://www.ingentaconnect.com/contentone/ist/ei/2017/00002017/00000003/art00009?crawler=true&mimetype=application/pdf

Kennedy, J. F. (1962). *Moon Speech*. Rice Stadium. Retrieved July 10, 2018 from https://er.jsc.nasa.gov/seh/ricetalk.htm

Kennedy, R. S., Berbaum, K. S., & Drexler, J. (1994, June). Methodological and measurement issues for identification of engineering features contributing to virtual reality sickness. In *Image 7*. Tucson, AZ: Conference.

Kerawalla, L., Luckin, R., Seljeflot, S., & Woolard, A. (2006). "Making it real": Exploring the potential of augmented reality for teaching primary school science. *Virtual Reality (Waltham Cross)*, *10*(3-4), 163–174. doi:10.100710055-006-0036-4

Keshav, N. U., Salisbury, J. P., Vahabzadeh, A., & Sahin, N. T. (2017). Social communication coaching smartglasses: Well tolerated in a diverse sample of children and adults with autism. *JMIR mHealth and uHealth*, *5*(9), e140. doi:10.2196/mhealth.8534 PMID:28935618

Key, A., George, C. L., Beattie, D., Stammers, K., Lacey, H., & Waller, G. (2002). Body image treatment within an inpatient program for anorexia nervosa: The role of mirror exposure in the desensitization process. *International Journal of Eating Disorders*, *31*(2), 185–190. doi:10.1002/eat.10027 PMID:11920979

Khanna, P. A. (2012). *Hybrid Reality. Thriving in the Emerging Human-Technology Civilization*. TED Books.

Kilgus, T., Heim, E., Haase, S., Prüfer, S., Müller, M., Seitel, A., ... Schlemmer, H.-P. (2015). Mobile markerless augmented reality and its application in forensic medicine. *International Journal of Computer Assisted Radiology and Surgery, 10*(5), 573–586. doi:10.100711548-014-1106-9 PMID:25149272

Kim, I.-J., Lee, H. J., & Kim, H.-G. (2004). Magic mirror: a new VR platform design and its applications. *Paper presented at the 2004 ACM SIGCHI International Conference on Advances in computer entertainment technology*, Singapore. 10.1145/1067343.1067394

Kim, K., Kim, S. I., Cha, K. R., Park, J., Rosenthal, M. Z., Kim, J. J., ... Kim, C. H. (2010). Development of a computer-based behavioral assessment of checking behavior in obsessive-compulsive disorder. *Comprehensive Psychiatry, 51*(1), 86–93. doi:10.1016/j.comppsych.2008.12.001 PMID:19932831

Kim, S. G., & Uĝurbil, K. (1997). Comparison of blood oxygenattion and cerebral blood flow effect in fMRI: Estimation of relative oxygen consumption change. *Magnetic Resonance in Medicine, 38*(1), 59–65. doi:10.1002/mrm.1910380110 PMID:9211380

King, S., Chambers, C. T., Huguet, A., MacNevin, R. C., McGrath, P. J., Parker, L., & MacDonald, A. J. (2011). The epidemiology of chronic pain in children and adolescents revisited: A systematic review. *Pain, 152*(12), 2729–2738. doi:10.1016/j.pain.2011.07.016 PMID:22078064

Kinsella, B. G., Chow, S., & Kushki, A. (2017). Evaluating the usability of a wearable social skills training technology for children with autism spectrum disorder. *Frontiers in Robotics and AI, 4*, 31. doi:10.3389/frobt.2017.00031

Kin, T., Nakatomi, H., Shono, N., Nomura, S., Saito, T., Oyama, H., & Saito, N. (2017, October 15). Neurosurgical Virtual Reality Simulation for Brain Tumor Using High-definition Computer Graphics: A Review of the Literature. *Neurologia Medico-Chirurgica, 57*(10), 513–520. doi:10.2176/nmc.ra.2016-0320 PMID:28637947

Kiryu, T., & So, R. H. (2007). Sensation of presence and cybersickness in applications of virtual reality for advanced rehabilitation. *Journal of Neuroengineering and Rehabilitation, 4*(1), 34. doi:10.1186/1743-0003-4-34 PMID:17894857

Kizony, R., Weiss, P. L., Harel, S., Feldman, Y., Obuhov, A., Zeilig, G., & Shani, M. (2017). Tele-rehabilitation service delivery journey from prototype to robust in-home use. *Disability and Rehabilitation, 39*(15), 1532–1540. doi:10.1080/09638288.2016.1250827 PMID:28004980

Klinger, E., Legeron, P., Roy, S., Chemin, I., Lauer, F., & Nugues, P. (2006). Virtual reality exposure in the treatment of social phobia. In G. Riva., C. Botella, P. Legeron & G. Optale (Eds.), Cybertherapy: Internet and Virtual Reality as Assessment and Rehabilitation Tools for Clinical Psychology and Neuroscience. Amsterdam: IOS Press.

Klopfer, E. (2008). *Augmented learning: Research and design of mobile educational games*. Cambridge, MA: MIT Press. doi:10.7551/mitpress/9780262113151.001.0001

Klopfer, E., & Sheldon, J. (2010). Augmenting your own reality: Student authoring of science-based augmented reality games. *New Directions for Youth Development, 2010*(128), 85–94. doi:10.1002/yd.378 PMID:21240956

Klopfer, E., & Squire, K. (2008). Environmental detectives: The development of an augmented reality platform for environmental simulations. *Educational Technology Research and Development, 56*(2), 203–228. doi:10.100711423-007-9037-6

Kokinsky, E., Enska, K., Nilsson, S., & Finnstro, B. (2009). The use of Virtual Reality for needle-related procedural pain and distress in children and adolescents in a paediatric oncology unit. *European Journal of Oncology Nursing, 13*, 102–109. doi:10.1016/j.ejon.2009.01.003

Korkman, M., Kirk, U., & Kemp, S. (2007). NEPSY–Second Edition (NEPSY-II). San Antonio, TX: The Psychological Corporation.

Kotranza, A., Lind, D. S., Pugh, C. M., & Lok, B. (2009). Real-time in-situ visual feedback of task performance in mixed environments for learning joint psychomotorcognitive tasks In *Mixed and Augmented Reality, 2009. ISMAR 2009. 8th IEEE International Symposium on* (pp. 125-134). IEEE. doi: 10.1109/ISMAR.2009.5336485

Kraus, R., Zack, J., & Stricker, G. (2004). *On line Counseling: a Handbook For Mental Health Professionals*. San Diego, CA: Elsevier.

Krepki, R., Blankertz, B., Curio, G., & Müller, K.-R. (2007). The Berlin Brain-Computer Interface (BBCI) – Towards a new communication channel for online control in gaming Applications. *Multimedia Tools and Applications*, *33*(1), 73–90. doi:10.100711042-006-0094-3

Krijn, M., Emmelkamp, P. M. G., Olafsson, R. P., & Biemond, R. (2004). Virtual reality exposure therapy of anxiety disorders: A review. *Clinical Psychology Review*, *24*(3), 259–281. doi:10.1016/j.cpr.2004.04.001 PMID:15245832

Kroker, A., & Weinstein, M. (1995). *Data Trash*. Montreal: New World Perspectives.

Krueger, M. W. (1983). *Artificial Reality*. Boston: Addison-Wesley.

Kugelmann, D., Stratmann, L., Nühlen, N., Bork, F., Hoffmann, S., Samarbarksh, G., ... Fallavollita, P. (2018). An Augmented Reality magic mirror as additive teaching device for gross anatomy. *Annals of Anatomy-Anatomischer Anzeiger*, *215*, 71–77. doi:10.1016/j.aanat.2017.09.011 PMID:29017852

Ku, J., Jang, H. J., Kim, K. U., Park, S. H., Kim, J. J., Kim, C. H., ... Kim, S. I. (2006). Pilot study for assessing the behaviors of patients with schizophrenia towards a virtual avatar. *Cyberpsychology & Behavior*, *9*(5), 531–539. doi:10.1089/cpb.2006.9.531 PMID:17034319

Kulman, R. (2018). *Virtual Reality (VR) assessment of ADHD*. Retrieved March, 5 2018, from http://learningworksforkids.com/2018/01/virtual-reality-vr-assessment-adhd

Kuriakose, S., Kunche, S., Narendranath, B., Jain, P., Sonker, S., & Lahiri, U. (2013). A step towards virtual reality based social communication for children with Autism. *2013 International Conference on Control, Automation, Robotics and Embedded Systems (CARE)*. 10.1109/CARE.2013.6733744

Kurzweil, R. (2005). *The Singularity Is Near: When Humans Transcend Biology*. New York: Viking Books.

Kwon, C. (in press). Verification of the possibility and effectiveness of experiential learning using HMD-based immersive VR technologies. *Virtual Reality (Waltham Cross)*.

Lack, C. W., & Storch, E. A. (2008). The use of computers in the assessment and treatment of obsessive-compulsive disorder. *Computers in Human Behavior*, *24*(3), 917–929. doi:10.1016/j.chb.2007.02.010

Lahiri, U., Bekele, E., Dohrmann, E., Warren, Z., & Sarkar, N. (2015). A physiologically informed virtual reality based social communication system for individuals with autism. *Journal of Autism and Developmental Disorders*, *45*(4), 919–931. doi:10.100710803-014-2240-5 PMID:25261247

Lahiri, U., Welch, K. C., Warren, Z., & Sarkar, N. (2011). Understanding psychophysiological response to a Virtual Reality-based social communication system for children with ASD. *2011 International Conference on Virtual Rehabilitation*. 10.1109/ICVR.2011.5971841

Lamson, R., & Meisner, M. (1994, June). *The effects of virtual reality immersion in the treatment of anxiety, panic and phobia of heights. In Virtual reality and persons with disabilities*. Paper presented at the 2nd Annual International Conference, San Francisco, CA.

Lange, B. S., Flynn, S. M., Chang, K., Profitt, R., & Rizzo, A. (2010). Development of an interaction game-based rehabilitation tool for dynamic balance training. *Topics in Stroke Rehabilitation*, *17*(5), 345–352. doi:10.1310/tsr1705-345 PMID:21131259

Langton, G. L. (1997). *Artificial Life*. Boston: MIT Press.

Leblanc, F., Delaney, C. P., Ellis, C. N., Neary, P. C., Champagne, B. J., & Senagore, A. J. (2010). Hand-Assisted Versus Straight Laparoscopic Sigmoid Colectomy on a Training Simulator: What is the Difference? A Stepwise Comparison of Hand-Assisted Versus Straight Laparoscopic Sigmoid Colectomy Performance on an Augmented Reality Simulator. *World Journal of Surgery*, *34*(12), 2909–2914. doi:10.100700268-010-0765-0 PMID:20740283

Lee, J. M., Cho, B. H., Ku, J. H., Kim, J. S., Lee, J. H., Kim, I. Y., & Kim, S. I. (2001). A study on the system for treatment of ADHD using virtual reality. In *Engineering in Medicine and Biology Society. Proceedings of the 23rd Annual International Conference of the IEEE* (*vol. 4*, pp. 3754-3757). Istanbul: IEEE. 10.1109/IEMBS.2001.1019654

Lee, S. (2018). Suzanne Lee - Professional History. *LinkedIn*. Retrieved July 10, 2018 from https://www.linkedin.com/in/suzanne-lee/

Lee, I. J., Chen, C. H., & Chang, K. P. (2016). Augmented reality technology combined with three-dimensional holography to train the mental rotation ability of older adults. *Computers in Human Behavior*, *65*, 488–500. doi:10.1016/j.chb.2016.09.014

Lee, J. (1996). Charting the codes of cyberspace: a rethoric of electronic mail. In R. Strate, R. Jacobson, & S. Gibson (Eds.), *Communication and cyberspace: Social interaction in an electronic environment* (pp. 275–296). Hampton Press.

Lee, M., Pyun, S. B., Chung, J., Kim, J., Eun, S. D., & Yoon, B. (2016). A further step to develop patient-friendly implementation strategies for virtual reality-based rehabilitation in patients with acute stroke. *Physical Therapy*, *96*(10), 1554–1564. doi:10.2522/ptj.20150271 PMID:27149961

Leigh, J. P., & Du, J. (2015). Brief report: Forecasting the economic burden of autism in 2015 and 2025 in the United States. *Journal of Autism and Developmental Disorders*, *45*(12), 4135–4139. doi:10.100710803-015-2521-7 PMID:26183723

Lenhart, A., Purcell, K., & Smith, A. (2010). Social Media & Mobile Internet Use among Teens and Young Adults. *Pew Internet & American Life Project*. Retrieved from http://www.pewinternet.org/files/oldmedia/Files/Reports/2010/PIP_Social_Media_and_Young_Adults_Report_Final_with_toplines.pdf

Leo, T., Manganello, F., & Chen, N. S. (2010). From the learning work to the learning adventure. *Proceedings of EDEN 2010*.

Levin, M. F., Weiss, P. L., & Keshner, E. A. (2015). Emergence of virtual reality as a tool for upper limb rehabilitation: Incorporation of motor control and motor learning principles. *Physical Therapy*, *95*(3), 415–425. doi:10.2522/ptj.20130579 PMID:25212522

Leviski, Y. (n.d.). *AR and Healthcare: The Future Is Now*. Retrieved from https://appreal-vr.com/blog/augmented-reality-for-healthcare/

Lewin, J. E. (1986). Emergence: Labeled Autistic. *The American Journal of Occupational Therapy*, *40*(7), 503–503. doi:10.5014/ajot.40.7.503b

Lewis, C., & Griffin, M. (1997). Human factors consideration in clinical applications of virtual reality. *Studies in Health Technology and Informatics*, 35–58. PMID:10175342

Lewis, M. J., Davies, R., Jenkins, D., & Tait, M. I. (2005). A review of evaluative studies of computer-based learning in nursing education. *Nurse Education Today*, *25*(8), 586–597. doi:10.1016/j.nedt.2005.09.006 PMID:16289489

Li, A., Montaño, Z., Chen, V. J., & Gold, J. L. (2011). Virtual reality and pain management: Current trends and future directions. *Pain Management*, *1*(2), 147–157. doi:10.2217/pmt.10.15 PMID:21779307

Liao, Y.-Y., Yang, Y.-R., Cheng, S.-J., Wu, Y.-R., Fuh, J.-L., & Wang, R.-Y. (2015). Virtual reality–based training to improve obstacle-crossing performance and dynamic balance in patients with Parkinson's disease. *Neurorehabilitation and Neural Repair*, *29*(7), 658–667. doi:10.1177/1545968314562111 PMID:25539782

Liebermann, D. G., Berman, S., Weiss, P. L. T., & Levin, M. F. (2012). Kinematics of reaching movements in a 2-D virtual environment in adults with and without stroke. *IEEE Transactions on Neural Systems and Rehabilitation Engineering: A Publication of the IEEE Engineering in Medicine and Biology Society, 20*(6), 778-787. doi:10.1109/TNSRE.2012.2206117

Lim, T., Louchart, S., Suttie, N., Hauge, J. B., Stanescu, I. A., Ortiz, I. M., ... Ott, M. (2014). Narrative serious game mechanics (NSGM)–insights into the narrative-pedagogical mechanism. In *International Conference on Serious Games* (pp. 23-34). Springer. 10.1007/978-3-319-05972-3_4

Lin, C. S., Jeng, M. Y., & Yeh, T. M. (2018). The elderly perceived meanings and values of virtual reality leisure activities: A means-end chain approach. *International Journal of Environmental Research and Public Health*, *15*(4), 663. doi:10.3390/ijerph15040663 PMID:29614012

Lind, S. E., & Bowler, D. M. (2009). Delayed self-recognition in children with autism spectrum disorder. *Journal of Autism and Developmental Disorders*, *39*(4), 643–650. doi:10.100710803-008-0670-7 PMID:19051001

Liu, R., Salisbury, J. P., Vahabzadeh, A., & Sahin, N. T. (2017). Feasibility of an autism-focused augmented reality smartglasses system for social communication and behavioral coaching. *Frontiers in Pediatrics*, *5*, 145. doi:10.3389/fped.2017.00145 PMID:28695116

Liu, W., Cheok, A. D., Mei-Ling, C. L., & Theng, Y. L. (2007, September). Mixed reality classroom: learning from entertainment. In *Proceedings of the 2nd international conference on Digital interactive media in entertainment and arts* (pp. 65-72). ACM.

Lorenzo, G., Lledó, A., Pomares, J., & Roig, R. (2016). Design and application of an immersive virtual reality system to enhance emotional skills for children with autism spectrum disorders. *Computers & Education*, *98*, 192–205. doi:10.1016/j.compedu.2016.03.018

Lozano, J. A., Montesa, J., Juan, M. C., Alcañiz, M., Rey, B., Gil, J., . . . Morganti, F. (2005). VR-mirror: a virtual reality system for mental practice in post-stroke rehabilitation. *Paper presented at the International Symposium on Smart Graphics*. 10.1007/11536482_23

Lozano-Quilis, J.-A., Gil-Gomez, H., Gil-Gómez, J.-A., Albiol-Perez, S., Palacios, G., Fardoum, H. M., & Mashat, A. S. (2013). Virtual reality system for multiple sclerosis rehabilitation using KINECT. *Paper presented at the 2013 7th International Conference on Pervasive Computing Technologies for Healthcare (PervasiveHealth)*. 10.4108/icst.pervasivehealth.2013.252208

Lozano-Quilis, J.-A., Gil-Gómez, H., Gil-Gómez, J.-A., Albiol-Pérez, S., Palacios-Navarro, G., Fardoun, H. M., & Mashat, A. S. (2014). Virtual rehabilitation for multiple sclerosis using a kinect-based system: randomized controlled trial. *JMIR serious games, 2*(2).

Luciano, C. J., Banerjee, P. P., Bellotte, B., Oh, G. M., Lemole, M. Jr, Charbel, F. T., & Roitberg, B. (2011). Learning Retention of Thoracic Pedicle Screw Placement Using a High-Resolution Augmented Reality Simulator With Haptic Feedback. *Neurosurgery*, *69*, 14–19. doi:10.1227/NEU.0b013e31821954ed PMID:21471846

Luethcke, C. A., McDaniel, L., & Becker, C. B. (2011). A comparison of mindfulness, nonjudgmental, and cognitive dissonance-based approaches to mirror exposure. *Body Image*, *8*(3), 251–258. doi:10.1016/j.bodyim.2011.03.006 PMID:21561817

Lu, Y., Waltz, S., Stenzel, K., Muhle, H., & Stephani, U. (2008). Photosensitivity in epileptic syndromes of childhood and adolescence. *Epileptic Disorders*, *10*(2), 136–143. PMID:18539564

Lyons, V., & Fitzgerald, M. (2013). Atypical sense of self in autism spectrum disorders: a neuro-cognitive perspective. In M. Fitzgerald (Ed.), *Recent Advances in Autism Spectrum Disorders* (vol. 1). INTECH Open Access Publisher. Retrieved April 9, 2018 from https://mts.intechopen.com/books/recent-advances-in-autism-spectrum-disorders-volume-i/atypical-sense-of-self-in-autism-spectrum-disorders-a-neuro-cognitive-perspective

Lyons, V., & Fitzgerald, M. (2013). Atypical sense of self in autism spectrum disorders: a neuro-cognitive perspective. In M. Fitzgerald (Ed.), *Recent Advances in Autism Spectrum Disorders* (vol. 1). INTECH Open Access Publisher. Retrieved April 9, 2018, from https://mts.intechopen.com/books/recent-advances-in-autism-spectrum-disorders-volume-i/atypical-sense-of-self-in-autism-spectrum-disorders-a-neuro-cognitive-perspective

Maglione, M. A., Gans, D., Das, L., Timbie, J., & Kasari, C. (2012). Nonmedical interventions for children with ASD: Recommended guidelines and further research needs. *Pediatrics*, *130*(Suppl. 2), S169–S178. doi:10.1542/peds.2012-0900O PMID:23118248

Magora, F., Cohen, S., Shochina, M., & Dayan, E. (2006). Virtual reality immersion method of distraction to control experimental ischemic pain. *The Israel Medical Association Journal*, *8*(4), 261–265. PMID:16671363

Mahrer, N. E., & Gold, J. I. (2009). The use of virtual reality for pain control: A review. *Current Pain and Headache Reports*, *13*(2), 100–109. doi:10.100711916-009-0019-8 PMID:19272275

Maillot, P., Dommes, A., Dang, N. T., & Vienne, F. (2017). Training the elderly in pedestrian safety: Transfer effect between two virtual reality simulation devices. *Accident; Analysis and Prevention*, *99*, 161–170. doi:10.1016/j.aap.2016.11.017 PMID:27898369

Mairs, J. (2018). New virtual reality tool helps architects create dementia-friendly environments. *Dezeen*. Retrieved July 10, 2018 from https://www.dezeen.com/2017/02/22/virtual-reality-empathy-platform-tool-help-architects-create-dementia-friendly-environments-david-burgher-aitken-turnbull-wireframe-immersive/

Malloy, K. M., & Milling, L. S. (2010). The effectiveness of virtual reality distraction for pain reduction: A systematic review. *Clinical Psychology Review*, *30*(8), 1011–1018. doi:10.1016/j.cpr.2010.07.001 PMID:20691523

Manera, V., Chapoulie, E., Bourgeois, J., Guerchouche, R., David, R., Ondrej, J., ... Robert, P. (2016). A feasibility study with image-based rendered virtual reality in patients with mild cognitive impairment and dementia. *PLoS One*, *11*(3), e0151487–e0151487. doi:10.1371/journal.pone.0151487 PMID:26990298

Maraj, C. S., Martinez, S. G., Badillo-Urquiola, K. A., Stevens, J. A., & Maxwell, D. B. (2016). Preliminary review of a virtual world usability questionnaire. In S. Lackey & R. Shumaker (Eds.), Lecture Notes in Computer Science: Vol. 9740. *Virtual, Augmented and Mixed Reality. VAMR 2016* (pp. 35–46). Cham: Springer. doi:10.1007/978-3-319-39907-2_4

Maran, N. J., & Glavin, R. J. (2003). Low- to high-fidelity simulation – a continuum of medical education? *Medical Education*, *37*(1), 22–28. doi:10.1046/j.1365-2923.37.s1.9.x PMID:14641635

Marcelino, I., Laza, R., Domingues, P., Gómez-Meire, S., Fdez-Riverola, F., & Pereira, A. (2018). Active and assisted living ecosystem for the elderly. *Sensors (Basel)*, *18*(4), 1246. doi:10.339018041246 PMID:29673234

Marescaux, J., Rubino, F., Arenas, M., Mutter, D., & Soler, L. (2004, November 10). Augmented-reality-assisted laparoscopic adrenalectomy. *Journal of the American Medical Association*, *292*(18), 2214–2215. PMID:15536106

Martinez, L. (2010). *Getting there*. Bloomington, IN: Xlibris Corporation.

Mason, B. (2017). *Virtual reality has a motion sickness problem*. Retrieved April 29, 2018 from https://www.sciencenews.org/article/virtual-reality-has-motion-sickness-problem

Mason, B. (2017). *Virtual reality has a motion sickness problem*. Retrieved April 29, 2018, from https://www.sciencenews.org/article/virtual-reality-has-motion-sickness-problem

Massumi, B. (1998). From Hypersurface Architecture. *Architectural Design*, *68*(5/6), 16–24.

Massumi, B. (2002). *Parables for the virtual: movement, affect, sensation*. Durham, NC: Duke University. doi:10.1215/9780822383574

Mathur, A. S. (2015). Low cost virtual reality for medical training. *Paper presented at the 2015 IEEE Virtual Reality (VR)*. 10.1109/VR.2015.7223437

Matson, J. L., Rivet, T. T., Fodstad, J. C., Dempsey, T., & Boisjoli, J. A. (2009). Examination of adaptive behavior differences in adults with autism spectrum disorders and intellectual disability. *Research in Developmental Disabilities*, *30*(6), 1317–1325. doi:10.1016/j.ridd.2009.05.008 PMID:19540717

Mattan, B. D., Quinn, K. A., Acaster, S. L., Jennings, R. M., & Rotshtein, P. (2017). Prioritization of self-relevant perspectives in ageing. *Quarterly Journal of Experimental Psychology*, *70*(6), 1033–1052. doi:10.1080/17470218.2015.1127399 PMID:26652616

Maturana, R. H., & Varela, F. (1980). *Autopoiesis and Cognition. The Realization of the Living*. Dordrecht: Reidel Publishing Company. doi:10.1007/978-94-009-8947-4

Mayes, S. D., Calhoun, S. L., Aggarwal, R., Baker, C., Mathapati, S., Molitoris, S., & Mayes, R. D. (2013). Unusual fears in children with autism. *Research in Autism Spectrum Disorders*, *7*(1), 151–158. doi:10.1016/j.rasd.2012.08.002

McCaul, K. D., & Malott, J. M. (1984). Distraction and coping with pain. *Psychological Bulletin*, *95*(3), 516–533. doi:10.1037/0033-2909.95.3.516 PMID:6399756

McCleery, J. P. (2015). Comment on technology-based intervention research for individuals on the autism spectrum. *Journal of Autism and Developmental Disorders*, *45*(12), 3832–3835. doi:10.100710803-015-2627-y PMID:26537909

McCue, L. M., Flick, L. H., Twyman, K. A., Xian, H., & Conturo, T. E. (2016). Prevalence of non-febrile seizures in children with idiopathic autism spectrum disorder and their unaffected siblings: A retrospective cohort study. *BMC Neurology*, *16*(1), 245. doi:10.118612883-016-0764-3 PMID:27894273

McDonald, D. D., Walsh, S., Vergara, C., & Gifford, T. (2013). Effect of a virtual pain coach on pain management discussions: A pilot study. *Pain Management Nursing: Official Journal of The American Society of Pain Management Nurses*, *14*(4), 200–209. doi:10.1016/j.pmn.2011.03.004 PMID:24315243

McLuhan, M. (1964). *Understanding Media*. New York: Graw-Hill Book Company.

McWilliam, D. (2018). *The Product. V Store*. Retrieved July 10, 2018 from http://www.vitaevr.com/the-product/

Melzack, R. (1999). From the gate to the neuromatrix. *Pain*, *82*, S121–S126. doi:10.1016/S0304-3959(99)00145-1 PMID:10491980

Melzack, R. (2001). Pain and the neuromatrix in the brain. *Journal of Dental Education*. PMID:11780656

Melzack, R., & Wall, P. D. (1965). Pain mechanisms: A new theory. *Science*, *150*(3699), 971–978. doi:10.1126cience.150.3699.971 PMID:5320816

Menzies, R. J., Rogers, S. J., Phillips, A. M., Chiarovano, E., de Waele, C., Verstraten, F. A., & MacDougall, H. (2016). An objective measure for the visual fidelity of virtual reality and the risks of falls in a virtual environment. *Virtual Reality (Waltham Cross)*, *20*(3), 173–181. doi:10.100710055-016-0288-6

Merleau-Ponty, M. (2003). *Nature: Course Notes from the Collège de France*. Evanston, IL: Northwestern University Press.

Merleau-Pounty, M. (1962). *Phenomenology of Perception*. London: Routledge and Kegan Paul.

Merleau-Pounty, M. (1968). *The Visible and the Invisible*. Evanston, IL: Northwestern University Press.

Mikropoulos, T. A., & Natsis, A. (2011). Educational virtual environments: A ten-year review of empirical research (1999–2009). *Computers & Education*, *56*(3), 769–780. doi:10.1016/j.compedu.2010.10.020

Miller, K. J., Adair, B. S., Pearce, A. J., Said, C. M., Ozanne, E., & Morris, M. M. (2014). Effectiveness and feasibility of virtual reality and gaming system use at home by older adults for enabling physical activity to improve health-related domains: A systematic review. *Age and Ageing*, *43*(2), 188–195. doi:10.1093/ageing/aft194 PMID:24351549

Millett, C. J., Fish, D. R., Thompson, P. J., & Johnson, A. (1999). Seizures During Video-Game Play and Other Common Leisure Pursuits in Known Epilepsy Patients Without Visual Sensitivity. *Epilepsia*, *40*(s4), 59–64. doi:10.1111/j.1528-1157.1999.tb00908.x PMID:10487175

Milne, E., Griffiths, H., Buckley, D., & Scope, A. (2009). Vision in children and adolescents with autistic spectrum disorder: Evidence for reduced convergence. *Journal of Autism and Developmental Disorders*, *39*(7), 965–975. doi:10.100710803-009-0705-8 PMID:19224351

Mineo, B. A., Ziegler, W., Gill, S., & Salkin, D. (2009). Engagement with electronic screen media among students with autism spectrum disorders. *Journal of Autism and Developmental Disorders*, *39*(1), 172–187. doi:10.100710803-008-0616-0 PMID:18626761

Miranda, E., & Brouse, A. (2005). Toward direct brain-computer musical interfaces. In *Proceedings of the 2005 Conference on New Interfaces for Musical Expression* (pp. 216-219). National University of Singapore.

Mirelman, A., Rochester, L., Maidan, I., Del Din, S., Alcock, L., Nieuwhof, F., ... Hausdorff, J. M. (2016). Addition of a non-immersive virtual reality component to treadmill training to reduce fall risk in older adults (V-TIME): A randomised controlled trial. *Lancet*, *388*(10050), 1170–1182. doi:10.1016/S0140-6736(16)31325-3 PMID:27524393

Mirelman, A., Rochester, L., Reelick, M., Nieuwhof, F., Pelosin, E., Abbruzzese, G., ... Hausdorff, J. M. (2013). V-TIME: A treadmill training program augmented by virtual reality to decrease fall risk in older adults: Study design of a randomized controlled trial. *BMC Neurology*, *13*(1), 15–15. doi:10.1186/1471-2377-13-15 PMID:23388087

Mitchell, A. J., Chan, M., Bhatti, H., Halton, M., Grassi, L., Johansen, C., & Meader, N. (2011). Prevalence of depression, anxiety, and adjustment disorder in oncological, haematological, and palliative-care settings: A meta-analysis of 94 interview-based studies. *The Lancet Oncology*, *12*(2), 160–174. doi:10.1016/S1470-2045(11)70002-X PMID:21251875

Mitchell, P., Parsons, S., & Leonard, A. (2007). Using virtual environments for teaching social understanding to 6 adolescents with autistic spectrum disorders. *Journal of Autism and Developmental Disorders*, *37*(3), 589–600. doi:10.100710803-006-0189-8 PMID:16900403

Mitgutsch, K. (2011). Serious learning in serious games. In M. Ma, A. Oikonomou, & L. C. Jain (Eds.), *Serious Games and Edutainment Applications* (pp. 45–58). Springer London. doi:10.1007/978-1-4471-2161-9_4

Mitha, A. P., Almekhlafi, M. A., Janjua, M. J. J., Albuquerque, F. C., & McDougall, C. G. (2013). Simulation and augmented reality in endovascular neurosurgery: Lessons from aviation. *Neurosurgery*, *72*(1), 107–114. doi:10.1227/NEU.0b013e31827981fd PMID:23254798

Moayedi, M., & Davis, K. D. (2013). Theories of pain: From specificity to gate control. *Journal of Neurophysiology*, *109*(1), 5–12. doi:10.1152/jn.00457.2012 PMID:23034364

Mogk, C. (2017, June). *Virtual Reality in Health Care Makes Medical Reality Easier to Endure*. Retrieved from https://www.autodesk.com/redshift/virtual-reality-in-health-care/

Mohammadi, A., Kargar, M., & Hesami, E. (2018). Using virtual reality to distinguish subjects with multiple- but not single-domain amnestic mild cognitive impairment from normal elderly subjects. *Psychogeriatrics: The Official Journal of the Japanese Psychogeriatric Society*, *18*(2), 132–142. doi:10.1111/psyg.12301 PMID:29409155

Mölbert, S., Thaler, A., Mohler, B., Streuber, S., Romero, J., Black, M., ... Giel, K. (2018). Assessing body image in anorexia nervosa using biometric self-avatars in virtual reality: Attitudinal components rather than visual body size estimation are distorted. *Psychological Medicine*, *48*(4), 642–653. doi:10.1017/S0033291717002008 PMID:28745268

Molina, K. I., Ricci, N. A., de Moraes, S. A., & Perracini, M. R. (2014). Virtual reality using games for improving physical functioning in older adults: A systematic review. *Journal of Neuroengineering and Rehabilitation*, *11*(1), 156–156. doi:10.1186/1743-0003-11-156 PMID:25399408

Monguet, J. M., Costa, J., Gaspar, P., & Costa, R. (2009). Web Based Learning Environment for medical education: E-fer, a practical tool for diagnosis and treatment of chronic wounds. In M. Manuela Cunha, A. Tavares, & R. Simões (Eds.), *Handbook of Research on Developments in e-Health and Telemedicine: Technological and Social Perspectives* (pp. 728–755). Hershey, PA: IGI Global.

Monkman, H., & Kushniruk, A. W. (2015). A see through future: Augmented reality and health information systems. *Studies in Health Technology and Informatics*, *208*, 281–285. PMID:25676988

Monteiro-Junior, R. S., da Silva Figueiredo, L. F., Maciel-Pinheiro, P. T., Abud, E. L. R., Braga, A. E. M. M., Barca, M. L., ... Laks, J. (2017). Acute effects of exergames on cognitive function of institutionalized older persons: A single-blinded, randomized and controlled pilot study. *Aging Clinical and Experimental Research*, *29*(3), 387–394. doi:10.100740520-016-0595-5 PMID:27256080

Montero-Alia, P., Munoz-Ortiz, L., Jimenez-Gonzalez, M., Benedicto-Pañell, C., Altimir-Losada, S., López-Colomer, Y., ... Torán-Monserrat, P. (2016). Study protocol of a randomized clinical trial evaluating the effectiveness of a primary care intervention using the Nintendo Wii console to improve balance and decrease falls in the elderly. *BMC Geriatrics*, *16*(1), 8. doi:10.118612877-015-0178-x PMID:26796956

Moore, D., Cheng, Y., McGrath, P., & Powell, N. (2005). Collaborative virtual environment technology for people with autism. *Focus on Autism and Other Developmental Disabilities*, *20*(4), 231–243. doi:10.1177/10883576050200040501

Morina, N., Ijntema, H., Meyerbröker, K., & Emmelkamp, P. M. (2015). Can virtual reality exposure therapy gains be generalized to real-life? A meta-analysis of studies applying behavioral assessments. *Behaviour Research and Therapy*, *74*, 18–24. doi:10.1016/j.brat.2015.08.010 PMID:26355646

Moro, C., Stromberga, Z., & Stirling, A. (2017). Virtualisation devices for student learning: Comparison between desktop-based (Oculus Rift) and mobile-based (Gear VR) virtual reality in medical and health science education. *Australasian Journal of Educational Technology*, *33*(6). doi:10.14742/ajet.3840

Morris, L. D., Louw, Q. A., & Grimmer-Somers, K. (2009). The effectiveness of virtual reality on reducing pain and anxiety in burn injury patients: A systematic review. *The Clinical Journal of Pain*, *25*(9), 815–826. doi:10.1097/AJP.0b013e3181aaa909 PMID:19851164

Morrongiello, B. A., Corbett, M., Foster, A., & Koutsoulianos, S. (2018). *Using Virtual Reality to Examine the Effects of Peer Modeling on Child Pedestrian Behavior.* Retrieved from https://trid.trb.org/view/1494797

Moseley, G. L., Gallace, A., & Spence, C. (2012). Bodily illusions in health and disease: Physiological and clinical perspectives and the concept of a cortical "body matrix.". *Neuroscience and Biobehavioral Reviews*, *36*(1), 34–46. doi:10.1016/j.neubiorev.2011.03.013 PMID:21477616

Mostafa, A. E., Ryu, W. H. A., Chan, S., Takashima, K., Kopp, G., Sousa, C. M., & Sharlin, E. (2017). *Designing NeuroSimVR: A Stereoscopic Virtual Reality Spine Surgery Simulator.* Retrieved from https://prism.ucalgary.ca/handle/1880/52230

Moult, E., Ungi, T., Welch, M., Lu, J., McGraw, R. C., & Fichtinger, G. (2013). Ultrasound-guided facet joint injection training using Perk Tutor. *International Journal of Computer Assisted Radiology and Surgery*, *8*(5), 831–836. doi:10.100711548-012-0811-5 PMID:23329279

Mouraux, D., Brassinne, E., Sobczak, S., Nonclercq, A., Warzée, N., Sizer, P. S., ... Penelle, B. (2017). 3D augmented reality mirror visual feedback therapy applied to the treatment of persistent, unilateral upper extremity neuropathic pain: A preliminary study. *The Journal of Manual & Manipulative Therapy*, *25*(3), 137–143. doi:10.1080/10669817.2016.1176726 PMID:28694676

Mühlberger, A., Jekel, K., Probst, T., Schecklmann, M., Conzelmann, A., Andreatta, M., ... Romanos, M. (2016). The influence of methylphenidate on hyperactivity and attention deficits in children with ADHD: A virtual classroom test. *Journal of Attention Disorders*. doi:10.1177/1087054716647480 PMID:27178061

Mukamal, R. (2017). Are virtual reality headsets safe for eyes? Retrieved July 10, 2018 from https://www.aao.org/eye-health/tips-prevention/are-virtual-reality-headsets-safe-eyes

Mukamal, R. (2017). *Are virtual reality headsets safe for eyes?* Retrieved July 5, 2018 from https://www.aao.org/eye-health/tips-prevention/are-virtual-reality-headsets-safe-eyes

Müller, H., Michoux, N., Bandon, D., & Geissbuhler, A. (2004). A review of content-based image retrieval systems in medical applications—clinical benefits and future directions. *International Journal of Medical Informatics*, *73*(1), 1–23. doi:10.1016/j.ijmedinf.2003.11.024 PMID:15036075

Muneer, R., Saxena, T., & Karanth, P. (2015.). *Virtual Reality Games as an Intervention for Children: A Pilot Study.* Retrieved July 5, 2018 from http://dcidj.org/article/view/456

Munkhaugen, E. K., Gjevik, E., Pripp, A. H., Sponheim, E., & Diseth, T. H. (2017). School refusal behaviour: Are children and adolescents with autism spectrum disorder at a higher risk? *Research in Autism Spectrum Disorders*, *41*, 31–38. doi:10.1016/j.rasd.2017.07.001

Murphy, K. (2015). *Feeling woozy? It may be cyber sickness.* Retrieved April 29, 2018, from https://well.blogs.nytimes.com/2015/11/14/feeling-woozy-it-may-be-cyber-sickness

Murphy, L., & Mitchell, D. (1998). When writing help to heal: E-mail as therapy. *British Journal of Guidance & Counselling*, (3): 377–386.

Murray, C. D., Pettifer, S., Howard, T., Patchick, E. L., Caillette, F., Kulkarni, J., & Bamford, C. (2007). The treatment of phantom limb pain using immersive virtual reality: Three case studies. *Disability and Rehabilitation*, *29*(18), 1465–1469. doi:10.1080/09638280601107385 PMID:17729094

Murray, C. D., Pettifer, S., Howard, T., Patchick, E., Caillette, F., & Murray, J. (2009). *Virtual solutions to phantom problems: Using immersive virtual reality to treat phantom limb pain. In Amputation, Prosthesis Use, and Phantom Limb Pain* (pp. 175–196). Springer.

Napoli, P. M. (2011). *Audience evolution: New technologies and the transformation of media audiences*. Columbia University Press.

National Autism Center. (2015). *Findings and conclusions: National standards project, phase 2*. Randolph, MA: Author.

National Child Traumatic Stress Network (NCTSN). (n.d.) Retrieved from https://www.nctsn.org/

National Institute of Mental Health (NIMH). (n.d.) Retrieved from https://www.nimh.nih.gov/

National Research Council. (2001). *Educating children with autism*. National Academies Press.

Neisser, U. (1982). Memory: What are the important questions. *Memory observed: Remembering in natural contexts*, 3-19.

Nepal, C. G., & Tang, S. (2017). *Virtual Reality Components*. Retrieved from http://web.tecnico.ulisboa.pt/ist188480/cmul/about.html

Neufeld, N. J., Elnahal, S. M., & Alvarez, R. H. (2017). Cancer pain: A review of epidemiology, clinical quality and value impact. *Future Oncology (London, England)*, *13*(9), 833–841. doi:10.2217/fon-2016-0423 PMID:27875910

Neugebauer, V., Li, W., Bird, G. C., & Han, J. S. (2004). The amygdala and persistent pain. *The Neuroscientist*, *10*(3), 221–234. doi:10.1177/1073858403261077 PMID:15155061

Neut, D., Fily, A., Cuvellier, J. C., & Vallée, L. (2012). The prevalence of triggers in paediatric migraine: A questionnaire study in 102 children and adolescents. *The Journal of Headache and Pain*, *13*(1), 61–65. doi:10.100710194-011-0397-2 PMID:22042255

Newbutt, N., Sung, C., Kuo, H. J., Leahy, M. J., Lin, C. C., & Tong, B. (2016). Brief report: A pilot study of the use of a virtual reality headset in autism populations. *Journal of Autism and Developmental Disorders*, *46*(9), 3166–3176. doi:10.100710803-016-2830-5 PMID:27272115

Nichols, S., & Patel, H. (2002). Health and safety implications of virtual reality: A review of empirical evidence. *Applied Ergonomics*, *33*(3), 251–271. doi:10.1016/S0003-6870(02)00020-0 PMID:12164509

Niolu, C., De Lorenzo, V., Stella, G., Di Lorenzo, G., Mastrofini, F., Modugno, L., ... Siracusano, A. (2017). Tor Vergata Virtual Reality Rehub. *Proceedings of the 21th National Congress of the Italian Society of Psychopathology*.

Nir-Hadad, S. Y., Weiss, P. L., Waizman, A., Schwartz, N., & Kizony, R. (2017). A virtual shopping task for the assessment of executive functions: Validity for people with stroke. *Neuropsychological Rehabilitation*, *27*(5), 808–833. doi:10.1080/09602011.2015.1109523 PMID:26558414

Norman, K. L. (2017). *Cyberpsychology: An introduction to human-computer interaction*. Cambridge University Press. doi:10.1017/9781316212554

Norrholm, S. D., Jovanovic, T., Gerardi, M., Breazeale, K. G., Price, M., Davis, M., ... Tuerk, P. W. (2016). Baseline psychophysiological and cortisol reactivity as a predictor of PTSD treatment outcome in virtual reality exposure therapy. *Behaviour Research and Therapy*, *82*, 28–37. doi:10.1016/j.brat.2016.05.002 PMID:27183343

North, M. M., North, S. M., & Coble, J. R. (1997). Virtual reality therapy: An effective treatment for psychological disorders. *Studies in Health Technology and Informatics*, *44*, 59–70. PMID:10175343

North, M., & North, S. (1994). Relative effectiveness of virtual environment desensitization and imaginal desensitization in the treatment of aerophobia. *Electronic Journal of Virtual Culture*, *2*(4), 37–42.

North, M., & North, S. (1994). Virtual environments and psychological disorders. *Electronic Journal of Virtual Culture*, *2*(4), 37–42.

Nugent, E., Shirilla, N., Hafeez, A., O'Riordain, D. S., Traynor, O., Harrison, A. M., & Neary, P. (2013). Development and evaluation of a simulator-based laparoscopic training program for surgical novices. *Surgical Endoscopy and other Interventional Techniques, 27*(1), 214-221. doi:10.100700464-012-2423-0

Nunes, M. (1995). Jean Baudrillard in cyberspace: Internet, virtuality, and postmodernity. *Style (Fayetteville)*, (29), 314–327.

Odom, S. L., Boyd, B. A., Hall, L. J., & Hume, K. (2010). Evaluation of comprehensive treatment models for individuals with autism spectrum disorders. *Journal of Autism and Developmental Disorders*, *40*(4), 425–436. doi:10.100710803-009-0825-1 PMID:19633939

Odom, S. L., Thompson, J. L., Hedges, S., Boyd, B. A., Dykstra, J. R., Duda, M. A., ... Bord, A. (2015). Technology-aided interventions and instruction for adolescents with autism spectrum disorder. *Journal of Autism and Developmental Disorders*, *45*(12), 3805–3819. doi:10.100710803-014-2320-6 PMID:25468409

Ofstedal, M. B., Zimmer, Z. S., & Lin, H. S. (1999). A comparison of correlates of cognitive functioning in older persons in Taiwan and the United States. *The Journals of Gerontology. Series B, Psychological Sciences and Social Sciences*, *54*(5), S291–S301. doi:10.1093/geronb/54B.5.S291 PMID:10542831

Oigara, J. N. (2018). Integrating virtual reality tools into classroom instruction. In J. Keengwe (Ed.), *Handbook of Research on Mobile Technology, Constructivism, and Meaningful Learning* (pp. 147–159). Hershey, PA: IGI Global. doi:10.4018/978-1-5225-3949-0.ch008

Oneal, B. J., Patterson, D. R., Soltani, M., Teeley, A., & Jensen, M. P. (2008). Virtual reality hypnosis in the treatment of chronic neuropathic pain: A case report. *The International Journal of Clinical and Experimental Hypnosis*, *56*(4), 451–462. doi:10.1080/00207140802255534 PMID:18726807

Onken, L., & Shoham, V. (2014). Tecnhology and the Stage Model of Behavioral Intervention Development. In L. Marsch, S. Lord, & J. Dallery (Eds.), *Behavioral Healthcare and Technology. Using Science-Based Innovations to Trasform Practise* (pp. 3–12). Oxford, UK: Oxford Press. doi:10.1093/med/9780199314027.003.0001

Oostema, J. A., Abdel, M. P., & Gould, J. C. (2008). Time-efficient laparoscopic skills assessment using an augmented-reality simulator. *Surgical Endoscopy and other Interventional Techniques, 22*(12), 2621-2624. doi:10.100700464-008-9844-9

Orange España. (2012). Pictogram Room: juegos educativos para autism [YouTube video]. Retrieved from https://www.youtube.com/watch?v=5B4mKPdBbtE

Ortiz-Catalan, M., Sander, N., Kristoffersen, B. M., Håkansson, Bo., & Brånemark, R. (2014). *Treatment of phantom limb pain (PLP) based on augmented reality and gaming controlled by myoelectric pattern recognition: a case study of a chronic PLP patient.* Retrieved from https://www.frontiersin.org/articles/10.3389/fnins.2014.00024/full

Ortiz-Catalan, M., Sander, N., Kristoffersen, M. B., Håkansson, B., & Brånemark, R. (2014). Treatment of phantom limb pain (PLP) based on augmented reality and gaming controlled by myoelectric pattern recognition: A case study of a chronic PLP patient. *Frontiers in Neuroscience*, *8*, 24. doi:10.3389/fnins.2014.00024 PMID:24616655

Osumi, M., Ichinose, A., Sumitani, M., Wake, N., Sano, Y., Yozu, A., ... Morioka, S. (2017). Restoring movement representation and alleviating phantom limb pain through short-term neurorehabilitation with a virtual reality system. *European Journal of Pain (London, England)*, *21*(1), 140–147. doi:10.1002/ejp.910 PMID:27378656

Oswald, D. P., & Sonenklar, N. A. (2007). Medication use among children with autism spectrum disorders. *Journal of Child and Adolescent Psychopharmacology*, *17*(3), 348–355. doi:10.1089/cap.2006.17303 PMID:17630868

Otten, L. J. & Rugg, M. D. (2005). Interpreting event-related brain potentials. *Event-Related Potentials: A Methods Handbook,* 3-16.

Oyama, H. (1998). Virtual reality for the palliative care of cancer. *Studies in Health Technology and Informatics*, *58*, 140–150. PMID:10350914

Palacio, R. R., Acosta, C. O., Cortez, J., & Morán, A. L. (2017). Usability perception of different video game devices in elderly users. *Universal Access in the Information Society*, *16*(1), 103–113. doi:10.100710209-015-0435-y

Palazzo, C., Klinger, E., Dorner, V., Kadri, A., Thierry, O., Boumenir, Y., ... Ville, I. (2016). Barriers to home-based exercise program adherence with chronic low back pain: Patient expectations regarding new technologies. *Annals of Physical and Rehabilitation Medicine*, *59*(2), 107–113. doi:10.1016/j.rehab.2016.01.009 PMID:27050664

Palermo, T. M., Eccleston, C., Lewandowski, A. S., Williams, A. C. de C., & Morley, S. (2010). Randomized controlled trials of psychological therapies for management of chronic pain in children and adolescents: An updated meta-analytic review. *Pain*. doi:10.1016/j.pain.2009.10.004 PMID:19910118

Pan, Z., Cheok, A. D., Yang, H., Zhu, J., & Shi, J. (2006). Virtual reality and mixed reality for virtual learning environments. *Computers & Graphics*, *30*(1), 20–28. doi:10.1016/j.cag.2005.10.004

Paquin, K., Crawley, J., Harris, J. E., & Horton, S. (2016). Survivors of chronic stroke - participant evaluations of commercial gaming for rehabilitation. *Disability and Rehabilitation*, *38*(21), 2144–2152. doi:10.3109/09638288.2015.1114155 PMID:26728133

Parent's Guide to Child Protective Services. (n.d.) Retrieved from https://www.dshs.wa.gov/sites/default/files/SESA/publications/documents/22-484.pdf

Parijat, P., Lockhart, T. E., & Liu, J. (2015). Effects of perturbation-based slip training using a virtual reality environment on slip-induced falls. *Annals of Biomedical Engineering*, *43*(4), 958–967. doi:10.100710439-014-1128-z PMID:25245221

Park, J.-Y., Chang, M., Kim, K.-M., & Kim, H.-J. (2015). The effect of mirror therapy on upper-extremity function and activities of daily living in stroke patients. *Journal of Physical Therapy Science*, *27*(6), 1681–1683. doi:10.1589/jpts.27.1681 PMID:26180297

Park, J., & Yim, J. (2016). A new approach to improve cognition, muscle strength, and postural balance in community-dwelling elderly with a 3-D virtual reality Kayak program. *The Tohoku Journal of Experimental Medicine*, *238*(1), 1–8. doi:10.1620/tjem.238.1 PMID:26656425

Park, Y. S., & Kim, H. J. (2005). Effects of a taping method on pain and ROM of the knee joint in the elderly. *Journal of Korean Academy of Nursing*, *35*(2), 372–381. doi:10.4040/jkan.2005.35.2.372 PMID:15860951

Parsons, S. (2016). Authenticity in Virtual Reality for assessment and intervention in autism: A conceptual review. *Educational Research Review*, *19*, 138–157. doi:10.1016/j.edurev.2016.08.001

Parsons, S., & Cobb, S. (2011). State-of-the-art of virtual reality technologies for children on the autism spectrum. *European Journal of Special Needs Education*, *26*(3), 355–366. doi:10.1080/08856257.2011.593831

Parsons, S., & Mitchell, P. (2002). The potential of virtual reality in social skills training for people with autistic spectrum disorders. *Journal of Intellectual Disability Research*, *46*(5), 430–443. doi:10.1046/j.1365-2788.2002.00425.x PMID:12031025

Parsons, S., Mitchell, P., & Leonard, A. (2004). The use and understanding of virtual environments by adolescents with autistic spectrum disorders. *Journal of Autism and Developmental Disorders*, *34*(4), 449–466. doi:10.1023/B:JADD.0000037421.98517.8d PMID:15449520

Parsons, T. D., & Barnett, M. (2017). Validity of a newly developed measure of memory: Feasibility study of the virtual environment grocery store. *Journal of Alzheimer's Disease*, *59*(4), 1227–1235. doi:10.3233/JAD-170295 PMID:28759971

Parsons, T. D., Carlew, A. R., Magtoto, J., & Stonecipher, K. (2017). The potential of function-led virtual environments for ecologically valid measures of executive function in experimental and clinical neuropsychology. *Neuropsychological Rehabilitation*, *27*(5), 777–807. doi:10.1080/09602011.2015.1109524 PMID:26558491

Parsons, T. D., Riva, G., Parsons, S., Mantovani, F., Newbutt, N., Lin, L., ... Hall, T. (2017). Virtual reality in pediatric psychology. *Pediatrics*, *140*(Suppl. 2), S86–S91. doi:10.1542/peds.2016-1758I PMID:29093039

Parsons, T. D., Rizzo, A. A., Rogers, S., & York, P. (2009). Virtual reality in paediatric rehabilitation: A review. *Developmental Neurorehabilitation*, *12*(4), 224–238. doi:10.1080/17518420902991719 PMID:19842822

Patient Protection and Affordable Care Act. (2010). Retrieved from https://www.healthcare.gov/glossary/patient-protection-and-affordable-care-act/

Paysant, J., Beis, J. M., Le Chapelain, L., & André, J. M. (2004). Mirror asomatognosia in right lesions stroke victims. *Neuropsychologia*, *42*(7), 920–925. doi:10.1016/j.neuropsychologia.2003.12.001 PMID:14998706

Perpiñá, C., Botella, C., & Baños, R. (2003). Virtual reality in eating disorders. *European Eating Disorders Review*, *11*(3), 261–278. doi:10.1002/erv.520

Perquin, C. W., Hazebroek-Kampschreur, A. A. J. M., Hunfeld, J. A. M., Bohnen, A. M., Van Suijlekom-Smit, L. W. A., Passchier, J., & Van Der Wouden, J. C. (2000). Pain in children and adolescents: A common experience. *Pain*, *87*(1), 51–58. doi:10.1016/S0304-3959(00)00269-4 PMID:10863045

Phillips, C. J., Humphreys, I., Fletcher, J., Harding, K., Chamberlain, G., & Macey, S. (2016). Estimating the costs associated with the management of patients with chronic wounds using linked routine data. *International Wound Journal*, *13*(6), 1193–1197. doi:10.1111/iwj.12443 PMID:25818405

Piaget, J. (1998). *The origin of intelligence in the child. Jean Piaget: Selected Works*. London: Routledge.

Pigford, T., & Andrews, A. W. (2010). Feasibility and benefit of using the Nintendo Wii Fit for balance rehabilitation in an elderly patient experiencing recurrent falls. *Journal of Student Physical Therapy Research*, *2*(1), 12–20.

Plancher, G., Tirard, A., Gyselinck, V., Nicolas, S., & Piolino, P. (2012). Using virtual reality to characterize episodic memory profiles in amnestic mild cognitive impairment and Alzheimer's disease: Influence of active and passive encoding. *Neuropsychologia*, *50*(5), 592–602. doi:10.1016/j.neuropsychologia.2011.12.013 PMID:22261400

Ploog, B. O., Scharf, A., Nelson, D., & Brooks, P. J. (2013). Use of computer-assisted technologies (CAT) to enhance social, communicative, and language development in children with autism spectrum disorders. *Journal of Autism and Developmental Disorders*, *43*(2), 301–322. doi:10.100710803-012-1571-3 PMID:22706582

Portalés Ricart, C. (2009). *Entornos multimedia de realidad aumentada en el campo del arte* [Doctoral Thesis]. Universidad Politécnica de Valencia, Valencia.

Portalés, C., Gimeno, J., Casas, S., Olanda, R., & Martínez, F. G. (2016). Interacting with Augmented Reality Mirrors. In Handbook of Research on Human-Computer Interfaces, Developments, and Applications (pp. 216–244). Hershey, PA: IGI Global.

Portalés, C., Alonso-Monasterio, P., & Viñals, M. J. (2017). 3D virtual reconstruction and visualisation of the archaeological site Castellet de Bernabé (Llíria, Spain). *Virtual Archaeology Review*, *8*(16). doi:10.4995/var.2017.5890

Powers, M. B., & Emmelkamp, P. M. (2008). Virtual reality exposure therapy for anxiety disorders: A meta-analysis. *Journal of Anxiety Disorders*, *22*(3), 561–569. doi:10.1016/j.janxdis.2007.04.006 PMID:17544252

Pravettoni, G. (2002). *Web Psychology*. Milan, Italy: Guerini e Associati.

Prensky, M. (2001). Digital natives, digital immigrants. *On the Horizon*, (5): 1–6.

Prensky, M. (2003). Digital game-based learning. *Computers in Entertainment*, *1*(1), 21–21. doi:10.1145/950566.950596

Probst, M. (2015). Body image therapy for patients with eating disorders: scientific and clinical perspectives.

Psychiatry Online | DSM Library. (n.d.). Retrieved May 20, 2018 from https://dsm.psychiatryonline.org/doi/book/10.1176/appi.books.9780890425596

Pull, C. B. (2005). Current status of virtual reality exposure therapy in anxiety disorders. *Current Opinion in Psychiatry*, *18*(1), 7–14. PMID:16639177

Radu, I. (2014). Augmented reality in education: A meta-review and cross-media analysis. *Personal and Ubiquitous Computing*, *18*(6), 1533–1543. doi:10.100700779-013-0747-y

Rahaman, S., Ansari, Z., Biswas, P., & Memon, S. B. (n.d.). *Virtual Reality for combating social awkwardness in Special Needs*. Retrieved March 10, 2018 from https://www.scitechnol.com/peer-review/virtual-reality-for-combating-social-awkwardness-in-special-needs-twPN.php?article_id=6674

Ramachandiran, C. R., Jomhari, N., Thiyagaraja, S., & Maria, M. (2015). Virtual reality based behavioural learning for autistic children. *The Electronic Journal of e-Learning*, *13*(5), 357-365.

Ramachandran, V. S. (1993). Behavioral and magnetoencephalographic correlates of plasticity in the adult human brain. *Proceedings of the National Academy of Sciences*. 10.1073/pnas.90.22.10413

Ramachandran, V. S., & Altschuler, E. L. (2009). The use of visual feedback, in particular mirror visual feedback, in restoring brain function. *Brain*, *132*(7), 1693–1710. doi:10.1093/brain/awp135 PMID:19506071

Ramachandran, V. S., & Rogers-Ramachandran, D. (2000). Phantom Limbs and Neural Plasticity. *Archives of Neurology*, *57*(3), 317. doi:10.1001/archneur.57.3.317 PMID:10714655

Ramachandran, V. S., Rogers-Ramachandran, D., & Cobb, S. (1995). Touching the phantom limb. *Nature*, *377*(6549), 489–490. doi:10.1038/377489a0 PMID:7566144

Ramachandran, V. S., Stewart, M., & Rogers-Ramachandran, D. C. (1992). Perceptual correlates of massive cortical reorganization. *Neuroreport*, *3*(7), 583–586. doi:10.1097/00001756-199207000-00009 PMID:1421112

Rand, D., Weingarden, H., Weiss, R., Yacoby, A., Reif, S., Malka, R., ... Zeilig, G. (2017). Self-training to improve UE function at the chronic stage post-stroke: A pilot randomized controlled trial. *Disability and Rehabilitation*, *39*(15), 1541–1548. doi:10.1080/09638288.2016.1239766 PMID:27793071

Rapport, M. D., Chung, K. M., Shore, G., Denney, C. B., & Isaacs, P. (2000). Upgrading the science and technology of assessment and diagnosis: Laboratory and clinic-based assessment of children with ADHD. *Journal of Clinical Child Psychology*, *29*(4), 555–568. doi:10.1207/S15374424JCCP2904_8 PMID:11126633

Ravindran, V., Sazawal, V., Solorzano, R., & Turnacioglu, S. (2017). Experiences with virtual reality-based training for joint attention: a usability and initial feasibility pilot of FloreoVR's Joint Attention Module in a special education school setting.

Reconnect Integrative Trauma Treatment Center. (2018). Retrieved from http://www.reconnectcenter.com/

Regenbrecht, H. T., Franz, E. A., McGregor, G., Dixon, B. G., & Hoermann, S. (2011). Beyond the Looking Glass: Fooling the Brain with the Augmented Mirror Box. *Presence*, *20*(6), 559–576. doi:10.1162/PRES_a_00082

Reid, G. J., Lang, B. A., & McGrath, P. J. (1997). Primary juvenile fibromyalgia: Psychological adjustment, family functioning, coping, and functional disability. *Arthritis and Rheumatism*, *40*(4), 752–760. doi:10.1002/art.1780400423 PMID:9125260

Reitinger, B., Bornik, A., Beichel, R., & Schmalstieg, D. (2006). Liver surgery planning using virtual reality. *IEEE Computer Graphics and Applications*, *26*(6), 36–47. doi:10.1109/MCG.2006.131 PMID:17120912

Rendon, A. A., Lohman, E. B., Thorpe, D., Johnson, E. G., Medina, E., & Bradley, B. (2012). The effect of virtual reality gaming on dynamic balance in older adults. *Age and Ageing*, *41*(4), 549–552. doi:10.1093/ageing/afs053 PMID:22672915

Renner, R., & Erfurt-Berge, C. (2017). Depression and quality of life in patients with chronic wounds: Ways to measure their influence and their effect on daily life. *Chronic Wound Care Management and Research*, *4*, 143–151. doi:10.2147/CWCMR.S124917

Rey, G., Visconti, A., Balaguer, E., & Martínez, J. (2006). Uso de simuladores en ginecología y obstetricia: Experiencia en la enseñanza de pregrado. *Educação Médica*, *9*(4b), 229–233.

Reynolds, L., Smith, M. E., Birnholtz, J. P., & Hancock, J. T. (2013). Butler lies from both sides: Actions and perceptions of unavailability management in texting. *Proceedings of the 2013 2nd ACM Conference on Computer Supported Cooperative Work*. 10.1145/2441776.2441862

Rhee, H. (2000). Prevalence and predictors of headaches in US adolescents. *Headache*, *40*(7), 528–538. doi:10.1046/j.1526-4610.2000.00084.x PMID:10940091

Richard, E., Billaudeau, V., Richard, P., & Gaudin, G. (2007, September 27-29). Augmented Reality for Rehabilitation of Cognitive Disabled Children: A Preliminary Study. *Paper presented at the Virtual Rehabilitation, 2007.*

Richards-Rissetto, H., Robertsson, J., von Schwerin, J., Agugiaro, G., Remondino, F., & Girardi, G. (2014). Geospatial virtual heritage: a gesture-based 3D GIS to engage the public with ancient maya archaeology. In Archaeology in the Digital Era (pp. 118-130).

Riva, G. (1999). Virtual reality as communication tool: A sociocognitive analysis. *Presence (Cambridge, Mass.)*, *8*(4), 462–468. doi:10.1162/105474699566341

Riva, G. (2005). Virtual Reality in Psychotherapy [Review]. *Cyberpsychology & Behavior*, *8*(3), 220–240. doi:10.1089/cpb.2005.8.220 PMID:15971972

Riva, G. (2007). Cyberterapia: Ambienti Reali, Emozioni Virtuali. *Psicologia Contemporanea*, *201*(3), 18–23.

Riva, G. (2014). *Nativi digitali. Crescere e apprendere nel mondo dei nuovi media*. Bologna, Italy: Il Mulino.

Riva, G., Waterworth, J. A., Waterworth, E. L., & Mantovani, F. (2009). From intention to action: The role of presence. *New Ideas in Psychology*, 1–14.

Riva, G., Bacchetta, M., Baruffi, M., & Molinari, E. (2001). Virtual reality based treatment of body image disturbances in anorexia and bulimia nervosa: two pilot studies. *European Psychotherapy.*, *2*(3), 17.

Riva, G., Bacchetta, M., Baruffi, M., & Molinari, E. (2001). Virtual reality–based multidimensional therapy for the treatment of body image disturbances in obesity: A controlled study. *Cyberpsychology & Behavior*, *4*(4), 511–526. doi:10.1089/109493101750527079 PMID:11708731

Rivoltella, P. C. (2012). *Neurodidattica. Insegnare al cervello che apprende.* Milan, Italy: Raffaello Cortina.

Rizzo, A, & Rothbaum, B. O. (2002). Ethical issues for the use of virtual reality in the psychological sciences. *Ethical issues in clinical neuropsychology*, 243.

Rizzo, A., & Kim, J.G. (2005). A SWOT Analysis of the Field of Virtual Reality Rehabilitation and Therapy. *Presence, 14*(2), 119–146.

Rizzo, P. (2011). *Accuracy of self-perceptions in children and adults with ADHD* (Unpublished doctoral dissertation). University of Zurich, Switzerland. Retrieved April, 7 2018, from http://www.zora.uzh.ch/id/eprint/52775/1/RizzoFinales_Manuskript_dez_2011.pdf

Rizzo, A. S., Difede, J., Rothbaum, B. O., Reger, G., Spitalnick, J., Cukor, J., & McLay, R. (2010). Development and early evaluation of the Virtual Iraq/Afghanistan exposure therapy system for combat-related PTSD. *Annals of the New York Academy of Sciences*, *1208*(1), 114–125. doi:10.1111/j.1749-6632.2010.05755.x PMID:20955333

Rizzo, A., Hartholt, A., Grimani, M., Leeds, A., & Liewer, M. (2014). Virtual reality exposure therapy for combat-related posttraumatic stress disorder. *Computer*, *47*(7), 31–37. doi:10.1109/MC.2014.199

Rizzo, A., & Kim, J. G. (2005). A SWOT analysis of the field of virtual reality rehabilitation and therapy. *Presence (Cambridge, Mass.)*, *14*(2), 119–146.

Rizzo, A., & Koenig, S. T. (2017). Is clinical virtual reality ready for primetime? *Neuropsychology*, *31*(8), 877–899. doi:10.1037/neu0000405 PMID:29376669

Robertson, A., Khan, R., Fick, D., Robertson, W. B., Gunaratne, D. G. R., & Yapa, S., … Rajan, R. (2017). *The effect of Virtual Reality in reducing preoperative anxiety in patients prior to arthroscopic knee surgery: A randomised controlled trial.* Paper presented at IEEE 5th International Conference on Serious Games and Applications for Health (SeGAH), Perth, Australia. 10.1109/SeGAH.2017.7939282

Rochat, P., & Zahavi, D. (2011). The uncanny mirror: A re-framing of mirror self-experience. *Consciousness and Cognition*, *20*(2), 204–213. doi:10.1016/j.concog.2010.06.007 PMID:20889353

Rodriguez, M. C., Aruanno, B., Bordegoni, M., Rossini, M., & Molteni, F. (2017). Immersive Virtual Reality System for Treatment of Phantom Limb Pain (PLP). *Paper presented at the ASME 2017 International Design Engineering Technical Conferences and Computers and Information in Engineering Conference.*

Roobsky, E. (2003). *E-mail and Ethics. Style and ethical relations in computer-mediated communication.* London: Routledge.

Roosink, M., Robitaille, N., McFadyen, B. J., Hébert, L. J., Jackson, P. L., Bouyer, L. J., & Mercier, C. (2015). Real-time modulation of visual feedback on human full-body movements in a virtual mirror: Development and proof-of-concept. *Journal of Neuroengineering and Rehabilitation*, *12*(1), 2. doi:10.1186/1743-0003-12-2 PMID:25558785

Rose, F. D., Brooks, B. M., & Rizzo, A. A. (2005). Virtual reality in brain damage rehabilitation [review]. *Cyberpsychology & Behavior*, *8*(3), 241–262. doi:10.1089/cpb.2005.8.241 PMID:15971974

Rossi, E. G. (2018). *Roy Ascott. Esperienze telematiche.* Retrieved July 8, 2018, from http://www.arshake.com/roy-ascott-esperienze-telematiche/

Rossiter, H. E., Borrelli, M. R., Borchert, R. J., Bradbury, D., & Ward, N. S. (2015). Cortical mechanisms of mirror therapy after stroke. *Neurorehabilitation and Neural Repair*, *29*(5), 444–452. doi:10.1177/1545968314554622 PMID:25326511

Rothbaum, O. B., Price, M., Jovanovic, T., Norrholm, S. D., Gerardi, M., Dunlop, B., … Ressler, J. K. (2014). *A Randomized, Double-Blind Evaluation of d-Cycloserine or Alprazolam Combined With Virtual Reality Exposure Therapy for Posttraumatic Stress Disorder in Iraq and Afghanistan War Veterans.* Retrieved from https://ajp.psychiatryonline.org/doi/abs/10.1176/appi.ajp.2014.13121625

Roth-Isigkeit, A. (2005). Pain Among Children and Adolescents: Restrictions in Daily Living and Triggering Factors. *Pediatrics*, *115*(2), e152–e162. doi:10.1542/peds.2004-0682 PMID:15687423

Roux, A. M., Shattuck, P. T., Rast, J. E., Rava, J. A., & Anderson, K. A. (2015). National Autism Indicators Report: Transition into Young Adulthood. Philadelphia, PA: Life Course Outcomes Research Program, A.J. Drexel Autism Institute, Drexel University.

Rubboli, G., Parra, J., Seri, S., Takahashi, T., & Thomas, P. (2004). EEG diagnostic procedures and special investigations in the assessment of photosensitivity. *Epilepsia*, *45*(s1), 35–39. doi:10.1111/j.0013-9580.2004.451002.x PMID:14706044

Rus-Calafell, M., Garety, P., Sason, E., Craig, T. J. K., & Valmaggia, L. R. (2018, February). Virtual reality in the assessment and treatment of psychosis: A systematic review of its utility, acceptability and effectiveness. *Psychological Medicine*, *48*(3), 362–391. doi:10.1017/S0033291717001945 PMID:28735593

Rus-Calafell, M., Gutiérrez-Maldonado, J., & Ribas-Sabaté, J. (2013). A virtual reality-integrated program for improving social skills in patients with schizophrenia: A pilot study. *Journal of Behavior Therapy and Experimental Psychiatry*, *45*(1), 81–89. doi:10.1016/j.jbtep.2013.09.002 PMID:24063993

Saadatzi, M. N., Pennington, R. C., Welch, K. C., & Graham, J. H. (2018). Small-Group Technology-Assisted Instruction: Virtual Teacher and Robot Peer for Individuals with Autism Spectrum Disorder. *Journal of Autism and Developmental Disorders*. doi:10.100710803-018-3654-2 PMID:29926295

Sahin, N. T., Keshav, N. U., Salisbury, J. P., & Vahabzadeh, A. (2017). An augmented reality social communication aid for children and adults with autism: User and caregiver report of safety and lack of negative effects.

Sahin, N. T., Keshav, N. U., Salisbury, J. P., & Vahabzadeh, A. (2017). Cool enough for school: Second version of Google Glass rated by children facing challenges to social integration as desirable to wear at school.

Saiano, M., Pellegrino, L., Casadio, M., Summa, S., Garbarino, E., Rossi, V., ... Sanguineti, V. (2015). Natural interfaces and virtual environments for the acquisition of street crossing and path following skills in adults with Autism Spectrum Disorders: A feasibility study. *Journal of Neuroengineering and Rehabilitation*, *12*(1), 17. doi:10.118612984-015-0010-z PMID:25885279

Saldana, S. J., Marsh, A. P., Rejeski, W. J., Haberl, J. K., Wu, P., Rosenthal, S., & Ip, E. H. (2017). Assessing balance through the use of a low-cost head-mounted display in older adults: A pilot study. *Clinical Interventions in Aging*, *12*, 1363–1370. doi:10.2147/CIA.S141251 PMID:28883717

Sas, C., & Chopra, R. (2015). MeditAid: A wearable adaptive neurofeedback-based system for training mindfulness state. *Personal and Ubiquitous Computing*, *19*(7), 1169–1182. doi:10.100700779-015-0870-z

Sastry, L., & Boyd, D. R. S. (1998). Virtual environments for engineering applications. *Virtual Reality (Waltham Cross), 3*(4), 226–234. doi:10.1007/BF01408704

Sato, H., Kitahara, I., & Ohta, Y. (2009). MR-mirror: a complex of real and virtual mirrors. *Paper presented at the International Conference on Virtual and Mixed Reality.* 10.1007/978-3-642-02771-0_54

Scapina, Q. S., Echevarría-Guaniloa, M. E., Fuculo, P. R. B., Jr., Gonçalvesa, N., Rochaa, P. K., & Coimbraa, R. (2018). *Virtual Reality in the treatment of burn patients: A systematic review.* Retrieved from https://www.sciencedirect.com/science/article/pii/S030541791

Schaaf, R. C., Toth-Cohen, S., Johnson, S. L., Outten, G., & Benevides, T. W. (2011). The everyday routines of families of children with autism: Examining the impact of sensory processing difficulties on the family. *Autism, 15*(3), 373–389. doi:10.1177/1362361310386505 PMID:21430016

Schrooten, I., Scholte, R. H., & Didden, R. (2017). Bullying Among Youth with Autism Spectrum Disorders. Handbook of Social Skills and Autism Spectrum Disorder, (1), 45.

Schultheis, M. T., Rizzo, A. A., & Himelstein, J. (2002). Virtual reality and neuropsychology: Upgrading the current tools. *The Journal of Head Trauma Rehabilitation, 17*(5), 378–394. doi:10.1097/00001199-200210000-00002 PMID:12802250

Scozzari, S., & Gamberini, L. (2011). Virtual Reality as a Tool for Cognitive Behavioral Therapy: A Review. In S. Brahnam & L. C. Jain (Eds.), *Advanced Computational Intelligence Paradigms in Healthcare 6. Virtual Reality in Psychotherapy, Rehabilitation, and Assessment. Studies in Computational Intelligence* (Vol. 337). Berlin: Springer. doi:10.1007/978-3-642-17824-5_5

Selwyn, N. (2009). The digital native–myth and reality. *Aslib Proceedings, 61*(4), 364–379. doi:10.1108/00012530910973776

Senson, A. (2016). Virtual reality therapy: Treating the global mental health crisis. *Tech Crunch.* Retrieved January 10, 2018 from https://techcrunch.com/2016/01/06/virtual-reality-therapy-treating-the-global-mental-health-crisis/

Shah, P., & Chong, B. S. (2018, March). 3D imaging, 3D printing and 3D virtual planning in endodontics. *Clinical Oral Investigations, 22*(2), 641–654. doi:10.100700784-018-2338-9 PMID:29330656

Shahrbanian, S., Ma, X., Aghaei, N., Korner-bitensky, N., & Simmonds, M. J. (2012). Use of virtual reality (immersive vs. non immersive) for pain management in children and adults: A systematic review of evidence from randomized controlled trials. *European Journal of Experimental Biology.*

Sharar, S. R., Carrougher, G. J., Nakamura, D., Hoffman, H. G., Blough, D. K., & Patterson, D. R. (2007). Factors Influencing the Efficacy of Virtual Reality Distraction Analgesia During Postburn Physical Therapy: Preliminary Results from 3 Ongoing Studies. *Archives of Physical Medicine and Rehabilitation, 88*(12), S43–S49. doi:10.1016/j.apmr.2007.09.004 PMID:18036981

Shields. (2016). Aristotle's Psychology. *The Stanford Encyclopedia of Philosophy (Winter 2016 Edition).* Retrieved July 10, 2018 from https://plato.stanford.edu/archives/win2016/entries/aristotle-psychology/

Shoja, M. M., Tubbs, R. S., Malekian, A., Jafari Rouhi, A. H., Barzgar, M., & Oakes, W. J. (2007). Video game epilepsy in the twentieth century: A review. *Child's Nervous System, 23*(3), 265–267. doi:10.100700381-006-0285-2 PMID:17211654

Shrum, L. (2009). Media consumption and perceptions of social reality: Effects and underlying processes. *Media Effects*, 66-89.

Shuhaiber, J. H. (2004). Augmented reality in surgery. *Archives of Surgery (Chicago, Ill.), 139*(2), 170–174. doi:10.1001/archsurg.139.2.170 PMID:14769575

Sielhorst, T., Feuerstein, M., & Navab, N. (2008). Advanced Medical Displays: A Literature Review of Augmented Reality. *Display Technology. Journalism*, *4*(4), 451–467. doi:10.1109/jdt.2008.2001575

Sillanpää, M., & Anttila, P. (1996). Increasing prevalence of headache in 7-year-old schoolchildren. *Headache*, *36*(8), 466–470. doi:10.1046/j.1526-4610.1996.3608466.x PMID:8824000

Sime, D. (2018). David Sime - Professional History. *LinkedIn*. Retrieved July 10, 2018 from https://www.linkedin.com/in/davidsime/

Simone, R. (2012). *Presi nella rete. La mente ai tempi del web*. Milan, Italy: Garzanti.

Singletary, C. (2016). Solis VR takes elderly patients to places long thought out of reach. Retrieved July 10, 2018 from https://uploadvr.com/patients-solis-vr-edlerly/

Siriaraya, P., & Ang, C. (2014). Recreating living experiences from past memories through virtual worlds for people with dementia. In *Proceedings of the SIGCHI Conference on Human Factors in Computing Systems (CHI '14)*. ACM. 10.1145/2556288.2557035

Skjæret, N., Nawaz, A., Morat, T., Schoene, D., Helbostad, J. L., & Vereijken, B. (2016). Exercise and rehabilitation delivered through exergames in older adults: An integrative review of technologies, safety and efficacy. *International Journal of Medical Informatics*, *85*(1), 1–16. doi:10.1016/j.ijmedinf.2015.10.008 PMID:26559887

Slater, M., Perez-Marcos, D., Ehrsson, H. H., & Sanchez-Vives, M. (2008). Towards a digital body: The virtual arm illusion. *Frontiers in Human Neuroscience*, *2*(8). PMID:18958207

Slater, M., Perez-Marcos, D., Ehrsson, H. H., & Sanchez-Vives, M. V. (2009). Inducing illusory ownership of a virtual body. *Frontiers in Neuroscience*, *3*(2), 214–220. doi:10.3389/neuro.01.029.2009 PMID:20011144

Slater, M., Spanlang, B., Sanchez-Vives, M. V., & Blanke, O. (2010). First person experience of body transfer in virtual reality. *PLoS One*, *5*(5), e10564. doi:10.1371/journal.pone.0010564 PMID:20485681

Smith, M. J., Ginger, E. J., Wright, K., Wright, M. A., Taylor, J. L., Humm, L. B., ... Fleming, M. F. (2014). Virtual reality job interview training in adults with autism spectrum disorder. *Journal of Autism and Developmental Disorders*, *44*(10), 2450–2463. doi:10.100710803-014-2113-y PMID:24803366

Smith, M. J., & Steel, M. J. (2001). *The use of virtual simulation for dismounted infantry training*. Shrivenham, UK: Cranfield University - Royal Militar College of Science.

Sohlberg, M. M., & Mateer, C. A. (2017). *Cognitive rehabilitation: An integrative neuropsychological approach*. Guilford Publications.

Soler, M. D., Kumru, H., Pelayo, R., Vidal, J., Tormos, J. M., Fregni, F., ... Pascual-Leone, A. (2010). Effectiveness of transcranial direct current stimulation and visual illusion on neuropathic pain in spinal cord injury. *Brain*, *133*(9), 2565–2577. doi:10.1093/brain/awq184 PMID:20685806

Songer, D. (2005). Psychotherapeutic Approaches in the Treatment of Pain. *Psychiatry*. PMID:21152145

Sotiriou, S., & Bogner, F. X. (2008). Visualizing the invisible: Augmented reality as an innovative science education scheme. *Advanced Science Letters*, *1*(1), 114–122. doi:10.1166/asl.2008.012

Spagnolli, A., & Gamberini, L. (2005). A Place for presence. Understanding the human involvement in mediated interactive environments. *PsychNology Journal*, *3*(1), 6–15. PMID:16190023

Spagnolli, A., Gamberini, L., Cottone, P., & Mantovani, G. (2003). Ergonomics of virtual environments for clinical use. *Studies in Health Technology and Informatics*, *99*, 217–230. PMID:15295153

Speyer, C., & Zack, J. (2010). *Online Counseling: Beyond the Pros and the Cons*. Retrieved from https://www.easna.org/wp-content/uploads/2010/08/WS2B-E-counselingBeyondthatProsandCons-Handout.pdf

Spinoza, B. (2007). *Opere*. Milano: Mondadori.

Squire, K., & Jan, M. (2007). Mad city mystery: Developing scientific argumentation skills with a place-based augmented reality game on handheld computers. *Journal of Science Education and Technology*, *16*(1), 5–29. doi:10.100710956-006-9037-z

Squire, K., & Klopfer, E. (2007). Augmented reality simulations on handheld computers. *Journal of the Learning Sciences*, *16*(3), 371–413. doi:10.1080/10508400701413435

Stanford, E. A., Chambers, C. T., Biesanz, J. C., & Chen, E. (2008). The frequency, trajectories and predictors of adolescent recurrent pain: A population-based approach. *Pain*, *138*(1), 11–21. doi:10.1016/j.pain.2007.10.032 PMID:18093737

Sterman, M. B., & Egner, T. (2006). Foundation and practice of neurofeedback for the treatment of epilepsy. *Applied Psychophysiology and Biofeedback*, *31*(1), 21–35. doi:10.100710484-006-9002-x PMID:16614940

Stevens, J. A., & Stoykov, M. E. P. (2003). Using Motor Imagery in the Rehabilitation of Hemiparesis 1. *Archives of Physical Medicine and Rehabilitation*, *84*(7), 1090–1092. doi:10.1016/S0003-9993(03)00042-X PMID:12881842

Stokes, T. F., & Baer, D. M. (1977). An implicit technology of generalization. *Journal of Applied Behavior Analysis*, *10*(2), 349–367. doi:10.1901/jaba.1977.10-349 PMID:16795561

Strain, P. S., Schwartz, I. S., & Bovey, E. H. (2008). Social competence interventions for young children with autism. *Social competence of young children: Risk, disability, and intervention*, 253-272.

Strickland, D. (1997). Virtual reality for the treatment of autism. *Studies in Health Technology and Informatics*, 81–86. PMID:10184809

Strickland, D. (1998). Virtual Reality for the Treatment of Autism. In G. Riva (Ed.), *Virtual reality in neuro-psycho-physiology* (pp. 81–86). Amsterdam: IOS Press.

Strickland, D. (2001, August). Virtual reality and multimedia applications for mental health assessment and treatment. *ACM SIGGRAPH 2001 Conference*.

Strickland, D. C., Coles, C. D., & Southern, L. B. (2013). JobTIPS: A transition to employment program for individuals with autism spectrum disorders. *Journal of Autism and Developmental Disorders*, *43*(10), 2472–2483. doi:10.100710803-013-1800-4 PMID:23494559

Strickland, D. C., McAllister, D., Coles, C. D., & Osborne, S. (2007). An evolution of virtual reality training designs for children with autism and fetal alcohol spectrum disorders. *Topics in Language Disorders*, *27*(3), 226–241. doi:10.1097/01.TLD.0000285357.95426.72 PMID:20072702

Strickland, D., Marcus, L. M., Mesibov, G. B., & Hogan, K. (1996). Brief report: Two case studies using virtual reality as a learning tool for autistic children. *Journal of Autism and Developmental Disorders*, *26*(6), 651–659. doi:10.1007/BF02172354 PMID:8986851

Sucar, L. E., Orihuela-Espina, F., Velazquez, R. L., Reinkensmeyer, D. J., Leder, R., & Hernández-Franco, J. (2014). Gesture therapy: An upper limb virtual reality-based motor rehabilitation platform. *IEEE Transactions on Neural Systems and Rehabilitation Engineering*, *22*(3), 634–643. doi:10.1109/TNSRE.2013.2293673 PMID:24760913

Suler, J. (2001). *The psychology of cyberspace*. Retrieved from http://users.rider.edu/suler/psycyher.html

Sutherland, C., Hashtrudi-Zaad, K., Sellens, R., Abolmaesumi, P., & Mousavi, P. (2013). An Augmented Reality Haptic Training Simulator for Spinal Needle Procedures. *IEEE Transactions on Biomedical Engineering*, *60*(11), 3009–3018. doi:10.1109/TBME.2012.2236091 PMID:23269747

Swaney, R. (2018). Virtual reality delivers real-world benefits to dementia patients. *Samsung*. Retrieved from https://insights.samsung.com/2018/03/13/virtual-reality-delivers-real-world-benefits-to-dementia-patients/

Sweller, J., Van Merrienboer, J. J., & Paas, F. G. (1998). Cognitive architecture and instructional design. *Educational Psychology Review*, *10*(3), 251–296. doi:10.1023/A:1022193728205

Székely, G., & Satava, R. M. (1999). *Virtual reality in medicine.* Retrieved from: https://www.ncbi.nlm.nih.gov/pmc/articles/PMC1129082/

Talamo, A., Camilli, M., Di Lucchio, L., & Ventura, S. (2017). Information from the past: How elderly people orchestrate presences, memories and technologies at home. *Universal Access in the Information Society*, *16*(3), 739–753. doi:10.100710209-016-0508-6

Tambovtsev, D., Floksy, N., & Peshé, O. (2016). *How to Avoid the Effect of Motion Sickness in VR*. Retrieved March 9, 2018, from https://vrscout.com/news/avoid-motion-sickness-developing-for-vr

Tang, S.-L., Kwoh, C.-K., Teo, M.-Y., Sing, N. W., & Ling, K.-V. (1998). Augmented reality systems for medical applications. *IEEE Engineering in Medicine and Biology Magazine*, *17*(3), 49–58. doi:10.1109/51.677169 PMID:9604701

Tapscott, D. (2008). *Grown up digital. How the net generation is changing your World.* New York, NY: Mac Graw Hill- Professional.

Taylor, R. H., & Stoianovici, D. (2003). Medical robotics in computer-integrated surgery. *IEEE Transactions on* Robotics and Automation, *19*(5), 765–781. doi:10.1109/tra.2003.817058

Temurnikar, A. (2018). *New age classrooms are the future of education (Interview).* Retrieved May 5, 2018, from http://bweducation.businessworld.in/article/New-Age-Classrooms-are-the-Future-of-Education-/10-04-2018-146020/

The Guardian. (2017). *The Party: a virtual experience of autism – 360 video*. Retrieved March 9, 2018, from https://www.theguardian.com/technology/2017/oct/07/the-party-a-virtual-experience-of-autism-360-video

The National Autistic Society. (2016). *Too much information.* Retrieved March, 9 2018, from http://www.autism.org.uk/vr

Thieme, H., Mehrholz, J., Pohl, M., Behrens, J., & Dohle, C. (2012). Mirror therapy for improving motor function after stroke. *Cochrane Database of Systematic Reviews*, *14*(3). PMID:22419334

Thieme, H., Mehrholz, J., Pohl, M., Behrens, J., & Dohle, C. (2013). Mirror therapy for improving motor function after stroke. *Stroke*, *44*(1), e1–e2. doi:10.1161/STROKEAHA.112.673087 PMID:23390640

Thomas, D. J. (2016). Augmented reality in surgery: The computer-aided medicine revolution. *International Journal of Surgery*, *36*, 25. doi:10.1016/j.ijsu.2016.10.003 PMID:27741424

Thomas, S., Hovinga, M. E., Rai, D., & Lee, B. K. (2017). Brief report: prevalence of co-occurring epilepsy and autism spectrum disorder: the US National Survey of Children's Health 2011–2012. *Journal of Autism and Developmental Disorders*, *47*(1), 224–229. doi:10.100710803-016-2938-7 PMID:27752862

Tiiro, A. (2018). *Effect of Visual Realism on Cybersickness in Virtual Reality* (Unpublished Master's thesis). University of Oulu, Finland. Retrieved July 16, 2018 from http://jultika.oulu.fi/files/nbnfioulu-201802091218.pdf

Toffler, A. (1980). *The Third Wave*. New York: William Morrow & C.

Tonioni, F. (2013). *Psicopatologia web-mediata. Dipendenza da internet e nuovi fenomeni dissociativi*. Milan, Italy: Springer. doi:10.1007/978-88-470-2817-3

Tribemix. (2017). *Commercial immersive virtual reality for people with dementia*. Retrieved August 10, 2017 from http://www.tribemix.co.uk/

Trindade, J., Kirner, C., & Fiolhais, C. (2004). Orbitário: Exploração de Orbitais Hidrogenoides com Realidade Aumentada. In J. Pérez, J. Pulido, M. Rodríguez, B. Manjón, J. Rodríguez (Eds.), Avances en Informática Educativa, artículos selecionados del VI Simpósio Internacional de Informática Educativa. Academic Press.

Trojan, J., Diers, M., Fuchs, X., Bach, F., Bekrater-Bodmann, R., Foell, J., ... Flor, H. (2014). An augmented reality home-training system based on the mirror training and imagery approach. *Behavior Research Methods*, *46*(3), 634–640. doi:10.375813428-013-0412-4 PMID:24338625

Tsakiris, M., & Haggard, P. (2005). The rubber hand illusion revisited: Visuotactile integration and self-attribution. *Journal of Experimental Psychology. Human Perception and Performance*, *31*(1), 80–91. doi:10.1037/0096-1523.31.1.80 PMID:15709864

Tsang, W. W. N., & Fu, A. S. N. (2016). Virtual reality exercise to improve balance control in older adults at risk of falling. *Hong Kong Medical Journal*, *22*(1 Suppl. 2), S19–S22. doi:10.12809/hkjr1615298 PMID:26908338

Tudor, S., Carey, S., & Dubey, R. (2015). Development and evaluation of a dynamic virtual reality driving simulator. *Paper presented at the 8th ACM International Conference on Pervasive Technologies Related to Assistive Environments*. 10.1145/2769493.2769593

Turk, D. C., & Okifuji, A. (2002). Psychological factors in chronic pain: Evolution and revolution. *Journal of Consulting and Clinical Psychology*, *70*(3), 678–690. doi:10.1037/0022-006X.70.3.678 PMID:12090376

Turk, D. C., Swanson, K. S., & Tunks, E. R. (2008). Psychological approaches in the treatment of chronic pain patients - When pills, scalpels, and needles are not enough. *Canadian Journal of Psychiatry*, *53*(4), 213–223. doi:10.1177/070674370805300402 PMID:18478824

Tzanavari, A., Charalambous-Darden, N., Herakleous, K., & Poullis, C. (2015). Effectiveness of an immersive virtual environment (CAVE) for teaching pedestrian crossing to children with PDD-NOS. In *2015 IEEE 15th International Conference on Advanced Learning Technologies (ICALT)* (pp. 423-427). IEEE.

Uddin, L. Q. (2011). The self in autism: An emerging view from neuroimaging. *Neurocase*, *17*(3), 201–208. doi:10.1080/13554794.2010.509320 PMID:21207316

Ungi, T., Sargent, D., Moult, E., Lasso, A., Pinter, C., McGraw, R. C., & Fichtinger, G. (2012). Perk Tutor: An Open-Source Training Platform for Ultrasound-Guided Needle Insertions. *IEEE Transactions on Biomedical Engineering*, *59*(12), 3475–3481. doi:10.1109/TBME.2012.2219307 PMID:23008243

United Nations. (n.d.). Virtual Reality. Retrieved from http://unvr.sdgactioncampaign.org/

Upton, D., & Hender, C. (2012). The cost of mood disorders in patients with chronic wounds. *Wounds UK*, *8*(1), 107–109.

Upton, D., Solowiej, K., & Woo, K. Y. (2014). A multinational health professional perspective of the prevalence of mood disorders in patients with acute and chronic wounds. *International Wound Journal*, *11*(6), 627–635. doi:10.1111/iwj.12018 PMID:23289905

Upton, D., Upton, P., & Alexander, R. (2015). The complexity of caring (Part 1): Detrimental health and well-being outcomes for caregivers of people with chronic wounds. *Wound Practice & Research: Journal of the Australian Wound Management Association*, *23*(3), 104.

Usability (Improving the User Experience). (2018). Retrieved July 10, 2018 from https://www.usability.gov/

Valet, M., Sprenger, T., Boecker, H., Willoch, F., Rummeny, E., & Conrad, B., … Tolle, T. R. (2004). Distraction modulates connectivity of the cingulo-frontal cortex and the midbrain during pain - An fMRI analysis. *Pain*. doi:10.1016/j.pain.2004.02.033

Valladares-Rodriguez, S., Perez-Rodriguez, R., Facal, D., Fernandez-Iglesias, M. J., Anido-Rifon, L., & Mourino-Garcia, M. (2017). Design process and preliminary psychometric study of a video game to detect cognitive impairment in senior adults. *PeerJ*, *5*, e3508. doi:10.7717/peerj.3508 PMID:28674661

Vallejo, V., Wyss, P., Rampa, L., Mitache, A. V., Müri, R. M., Mosimann, U. P., & Nef, T. (2017). Evaluation of a novel Serious Game based assessment tool for patients with Alzheimer's disease. *PLoS One*, *12*(5), e0175999. doi:10.1371/journal.pone.0175999 PMID:28472049

Valmaggia, L. (2017). *The use of virtual reality in psychosis research and treatment*. Retrieved from https://www.ncbi.nlm.nih.gov/pmc/articles/PMC5608845/

Vargas González, A. N., Kapalo, K., Koh, S., & LaViola, J. (2017). Exploring the virtuality continuum for complex rule-set education in the context of soccer rule comprehension. *Multimodal Technologies and Interaction*, *1*(4), 30. doi:10.3390/mti1040030

Vázquez, J., Vaca, V.L., Wiederhold, K.B., Miller, T.I., & Wiederhold, D.M. (2017). Virtual Reality Pain Distraction During Gynecological Surgery—A Report of 44 Cases. *Surgical Research Updates, 5,* 12-16 Doi:10.12970/2311-9888.2017.05.02

Vera, A. M., Russo, M., Mohsin, A., & Tsuda, S. (2014). Augmented reality telementoring (ART) platform: a randomized controlled trial to assess the efficacy of a new surgical education technology. *Surgical Endoscopy and other Interventional Techniques*, *28*(12), 3467-3472. doi:10.100700464-014-3625-4

Vidal, J. J. (1973). Toward direct brain-computer communication. *Annual Review of Biophysics and Bioengineering*, *2*(1), 157–180. doi:10.1146/annurev.bb.02.060173.001105 PMID:4583653

Vikal, S., U-Thainual, P., Carrino, J. A., Iordachita, I., Fischer, G. S., & Fichtinger, G. (2010). Perk Station-Percutaneous surgery training and performance measurement platform. *Computerized Medical Imaging and Graphics*, *34*(1), 19–32. doi:10.1016/j.compmedimag.2009.05.001 PMID:19539446

Villani, D., Cipresso, P., & Repetto, C. (2014). Coping with stress and anxiety: The role of presence in technology mediated environments. In Interacting with Presence: HCI and the Sense of Presence in Computer-Mediated Environments (pp. 139-151). De Gruyter Open Ltd. Doi:10.2478/9783110409697.9

Villani, D., Riva, F., & Riva, G. (2007). New technologies for relaxation: The role of presence. *International Journal of Stress Management*, *14*(3), 260–274. doi:10.1037/1072-5245.14.3.260

Vincelli, F., & Riva, G. (2007). La Realtà Virtuale come supporto alla psicoterapia cognitivo-comportamentale. In F. Vincelli, G. Riva, & E. Molinari (Eds.), *La realtà virtuale in psicologia clinica* (pp. 67–92). Milan, Italy: Mc Graw-Hill.

Vogt, B. A., Sikes, R. W., & Vogt, L. J. (1993). Anterior Cingulate Cortex and the Medial Pain System. In Neurobiology of Cingulate Cortex and Limbic Thalamus: A Comprehensive Handbook. Academic Press. doi:10.1007/978-1-4899-6704-6_11

Von Korff, M., Crane, P., Lane, M., Miglioretti, D. L., Simon, G., & Saunders, K. … Kessler, R. (2005). Chronic spinal pain and physical-mental comorbidity in the United States: Results from the national comorbidity survey replication. *Pain*. doi:10.1016/j.pain.2004.11.010

Vural, S. P., Yuzer, G. F. N., Ozcan, D. S., Ozbudak, S. D., & Ozgirgin, N. (2016). Effects of mirror therapy in stroke patients with complex regional pain syndrome type 1: A randomized controlled study. *Archives of Physical Medicine and Rehabilitation*, *97*(4), 575–581. doi:10.1016/j.apmr.2015.12.008 PMID:26723854

Wade, J., Zhang, L., Bian, D., Fan, J., Swanson, A., Weitlauf, A., ... Sarkar, N. (2016). A gaze-contingent adaptive virtual reality driving environment for intervention in individuals with autism spectrum disorders. *ACM Transactions on Interactive Intelligent Systems*, *6*(1), 3. doi:10.1145/2892636

Wainer, A. L., & Ingersoll, B. R. (2011). The use of innovative computer technology for teaching social communication to individuals with autism spectrum disorders. *Research in Autism Spectrum Disorders*, *5*(1), 96–107. doi:10.1016/j.rasd.2010.08.002

Walker, J., Pan, E., Johnston, D., Adler-Milstein, J., Bates, D. W., & Middleton, B. (2005). The Value of Health Care Information Exchange and Interoperability: There is a business case to be made for spending money on a fully standardized nationwide system. *Health Affairs*, 24–1.

Walker, L. S., & Greene, J. W. (1991). The functional disability inventory: Measuring a neglected dimension of child health status. *Journal of Pediatric Psychology*, *16*(1), 39–58. doi:10.1093/jpepsy/16.1.39 PMID:1826329

Walker, L. S., Guite, J. W., Duke, M., Barnard, J. A., & Greene, J. W. (1998). Recurrent abdominal pain: A potential precursor of irritable bowel syndrome in adolescents and young adults. *The Journal of Pediatrics*, *132*(6), 1010–1015. doi:10.1016/S0022-3476(98)70400-7 PMID:9627595

Wallace, J., Thieme, A., Wood, G., Schofield, G., & Olivier, P. (2012). Enabling self, intimacy and a sense of home in dementia: an enquiry into design in a hospital setting. In *Proceedings of the SIGCHI Conference on Human Factors in Computing Systems (CHI '12)*. ACM. 10.1145/2207676.2208654

Wallace, P. M. (2000). *La psicologia di Internet*. Milan, Italy: Cortina Editore.

Wallace, S., Parsons, S., Westbury, A., White, K., White, K., & Bailey, A. (2010). Sense of presence and atypical social judgments in immersive virtual environments: Responses of adolescents with Autism Spectrum Disorders. *Autism*, *14*(3), 199–213. doi:10.1177/1362361310363283 PMID:20484000

Waltemate, T., Gall, D., Roth, D., Botsch, M., & Latoschik, M. E. (2018). The impact of avatar personalization and immersion on virtual body ownership, presence, and emotional response. *IEEE Transactions on Visualization and Computer Graphics*, *24*(4), 1643–1652. doi:10.1109/TVCG.2018.2794629 PMID:29543180

Wang, P., & Spillane, A. (2009). Evidence-based social skills interventions for children with autism: A meta-analysis. *Education and Training in Developmental Disabilities*, 318–342.

Wang, S. Y., Cui, Y., & Parrila, R. (2011). Examining the effectiveness of peer-mediated and video-modeling social skills interventions for children with autism spectrum disorders: A meta-analysis in single-case research using HLM. *Research in Autism Spectrum Disorders*, *5*(1), 562–569. doi:10.1016/j.rasd.2010.06.023

Wann, J., & Mon-Williams, M. (1996). What does virtual reality NEED? Human factors issues in the design of three-dimensional computer environments. *International Journal of Human-Computer Studies*, *44*(6), 829–847. doi:10.1006/ijhc.1996.0035

Washington, P., Voss, C., Kline, A., Haber, N., Daniels, J., Fazel, A., ... Wall, D. (2017). SuperpowerGlass: A wearable aid for the at-home therapy of children with autism. *Proceedings of the ACM on Interactive, Mobile, Wearable and Ubiquitous Technologies, 1*(3), 112. 10.1145/3130977

Weibel, P. (1993). Mondi virtuali: i nuovi corpi dell'imperatore. In P. L. Capucci (Ed.), *Realtà del virtuale* (pp. 196–224). Bologna: CLUEB.

Wiederhold B. K., & Wiederhold, M. D. (2006). Virtual Reality as a Tool in Early Interventions. *Human Dimensions in Military Operations: Military Leaders' Strategies for Addressing Stress and Psychological Support*, 451-458.

Wiederhold, B. K., Gao, K., Sulea, C., & Wiederhold, M. D. (2014). Virtual Reality as a Distraction Technique in Chronic Pain Patients. *Cyberpsychology, Behavior, and Social Networking*, *17*(6), 346–352. doi:10.1089/cyber.2014.0207 PMID:24892196

Wiederhold, B. K., & Wiederhold, M. D. (2001). Virtual reality technology in the treatment of anxiety disorders. In M. Akay & A. Marsh (Eds.), *Information Technologies in Medicine*. London: John Wiley & Sons. doi:10.1002/0471206458.ch2

Wiederhold, B. K., & Wiederhold, M. D. (2005). *Virtual reality therapy for anxiety disorders: Advances in evaluation and treatment*. American Psychological Association. doi:10.1037/10858-000

Wikimedia Commons. (2016). *File:Orlan par Fabrice Lévêque*. Retrieved from https://commons.wikimedia.org/wiki/File:Orlan_par_Fabrice_L%C3%A9v%C3%AAque_1997-2.jpg

Williams, A., Eccleston, C., & Morley, S. (2012). Psychological therapies for the management of chronic pain (excluding headache) in adults. *Cochrane Database of Systematic Reviews*. doi:10.1002/14651858.CD007407.pub3 PMID:23152245

Williford, J. S., Hodges, L. F., North, M. M., & North, S. M. (1993). Relative effectiveness of virtual environment desensitization and imaginal desensitization in the treatment of acrophobia. In *Graphics interface* (pp. 162–162). Canadian Information Processing Society.

Wilson, S. (2010). *Art +Science Now*. London: Thames & Hundson.

Windheim, K., Veale, D., & Anson, M. (2011). Mirror gazing in body dysmorphic disorder and healthy controls: Effects of duration of gazing. *Behaviour Research and Therapy*, *49*(9), 555–564. doi:10.1016/j.brat.2011.05.003 PMID:21726855

Winn, W. (1993). A conceptual basis for educational applications of virtual reality. Human Interface Technology Laboratory, Washington Technology Center, University of Washington, USA.

Winn, W. (1993). A conceptual basis for educational applications of virtual reality. In Human Interface Technology Laboratory. Washington Technology Center, University of Washington.

Wollersheim, D., Merkes, M., Shields, N., Liamputtong, P., Wallis, L., Reynolds, F., & Koh, L. (2010). Physical and psychosocial effects of Wii video game use among older women. *International Journal of Emerging Technologies and Society*, *8*(2), 85–98.

Won, A. S., Bailey, J., Bailenson, J., Tataru, C., Yoon, I. A., & Golianu, B. (2017). Immersive virtual reality for pediatric pain. *Children*, *4*(7), 52. doi:10.3390/children4070052 PMID:28644422

Won, A. S., Tataru, C. A., Cojocaru, C. M., Krane, E. J., Bailenson, J. N., Niswonger, S. G. B., & Golianu, B. (2015). Two Virtual Reality Pilot Studies for the Treatment of Pediatric CRPS. *Pain Medicine*, *16*(8), 1644–1647. doi:10.1111/pme.12755 PMID:25930099

Wong, C., Odom, S. L., Hume, K. A., Cox, A. W., Fettig, A., Kucharczyk, S., ... Schultz, T. R. (2015). Evidence-based practices for children, youth, and young adults with autism spectrum disorder: A comprehensive review. *Journal of Autism and Developmental Disorders*, *45*(7), 1951–1966. doi:10.100710803-014-2351-z PMID:25578338

Wood, J. J., Drahota, A., Sze, K., Har, K., Chiu, A., & Langer, D. A. (2009). Cognitive behavioral therapy for anxiety in children with autism spectrum disorders: A randomized, controlled trial. *Journal of Child Psychology and Psychiatry, and Allied Disciplines*, *50*(3), 224–234. doi:10.1111/j.1469-7610.2008.01948.x PMID:19309326

Woodman, G. F. (2010). A brief introduction to the use of event-related potentials in studies of perception and attention. *Attention, Perception & Psychophysics*, *72*(8), 2031–2046. doi:10.3758/BF03196680 PMID:21097848

Wu, H. K., Lee, S. W.-L., Chang, H. Y., & Liang, J. C. (2013). Current status, opportunities and challenges of augmented reality in education. *Computers & Education*, *62*, 41–49. doi:10.1016/j.compedu.2012.10.024

Xu, G., Strathearn, L., Liu, B., & Bao, W. (2018). Prevalence of Autism Spectrum Disorder Among US Children and Adolescents, 2014-2016. *Journal of the American Medical Association*, *319*(1), 81–82. doi:10.1001/jama.2017.17812 PMID:29297068

Yang, T. T., Gallen, C., Schwartz, B., Bloom, F. E., Ramachandran, V. S., & Cobb, S. (1994). Sensory maps in the human brain. *Nature*, *368*(6472), 592–593. doi:10.1038/368592b0 PMID:8145842

Yang, Y. D., Allen, T., Abdullahi, S. M., Pelphrey, K. A., Volkmar, F. R., & Chapman, S. B. (2017). Brain responses to biological motion predict treatment outcome in young adults with autism receiving Virtual Reality Social Cognition Training: Preliminary findings. *Behaviour Research and Therapy*, *93*, 55–66. doi:10.1016/j.brat.2017.03.014 PMID:28384509

Yantaç, A. E., Çorlu, D., Fjeld, M., & Kunz, A. (2015). Exploring diminished reality (DR) spaces to augment the attention of individuals with autism. *Paper presented at the 2015 IEEE International Symposium on Mixed and Augmented Reality Workshops (ISMARW).*

Yardley, L., & Redfern, M. S. (2001). Psychological factors influencing recovery from balance disorders. *Journal of Anxiety Disorders*, *15*(1-2), 107–119. doi:10.1016/S0887-6185(00)00045-1 PMID:11388354

Yasuda, K., Muroi, D., Ohira, M., & Iwata, H. (2017). Validation of an immersive virtual reality system for training near and far space neglect in individuals with stroke: A pilot study. *Topics in Stroke Rehabilitation*, *24*(7), 533–538. doi:10.1080/10749357.2017.1351069 PMID:28701101

Yeo, C. T., Ungi, T., U-Thainual, P., Lasso, A., McGraw, R. C., & Fichtinger, G. (2011). The Effect of Augmented Reality Training on Percutaneous Needle Placement in Spinal Facet Joint Injections. *IEEE Transactions on Biomedical Engineering*, *58*(7), 2031–2037. doi:10.1109/TBME.2011.2132131 PMID:21435970

Yeşilyaprak, S. S., Yıldırım, M. Ş., Tomruk, M., Ertekin, Ö., & Algun, Z. C. (2016). Comparison of the effects of virtual reality-based balance exercises and conventional exercises on balance and fall risk in older adults living in nursing homes in Turkey. *Physiotherapy Theory and Practice*, *32*(3), 191–201. doi:10.3109/09593985.2015.1138009 PMID:27049879

Zablotsky, B., Black, L. I., Maenner, M. J., Schieve, L. A., & Blumberg, S. J. (2015). Estimated prevalence of autism and other developmental disabilities following questionnaire changes in the 2014 National Health Interview Survey (National health statistics reports; no 87). Hyattsville, MD: National Center for Health Statistics.

Zanfir, A.-M., Georgescu, D. I., Turturica, S. C., Eczedi, M., & Mironiuc, A. (2017). Immersive VR in phantom limb pain therapy of amputee patients due to critical limb ischemia. *Acta Medica Marisiensis*, *63*(3), 115–120. doi:10.1515/amma-2017-0031

Zarr, M. (1994). Computer-aided psychotherapy: Machine helping therapist. *Psychiatric Annals*, *24*(1), 42–46. doi:10.3928/0048-5713-19940101-13

Zhao, H., Swanson, A., Weitlauf, A., Warren, Z., & Sarkar, N. (2016). A Novel Collaborative Virtual Reality Game for Children with ASD to Foster Social Interaction. Universal Access in Human-Computer Interaction. Users and Context Diversity Lecture Notes in Computer Science, 276-288.

Zhou, F., Duh, H. B.-L., & Billinghurst, M. (2008). Trends in augmented reality tracking, interaction and display: A review of ten years of ISMAR. In *Proceedings of the 7th IEEE/ACM International Symposium on Mixed and Augmented Reality* (pp.193-202). IEEE Computer Society.

Zhu, E., Hadadgar, A., Masiello, I., & Zary, N. (2014). Augmented reality in healthcare education: An integrative review. *PeerJ*, *2*, e469. doi:10.7717/peerj.469 PMID:25071992

Zigmond, A. S., & Snaith, R. P. (1983). The hospital anxiety and depression scale. *Acta Psychiatrica Scandinavica*, *67*(6), 361–370. doi:10.1111/j.1600-0447.1983.tb09716.x PMID:6880820

Zimmerman, F., & Merci, J. A. (2010). A better start. Child maltreatment prevention as a public health priority. Retrieved July 18, 2018 from https://vetoviolence.cdc.gov/apps/phl/docs/A_Better_Start.pdf

Zinck, S., & Zinck, S. (2018). Virtual Reality: Not for Millennials only - Age and ability. *Age and Ability*. Retrieved July 10, 2018 from https://www.ibm.com/blogs/age-and-ability/2017/08/18/virtual-reality-not-millennials/

Zygouris, S., Giakoumis, D., Votis, K., Doumpoulakis, S., Ntovas, K., Segkouli, S., ... Tsolaki, M. (2015). Can a virtual reality cognitive training application fulfill a dual role? Using the virtual supermarket cognitive training application as a screening tool for mild cognitive impairment. *Journal of Alzheimer's Disease. JAD*, *44*(4), 1333–1347. doi:10.3233/JAD-141260 PMID:25428251

# About the Contributors

**Giuliana Guazzaroni** Technology Enhanced Learning Ph.D. She has developed EMMAP (Emotional Mapping of Museum Augmented Places) an interactive format for Museums. The Presidential Medal of the Italian Republic awarded her researches relating to "Quantum art, science and augmented reality: innovation synergies". She has been involved in e-moderating different online courses at the Università Ca' Foscari of Venice and the Università Politecnica delle Marche. She has used E-Learning environments, integrating learning objects with mobile devices, to create unique learning experiences where the participant interacts in a place, at the same time, authentic and augmented by the use of different media. She studies and develops virtual or augmented reality systems useful in treating mental health, including VR 360 movies. She has published and edited scientific articles on the themes of e-learning, augmented and virtual reality, virtual and augmented learning environments, virtual and augmented reality in mental health treatment. She has a degree in Foreign Languages (University of Macerata), a master degree in Technologies and Methodologies of E-Learning (University of Verona) and a Ph.D in Engineering Sciences, Curriculum E-Learning (Università Politecnica delle Marche).

* * *

**Simone Barbato** is Psychologist, enrolled in the Register of Psychologists of Lazio. Graduated in Clinical Psychology with the thesis: "Digital psychology as a support for the person", he specialized in "Human Performance Psychology" in Turin. He earned a Master in "Human Resources Management and Administration", with the thesis "Virtual Reality and Employer Branding: from innovation to new selection standard". He is Co-founder of IDEGO - Digital Psychology and currently works as Human Resoruce Advisor in the Training and Development department at Praxi S.p.a. in Rome. He is co-author along with Lorenzo Di Natale of the book "Finestre sul futuro. Fondamenti di Psicologia Digitale" ("A glimpse of the future. Fundamentals of Digital Psychology"), published by Alpes.

**Sergio Casas** has a master's degree in Computer Engineering and also a bachelor's degree in Telecommunications Engineering - Telematics Specialty. He received the Spanish National Award on University Studies in 2008. He received his PhD in Computational Mathematics at the University of Valencia in 2014. He works as a senior researcher in the Robotics Institute (IRTIC) of the University of Valencia, where he is also a part-time professor at the School of Engineering (ETSE). His expertise is in the simulation field with special focus on Virtual Reality, Augmented Reality and motion cueing.

**Brian Chau** is a Physical Medicine & Rehabilitation (PM&R) physician. Interested in improving function and health in patients through advances in technology, including virtual reality. http://brianchaumd.com.

**Giorgio Cipolletta** is a transdisciplinary artist and media-theorist. In 2012 he obtained a PhD in Information and Communication Theory at the University of Macerata where he is adjunct professor of Visual Art and Technology. He is member of the media editorial staff of Noema / mediaversi / Riviste di Scienze sociali. He works as freelancer layout designer for the University press of Macerata (eum). He writings appeared in many academic journals (Flusser Studies, Heteroglossia) and his first book is Metrobodily passages. For an aesthetics of transition, eum, Macerata 2014. He has won many international poem prizes. Besides, he's showed his multimedia installations and performances in many national exhibitions (Corpus 2012, Chaos 2013, Bookquake 2017, Mea Culpa, 2018, Soundscapes from Earth 2018). He is founding partner and vice-president of Crash (Creative Art Shocking, 2014).

**Lorenzo Di Natale** graduated in Economics, has worked for many years as Project Manager in International Cooperation and Development field, in particular in the Democratic Republic of Congo. He has a second degree in Development and Educational Psychology with the thesis "Cognitive, behavioral and emotional aspects of the relationship individual-physical environment". Co-founder and CEO of IDEGO - Digital Psychology, he leads the Research area. In this activity context, he has promoted partnerships with several Universities and Research Centres in order to develop software supporting mental health, among others with "TorVegata" University of Rome, the "Gabriele D'Annunzio" University of Chieti and Pescara and the Centre for Clinical Cognitivism of Florence. He is co-author along with Simone Barbato of the book "Finestre sul futuro. Fondamenti di Psicologia Digitale" ("A glimpse of the future. Fundamentals of Digital Psychology"), published by Alpes.

**Giacomo Ercolani** is a psychologist and cognitive psychotherapist in training. After he graduated from the University of Bologna, he served an internship at ANT Foundation, in 2016. Today he works for ANT, at the premises of Perugia, as a psychologist where he offers psychological support at-home to cancer patients and their relatives. In ANT he also carries out and research in order to improve patients and caregivers quality of life. He is a member of the Italian Society of Palliative Care.

**Pedro Gaspar** is associate professor at Polytechnic Institute of Leiria - School of Health Sciences; Reseracher at ciTechCare - Center for Innovative Care and Health Technology; Master in Communication and Education in Science - Universidade de Aveiro; Doctor in Communication Sciences (Multimedia Engineering) - Universidade Politécnica da Catalunha.

**Luca Golfari** has a degree in clinical psychology obtained at the University of Bologna (2017) and now he is doing an internship at the ANT Foundation. During the internship he takes part in different activities including participation in hosting interviews carried out at the ANT Institute with patients and relatives who wish to activate home care, he assists the psychologist tutor during the clinical support activity for patients and caregivers and he carries out activities in the Coordination Office of the Psychology and Training Unit of ANT Foundation.

**Nelson Jorge** holds a PhD in Education from Distance Education and Elearning Lab (LE@D) Universidade Aberta, Portugal, where he conducted research on the impact of augmented reality in e-learning. He has been working in the field of online education since 2007 and at the moment holds the position of Senior e-Learning Advisor at IHE Delft Institute of Water Education in the Netherlands.

**Franchini Luca** is a psychologist and cognitive psychotherapist in training. After he graduated from the University of Padua, he served an internship at ANT Foundation in 2017. Today he works in the Coordination Office of the Psychology and Training Unit at the ANT Foundation in Italy. His work at ANT includes the design and the implementation of projects in Italian schools about death education and cancer prevention. He cooperates to organize training course, both for professionals employed at the ANT Foundation as well as external, and works as a team in the selection and training of health personnel. He also carries out several researches in order to improve ANT patient and caregiver quality of life.

**Joseph McCleery**, Ph.D., is Assistant Professor in the Department of Psychology, and Executive Director of Academic Programs in the Kinney Center for Autism Education and Support, at Saint Joseph's University. He is also a Scientist in the Center for Autism Research at Children's Hospital of Philadelphia. Dr. McCleery earned an undergraduate degree in Psychology from Rutgers University, and both a Masters Degree and Ph.D. in Psychology from the University of California, San Diego. His research is focused along three major themes. The first theme involves examining and elucidating the mechanisms of social processing and perception in infants, children, and adults with and without Autism Spectrum Disorder (ASD). The second theme concerns the examination of genetic impacts on brain functioning, through the study of the relationships of normal genetic variation and rare genetic syndromes (e.g., mutations, microdeletions) with brain and behavioral functioning. The third theme involves the evaluation and development of behavioral and cognitive-behavioral interventions for individuals with ASD. Dr. McCleery has published his research and ideas in leading peer-reviewed journals in the fields of Clinical Psychology, Psychiatry, and Neuroscience; and his research has been supported by a number of organizations, including the National Institutes of Health, Autistica, Autism Speaks, the M.I.N.D. Institute, the Economic and Social Research Council, the Leverhulme Trust, and the McMorris Family Foundation. This includes serving as Principal Investigator for Research on a current, NIH-funded large-scale intervention research project designed to examine the safety, feasibility, and efficacy of a virtual reality intervention for adolescents and adults with ASD.

**Lina Morgado** holds a doctorate in Educacion (Online Education) from Universidade Aberta, Portugal (UAb), and a Master in Multimedia and Educational Communication from the same institution. She graduated with a bachelor's degree in Educational Psychology from the Institute of Educational Psychology of Lisbon (ISPA). Currently she is the director of the online Master's Degree in Elearning Pedagogy at Universidade Aberta (2006-2018), and member of the scientific council of the PhD in Education, branch of Distance Education and Elearning (2012-2018). She is co-author of Universidade Aberta's pedagogical model and was responsible for its development and for the implementation of the online teaching model. She coordinated the first institutional training program for University Teachers and Tutors for Elearning in Portugal (2007-2011), as well as the support systems for the teachers. She is a professor in the Distance Learning Department (1991-2018) and founder researcher of the Distance Education and Elearning Lab (LE@D) at Universidade Aberta. Her research interests include Open and Distance Education, Open Educational Resources, MOOCs, Elearning Models, Elearning Pedagogy and Educational Technology.

**Raffaella Pannuti** has an Industrial Chemistry degree. In 1998, she worked at ANT Foundation as Press Office Manager; in 2000 she became Segretary-General of ANT and since 2011 she is President of the Foundation. She is co-author of more than 20 national and international scientific paper and she participated as speaker in several national and international conference. She is member of European Union Action Groups.

**Julia Parish-Morris** is a Research Assistant Professor of Psychology in the Perelman School of Medicine at the University of Pennsylvania, and a Scientist with the Center for Autism Research at the Children's Hospital of Philadelphia. Her primary research interests are language development, social attention, and the interactive effects of language and social motivation on higher social cognition (e.g., Theory of Mind). Recent projects include assessing social motivation and language development using infrared eye tracking, studying growth trajectories of receptive and expressive language in preschoolers with autism spectrum disorder (ASD), examining the moderating effects of language on intervention outcomes in 3- to 5-year-olds with ASD, and applying computational linguistics methods to pinpoint a "linguistic signature" of autism. She is the recipient of numerous awards and honors, including a Presidential Fellowship, National Science Foundation Graduate Research Fellowship, American Psychological Association Dissertation Award, Autism Science Foundation Postdoctoral Fellowship, and an Award of Excellence from the Center for Autism Research. Her long-term research goals are to use cutting-edge technologies to identify the mechanisms that underlie pragmatic language impairment and social communication difficulty in neurodevelopmental disorders across the lifespan, chart relationships between these domains and functional impairment, inform individualized treatments, and contribute to early identification efforts.

**Cristina Portalés** (PhD in Surveying and Geoinformation, with specialization in Augmented Reality, 2008; IEEE Computer Society member) has been recently (2012-2015) a Juan de la Cierva post-doc fellow at the Institute of Robotics and Information and Communication Technology (IRTIC) at Universitat de València (Spain), where she currently works as full PhD senior researcher. She was formerly graduated with a double degree: Engineer in Geodesy and Cartography from the Universidad Politécnica de Valencia (Spain) and MSc in Surveying and Geoinformation from the Technische Universität Wien (Austria), with the specialization in photogrammetry/computer vision. She obtained her first diploma degree (Bachelor) with honours, for having the best academic record, being awarded with the San Isidoro prize. She was an ERASMUS, PROMOE and Leonardo da Vinci research fellow at the Institute of Photogrammetry and Remote Sensing (Vienna, 1999-2002), a PhD research fellow at the Mixed Reality Laboratory of the University of Nottingham (UK, 2005) and at the Interaction and Entertainment Research Centre of the Nanyang University of Singapore (2006). She received an outstanding PhD. Award by the UPV. First woman receiving the EH Thompson Award (best paper), given by the Remote Sensing and Photogrammetry Society (2010). During 2008-2010 she worked at the Photogrammetry and Laser Scanning Research Group (GIFLE) of the UPV, and during 2011-2012 she at the Technological Institute of Optics, Colour and Imaging (AIDO), being primarily involved in computer-vision related projects and in the project FP7-SYDDARTA, coordinating the technical work of the WP dedicated to software implementation and carrying out managerial tasks. She has been designed (since 2014) as the proposal coordinator for her research group (ARTEC). She is author of more than 60 scientific publications including international conferences, high impact journals, books and book chapters. She has been invited speaker by Univ. Granada, Aula Natura, UNITEC (Honduras), RUVID & Univ. Gjøvik (Norway). She is S&T program committee of diverse international conferences (e.g. ACM SIGCHI ACE, GECCO), highlighting her involvement in the IEEE ISMAR (CORE A*) for taking decisions on the selected papers. She is also reviewer of scientific journals with impact factors (e.g. MDPI Sensors, Springer Journal of Digital Imaging, Elsevier Computers in Industry). Cristina has co-organized the successful ACM Advances in Computer Entertainment Technology Conference 2005. Expert evaluator of FP7 and H2020 proposals. She is Deputy Editor-in-Chief of the scientific journal Multimodal Technologies and Interaction (MTI), and Editor-in-Chief of the International Journal of Virtual and Augmented Reality.

**José Vicente Riera** was born in Valencia in 1984. He received the Degree in Computer Science Engineering and Technical Telecommunication Engineering by the University of Valencia both in 2009. He has also completed the Master in Advanced Computing and Intelligent System in 2011. In 2008 he received a Collaboration Fellowship from the Ministry of Education and Science, and in 2009 a Research Fellowship from the University of Valencia. Since 2015 is associated professor at the University of Valencia. Since 2008 he has been involved in a number of scientific and technical projects on virtual reality and different kind of simulators (immersive systems, visual systems, motion platforms, etc). He worked in these projects as researcher at the Robotics Institute of the University of Valencia, and more concretely, at the Artec Research Group of that Institute, where he is actually working. His current research interests include the simulation hardware for all kind of vehicles (cars, trucks, heavy machinery, cranes, planes, helicopters, etc.), motion cueing algorithms and especially motion platform systems. The latter is the main focus of the PhD thesis that he is actually writing.

**Daniele Roganti** is a psychologist, psychotherapist specialized in health psychology and has a PhD in psychological sciences. He integrated psychological training with practice in yoga, mindfulness meditation and relaxation techniques, aimed to manage patients' stress, anxiety and pain. For ANT he provides psychotherapy and psychological support for cancer patients and their relatives in home-care setting and carries out researches about patients and caregivers quality of life, in order to develop innovative solutions. He is a member of the Italian Society of Palliative Care.

**Vibha Sazawal** is a Lecturer of Computer Science at the University of Maryland, College Park. She received her PhD in Computer Science and Engineering at the University of Washington in 2005.

**Vittoria Sichi** is a psychologist and family psychotherapist in training. After she graduated from the University of Bologna, she served an internship at ANT Foundation, in 2012. Today she works for ANT as psychologist where she offers psychological support at-home to cancer patients and their relatives. In ANT she also carries out research in order to improve patients and caregivers quality of life. She is a member of the Italian Society of Palliative Care.

**David Sime**, with over 18 years of digital media experience, delivers promotion and analysis at strategic, tactical and operational levels. Disciplines include Virtual Reality, Augmented Reality and targeted Online Video, across social media, mobile, pay per click, smart TV and out-of-home mediums. A qualified lecturer, David works with Google and the Chartered Institute of Marketing to deliver state of the art digital marketing and business development training for delegates at all levels from undergraduate to professional level. David directs the award winning team at Oncor Video. Based in London and Scotland this multimedia team delivers results-based immersive media solutions across engineering, construction, hospitality and luxury retail sectors all over the world. Experienced in coordinating specialist teams across widely differing disciplines, David enables clear communication and awareness of common strategic goals and is skilled in communicating complex technical information clearly and simpmy to stakeholders of all levels and disciplines. David has been recognised by Google and the Chartered Institute of Marketing for his skills in marketing leadership and planning, corporate reputation management, strategic analysis and decision-making, and emerging social and technological trends.

**Rita Solorzano** is a Speech Language Pathologist. She has worked extensively with students with autism. Throughout her career, she has been a participant in and witness to the evolving role of technology in creating therapies to address developmental issues. She is currently serving as Director of Therapy Content for Floreo, Inc., creating and overseeing the development of virtual reality therapies to address social communication and sensory/regulation needs of children and adults with autism.

**Sinan Turnacioglu**, M.D., is the Chief Medical Officer at Floreo, Inc. He is a board-certified physician with formal training in pediatrics and neurodevelopmental disabilities.

**Silvia Varani** is a psychologist and psychotherapist. Since 2001 she works in ANT Foundation as psychologist. Today she is the Head of the Psychology and Training Unit at the ANT Foundation in Italy. She is member of the Regional Executive Council of the Region of Emilia Romagna within the Italian Society of Palliative Care and the Italian Society of Psycho-Oncology. Her work includes coordinating the selection and training of health personnel and she is also responsible for training courses, both for professionals employed at the ANT Foundation as well as external. She has published a number of national and international scientific papers.

**Lucia Vera** graduated in Computer Science from the University of Valencia (Spain) in 1999. She received an extraordinary prize by the University of Valencia for the best academic record of the Computer Engineering promotion in 1999. Also she has an Executive Master in Project Management by the University of Valencia. She works as a senior researcher in the Robotics Institute (IRTIC) of the University of Valencia. Her expertise is in virtual characters and in the development of applications for simulation, training or learning mainly in the areas of Virtual and Augmented Reality.

# Index


3D 10, 20-21, 24, 26, 31, 41, 54, 59, 77, 81-83, 99-100, 103, 129, 141, 162, 177-179, 242, 244-246, 249-250, 253, 265

## A

Alzheimer's Disease 80, 93
ANT Foundation 262, 268
Anxiety 17, 21-22, 26-27, 64-65, 69-70, 72, 84, 97, 119, 127, 142, 159-162, 175, 178-179, 183-184, 186-187, 209-210, 212, 215, 222, 229-230, 243-244, 262-263, 266-268, 270
Anxiety Disorders 65, 97, 162, 175, 210, 222, 263
Art 2-5, 9-10, 13, 16-17, 33, 95-96, 185, 190, 268
Ascott 2-5, 16
ASD 24, 51-53, 55, 96, 103-105, 118-123, 126-133, 141-147, 149-150, 157, 159, 161-171, 176-180, 182-189, 191, 198
Attention-Deficit 176-177, 198
Augmented Reality (AR) 21-22, 31, 51, 58, 77, 81, 96, 118-119, 121, 157, 198, 241-242
Augmented Reality Mirror 117
Autism 20, 24, 35, 37, 51, 53, 64, 96, 103-104, 118-122, 139, 141-147, 149-150, 157, 159, 161, 166, 171, 175-177, 179-180, 183, 185-186, 188-189, 198, 211
Autism Spectrum Disorder (ASD) 51, 118-120, 141, 157, 159, 176, 198
Avatars 10, 53, 81, 102, 126, 140, 143, 145, 150, 162-163, 170, 179, 202, 231

## B

Balance 27, 79-82, 84-85, 102, 168, 224, 268
Behavioral Change 63
Biopsychosocial 240
Body 1-2, 4-10, 12-14, 16, 21, 23, 31, 46, 59, 61, 63, 77, 82-83, 96-97, 101-102, 104, 106, 121, 123, 133, 140, 146, 149, 162, 170, 178, 182, 205-206, 211, 220, 223, 225-228, 264
Brain-Computer Interfacing (BCI) 32-35, 49
Breakthrough Cancer Pain (BTcP) 270

## C

Cancer 21, 62, 102, 229, 262-264, 266, 268, 270
Cave Automatic Virtual Environments 81, 161, 175
CBT 64, 161, 166, 223, 229-230
Chat Therapy 199, 203, 205, 220
Chronic Pain 221-224, 226-232, 240, 263, 267
Clinical 24-25, 60, 64-65, 67, 80, 119-120, 123, 131, 133, 166, 183, 199-200, 202-203, 205, 209-211, 215, 226, 230-231, 241-243, 245, 248-251, 253, 261, 263, 268
Clinical Decision Making 261
Computer-Assisted Learning 121
Cortical Reorganization 240
Counseling 22, 199, 202, 206-209
Cyberception 2, 4, 16
Cybersickness 77, 123-124, 129, 139, 147-148, 157, 170, 190

## D

Dementia 51-52, 54-56, 58, 67, 80, 84
Dentistry 24
Depression 21, 27-28, 66, 68, 70, 119, 159-160, 203, 222, 229-230, 243-244, 262-263, 266-267
Diagnosis 17, 35, 51, 55-56, 60, 66-67, 84, 183, 211-212, 241, 243, 245, 249, 252-253, 261, 263, 267
Digital Learning 261
Digital Native 167, 220
Digital Natives 38, 201-202, 215
Disembodied 8

## E

Ecological Validity 80, 82, 84, 93, 121, 124, 144, 166-167
Educational Game 38

EEG or Electroencephalogram 35, 49
Elderly 79, 81-86
Emotional Security 62
Empathy 54, 61, 63, 68, 72, 142, 149, 176-177, 189, 192
End-of-Life Care 270
ERP or Event-Related Potential 36, 49
Evidence-Based Interventions 119, 132, 160, 169, 175
Exergame 81, 93
Exposure Therapy 21, 27, 31, 59, 64, 77, 162, 167-168, 175, 210, 263

## F

Face-to-Face 53, 100, 117, 203, 220, 245-246
Face-To-Face Interaction 100, 117
Fall 78, 80, 82
Flusser 8
Fourth VR (4VR) 16
Functional Magnetic Resonance Imaging or fMRI 35, 49
Fusion Imaging 26, 31

## G

Game 2, 10, 12, 22, 32-34, 36-40, 42, 44-47, 80, 82-83, 85, 93, 124, 130, 170
Giuseppe Riva 211

## H

Head-Mounted Display (HMD) 18, 123, 146, 157
Healthcare 17, 20, 26, 28, 51-52, 62, 67, 69-70, 78, 170, 222, 242-243, 249, 261, 264
Hierarchal Rehearsal 161, 175
Home Oncological Clinic 270
Hyperactivity Disorder 119, 167, 176-177, 198

## I

Image Blending 117
Immersive Interactive Simulation System 26, 31, 58
Immersive Learning Environment 142, 157, 198
Immersive Reminiscence 55, 58
Immersive Virtual Reality 22, 24, 61, 119, 140, 175, 240
Immersivity 220
Information Technologies 96, 98
Injury 23, 66-69, 226, 228
Interactive Environments 54, 186
International Society for Mental Health Online 203
In-Vivo Exposure Therapy 162, 175

## L

Learning 4, 20, 23-25, 32-34, 37-38, 40-44, 46-47, 49, 53-54, 61, 63, 65, 72, 79, 83-84, 86, 93, 98-99, 121, 123-124, 127, 131, 133, 141-146, 148-150, 157-158, 161-163, 166-168, 176-183, 185, 187-192, 198, 201, 212, 214, 241-249, 253, 261
Learning Adventure 149, 158, 182, 198
Learning Environment 63, 142-143, 145, 149, 157-158, 177-178, 181-183, 191-192, 198, 253
LPDT (La Plissure du Texte 16

## M

Maladaptive Behavior 161, 175
Mark Prensky 201, 220
Medical Education 242-243, 245-246, 248, 253, 261
Meditation 32-34, 37-47, 49, 65, 102, 223, 270
Medium-Transparency 220
Mental Health 20, 25, 33-34, 51, 62, 64-68, 72, 95-96, 98, 102-105, 119, 132-133, 200, 203, 207, 215, 221-223, 230, 243-244
Mental Illness 32, 35, 62, 244, 270
Metrobodily 1, 5, 12
Metrobody 1, 10, 12-13, 16
Mild Cognitive Impairment 80, 93
Mindfulness 37, 40, 46, 263, 270
Mirror Therapy 22, 96-98, 103, 105, 226
Mixed Approaches 36, 50
Mixed Reality (MR) 31, 59, 77
Moistmedia 4, 16
Motion Sickness 22, 129, 170, 190, 231, 265
Motivation 80, 85, 103, 131, 143, 160, 167-168, 181, 186, 222, 241, 247, 251, 253

## N

Neglect 60-62, 79-80, 82
Neurodevelopmental 118-119, 139, 145, 160
Neuroplasticity 80, 226, 228, 240
Non-Immersive 82, 84, 124-126, 140, 163, 227, 231
Non-Immersive Virtual Reality 140
Non-Verbal Cues 202-203, 206, 220

## P

Pain Relief 22, 96-97, 225
Pain Symptoms 262
Palliative Care (PC) 270
Peer-Mediated Interventions 160-161, 169

Perception 4, 6-7, 10, 54, 82, 98, 149, 181, 186, 221, 223-225, 228, 240, 244, 247, 264
Performance 9-10, 12, 18, 25, 79, 81, 83-84, 86, 102, 125-128, 142, 145-146, 162, 164, 168-169, 177, 179-180, 188, 190, 208, 229, 241, 245, 249-253, 266
Phobias 31, 65, 72, 77, 96, 102, 105, 162, 212
Physical Activity 78
Physical Illness 69
Physical therapy 21-23, 27
Post-Traumatic Stress Disorder 31, 63, 210, 212, 222
Protective Shield 205-206, 220
Psychological 22-23, 28, 34, 52, 60, 62-66, 68-70, 79, 82, 96, 102, 147, 171, 179, 199-200, 202-209, 215, 220-221, 244, 263-264, 268, 270
Psychological Disorders 28, 96, 215
Psychological Distress (Distress) 270

# Q

Quality of Life 78, 84, 150, 230, 243-244, 262-263, 265, 270

# R

Regular Mirror 96, 100, 117
Rehabilitation 17, 20-23, 25-27, 80-85, 96-97, 99, 102, 123, 177-179, 190, 200, 211-214, 227
Rubber Hand Illusion 225

# S

Science 10, 13, 33-35, 62, 98, 170, 243, 245, 247
Seamless Interaction 117
Sensation 6, 8-9, 16, 98, 223-224, 226, 231, 240
Serious Games 32-34, 37-38, 40-42, 46-47, 49-50, 79, 84, 246
Simulator 26, 77, 82-83, 98, 125-126, 128-129, 139, 157, 179, 241, 243, 249-251, 253, 261
Situated 38, 40-41, 244-245, 248, 261
Situated Learning 38, 40-41, 244-245, 248, 261
Skill Transfer 84, 93
Social Skills 25, 121-123, 126, 141-142, 145, 150, 159-167, 169, 179-180, 188, 212-213
Social Stories 160-161, 165-167, 169
Socio-Economic Costs 175
Special Education 132, 182, 186
Stimulate 146, 186, 188, 191, 214
Stress 20-21, 23, 26, 31, 37, 60-67, 69, 72, 77, 82, 101-102, 123, 210, 212, 222, 225, 244, 263
Stroke 23, 26, 80, 82-84, 97, 101
Surgery 10, 17, 20-22, 24-27, 31, 34-35, 101, 242-243
System Usability Scale (SUS) 50

# T

Technology-Based Intervention 119-120
Therapeutic 51, 53-56, 63, 120, 127-129, 146, 167, 171, 202, 205, 209, 213-215, 221, 223
Three Virtual Realities (3VRs) 16
Transfer of Knowledge 161, 164, 175
Trauma 23, 62-63, 66-72
Traumatic Stress 23, 62-63, 66, 77
Treatment 17, 20-28, 51-52, 55-56, 60, 62, 64-65, 70, 80, 86, 95-99, 101-103, 105-106, 119, 123, 125-127, 129, 142, 166, 168, 171, 177, 179, 190, 203, 210-213, 215, 221-223, 225, 229-230, 232, 241, 243-245, 249, 251-253, 261, 263, 270

# U

Ubiquitous Bodies 1, 9, 13-14, 16
Ubiquity 1, 12, 16
Uncanny 96, 98, 117
Usability 41-43, 46, 50, 78, 83, 122-123, 127, 171, 241, 247, 251, 253

# V

VE 123-128, 131-132, 140, 186, 209
Video-Modelling 161
Virtual Environments 6, 16, 21, 25, 53, 55, 58, 65, 81, 84, 145-146, 148, 161-163, 166-170, 175-176, 181, 186, 190, 209, 211, 215, 231
Virtual Reality (VR) 5, 16-18, 22, 24, 26, 31-32, 51, 59-60, 77-79, 96, 118-119, 121, 141, 158-159, 176, 198-200, 209, 221, 242, 262-263, 270
Virtual Reality Environments 51, 190
Virtual Reality Exposure Therapy (VRET) 21, 31, 59, 77, 210
Virtual Reality Mirror 117
Virtual Surgery 20-21, 26, 31
Virtual Worlds, 142, 176, 246
Vive Base-Station Area 164, 175

# W

Wearable Technology 140
Web-Based Learning Simulator (e-FER) 261
Well-Being 14, 33, 62, 64, 69-72, 133, 200, 208, 243-244, 267

www.ingramcontent.com/pod-product-compliance
Lightning Source LLC
LaVergne TN
LVHW060418300926
849162LV00006B/1462